UNITED STATES ARMY
INSTITUTE FOR MILITARY ASSISTANCE

ST 31-91B

US ARMY SPECIAL FORCES MEDICAL HANDBOOK

1 MARCH 1982

SPECIAL FORCES MEDICAL HANDBOOK

CONTENTS

PREFACE

This book is designed to serve as a ready reference and review for Special Forces (SF) medics. It covers diseases and medical problems that SF medics may encounter in various areas of the world. It does not, however, take the place or eliminate the need for a comprehensive medical area study.

Many treatments given in this handbook would best be given in a hospital where a laboratory and special equipment are available, and personnel with serious injuries or illnesses should be evacuated to such a hospital if at all possible. Know your limitations and do not exceed them. Remember the maxim "First thou shall do no harm" and seek the assistance of more competent medical authority whenever possible.

Since we want to use as few pages as possible in presenting this information, we use common medical abbreviations throughout. For example,

A. - analysis
ABE - acute bacterial endocarditis
ad - up to
A.M. - ante meridiem
BBT - basal body temperature
b.i.d. - twice a day
B.P. - blood pressure
BUN - blood urea nitrogen
BW - biological warfare
C. - Celsius, centigrade
CBC - complete blood count
cc. - cubic centimeter
CHF - congestive heart failure
cm. - centimeter
C.N.S. - central nervous system
COPD - chronic obstructive pulmonary disease
CPR - cardiopulmonary resuscitation
CT - clotting time
C.V.A. - costovertebral angle; cerebrovascular accident
d. - day; daily
D&C - dilatation and curretage
DTR - deep tendon reflex
Dx - diagnosis
E. coli - Escherichia coli
e.g. - for example
F. - Fahrenheit
G.I. - gastrointestinal
gm - gram
gr. - grain
gtt. - drops
GU - genitourinary
h. - hour
HB - hemoglobin
HCl - hydrochloride
HCT - hematocrit
HEENT - head, eye, ear, nose & throat
Hg - mercury
h.s. - at bedtime
Hx - history
ID - intradermal
I&D - incise & drain
i.e. - that is
IM - intramuscular
IV - intravenous
IU - international unit
kg. - kilogram
L. - liter
lab - laboratory
lb - pound(s)
LLQ - left lower quadrant
MCL - mid clavicular line
med - medication; medical; medicine
mEq. - milliequivalent
mg. - milligram
Mg - magnesium
MI - myocardial infarction
MIF - merthiolate/iodine/formaline solution
min - minute
ml. - milliliter
mm. - millimeter
M.U. - million units

Na - sodium (natrium)
NBC - nuclear, biological, chemical
NG - nasogastric
NPN - nonprotein nitrogen
N.P.O. - nothing by mouth
N&V - nausea & vomiting
O. - objective findings
OD - overdose
oz. - ounce
P. - plan of treatment
p.c. - after meals
P.E. - physical exam
pH - hydrogen in concentration
PID - pelvic inflammatory disease
PM - preventive medicine
P.M.I. - point of maximum impulse
P.M.N. - polymorphonuclear neutrophil leukocytes
P.O. - by mouth
pO_2 - partial pressure oxygen
PP - pulsus paradoxus
P.P.D. - purified protein derivative
ppm. - parts per million
p.r.n. - as required or as needed
psi - pounds per square inch
PTB - primary tuberculosis
p.v. - through the vagina
q. - every
q.d. - every day
q. h. - every ___ hours
q.i.d. - four times a day
q.s. - sufficient quantity
qt. - quart

S. - subject findings
SBE - subacute bacterial endocarditis
sec - second
sed. - sedimentation
SLR - straight leg raise
sp. gr. - specific gravity
spp. - species
SQ - subcutaneous
S and S - signs and symptoms
stat. - immediately
STS - serologic test for syphilis
Sx - symptoms
T. - temperature
tab. - tablet
TB - tuberculosis
t.i.d. - three times a day
Tx - treatment
U. - unit
URI - upper respiratory infection
U.S.P. - United States Pharmacopeia
VD - venereal disease
VS - vital signs
W.B.C. - white blood cell, white blood count
W.H.O. - World Health Organization
wo - without
wt. - weight

SYMBOLS

- increase

- decrease

- greater than

- less than

14 July 1982

Holders of ST 31-91B, Special Forces Medical Handbook, should add to/change the text as follows:

Page

iv — bottom right column, under SYMBOLS, add

- $\uparrow$ - increase
- $\downarrow$ - decrease
- $>$ - greater than
- $<$ - less than

1-15 — line 2, add $\downarrow$ before or in center and right columns

line 11 (Breath sounds & voice), same as for line 2

1-21 — bottom page, 2d para from bottom under O, add $\uparrow$ before W.B.C. and $>$ before 20,000

1-73 — para 1-51 O., first line, add $\downarrow$ before B.P.

2-17 — mid page, last para before A., 2d & 3d lines, add + sign over -; should read $89^{\pm}27$ & $124^{+}68$

D-2 — para D-4c, line 3, add ~ over =; should read W.B.C. $\cong$ 4,500

In addition to the above, users should be aware that superscripts and subscripts in the text are sometimes out of line due to mechanical error.

CHAPTER 1

BODY SYSTEMS

Section I - Integumentary System

1-1. SKIN. Tough elastic structure covering the entire body consisting of two layers: the epidermis and the dermis.

1-2. DIAGNOSIS OF SKIN DISEASES BY PHYSICAL EXAMINATION.

a. Primary lesion. Earliest changes to appear:

(1) Macule. Flat discolored spot of varied size 10 mm. or smaller.

(2) Patch. Flat discolored spot of varied size 10 mm. or larger.

(3) Papule. Solid elevated lesion 10 mm. or smaller.

(4) Plaque. A group of confluent papules.

(5) Nodule. Palpable solid lesion 5-10 mm. (may or may not be elevated).

(6) Tumors. Larger nodules usually 20 mm. or larger.

(7) Vesicle. Circumscribed elevated lesion 5 mm. or smaller containing serous fluid.

(8) Bulla. Circumscribed elevated lesion 5 mm. or larger.

(9) Pustule. Superficial elevated lesion containing pus.

(10) Wheal. Transient elevated lesion caused by local edema.

b. Secondary lesions result from either evolution (natural) of the primary lesions or patient manipulation of primary lesions.

(1) Scales. Heaped up parts of epithelium.

(2) Crusts (Scab). Dried serum, blood, or pus.

(3) Erosion. Loss of part or all of the epidermis.

(4) Ulcer. Loss of epidermis and at least part of dermis.

(5) Excoriation. Linear or hollowed-out crusted area caused by scratching, rubbing, or picking.

(6) Lichenification. Thickening of the skin with accentuation of the skin markings.

(7) Atrophy. Thinning and wrinkling of the skin resembling cigarette paper.

(8) Scar. The result of healing after destruction of the dermis.

1-3. SKIN DISORDERS.

a. Pruritus (Itching).

S. Compulsive itching accompanies primary skin disease or may be the only signs and symptoms.

O. Redness, uticarial papules, excoriated papules, fissures, crusting, etc.

A. Pruritus/Pruritus secondary to __________ skin disease.

P. Correct the skin disease, or discontinue using irritating substance, e.g., soap, clothing, chemical, etc. Use of mild tranquilizers: Valium, Vistiral. Use of major tranquilizers: Thorazine. Use of antihistamines: Benadryl 50 mg. t.i.d.

b. Contact dermatitis is divided into two types:

(1) Primary irritant contact dermatitis. Develops within a few hours, reaches peak severity in 24 hours then disappears; caused by contact with a chemical irritant.

(2) Allergic eczematous contact dermatitis. Has a delayed onset of about 18 hours, peaks in 48-72 hours, and often lasts 2-3 weeks after discontinuing exposure to the offending antigen. (Poison ivy, oak, or sumac or allergy to clothing, etc.)

(3) Symptoms vary from minor itching and redness to vesicles, redness, edema, oozing, crusting, and scaling; itching is usually sharply demarcated.

(4) Remove offending agent. Use tap water, soaks, or compresses. Blisters may be drained but leave the tops on. Oral corticosteriods - Prednisone 40-60 mg./day x 10-14 days in severe cases. Topical corticosteriods are not effective in acute phase. Antihistamines - Benadryl 50 mg. t.i.d.

1-4. BACTERIAL SKIN INFECTIONS.

a. Impetigo/Ecthyma. Superficial vesiculopustular skin infection seen chiefly in children. Ecthyma is an ulcerative form of impetigo.

S. Group A B-hemolytic streptococcus is usual cause, but Staphylococcus aureus may be cultured also.

O. Usually affects arms, legs, and face, with the legs being more susceptible to ecthyma than unexposed areas. Both may follow superficial trauma or may be secondary to skin disease or insect bites, but it is not uncommon for it to arise on normal skin.

Lesions vary from pea-sized vesicopustules to large bizarre circinate ringwormlike lesions that progress rapidly from maculopapules to vesicopustules or bullae to exudative and then to heavily crusted circinate lesions. Ecthyma is characterized by small, purulent, shallow ulcers covered with crusts. Itching is common and scratching can spread the infection.

A. Impetigo/ecthyma.

P. Systemic antibiotics are superior to topical antibiotics. Penicillin is the drug of choice; second choice is erythromycin.

	IM Penicillin	ORAL Penicillin	Erythromycin
Child	600,000 U. Pen G	125 mg. q.i.d. x 10 days	125 mg. q.i.d. x 10 days
Adult	1.2 mil U. Pen G	250 mg. q.i.d. x 10 days	250 mg. q.i.d. x 10 days

In secondary impetigo, the underlying cause should be treated also. Neglected infection may result in cellulitis, lymphangitis, or furunculosis in adults or acute glomerulonephritis in children.

b. Erysipelas. A superficial cellulitis caused by Group A B-hemolytic streptococci.

S. The face (bilaterally), an arm, or a leg is most often involved.

O. Lesion is well demarcated, shiny, red, edematous, and tender; vesicles and bullae often develop. Patches of peripheral redness and regional lymphadenopathy are seen occasionally; high fever, chills, and malaise are common. It may be recurrent and may result in chronic lymphedema. The causative agent may be difficult to culture from the lesion, but it may be cultured from the blood.

A. Erysipelas. NOTE: Erysipelas of the face must be differentiated from herpes zoster; contact dermatitis and angioneurotic edema may also be mistaken for erysipelas.

P. Pen VK or erythromycin 250 mg. q.i.d. x 14 days. In acute cases Pen G 1.2 million U. IV q.6h. x 36-48 hrs then start Pen VK. Local discomfort may be relieved by cold packs and/or 600 mg. aspirin with 30 mg. codeine.

c. Cellulitis. Has the same S and S and is treated the same as erysipelas. The only difference is cellulitis involves deeper tissue.

d. See Chapter 2, Section III, Bacterial, for typhoid fever, gas gangrene, anthrax, tularemia, plague, leprosy, and scarlet fever.

1-5. SUPERFICIAL FUNGAL INFECTIONS.

a. See Chapter 2, Section II, Mycotic, for coccidioidomycosis, North American blastomycosis, and Paracoccidioidomycosis (South American blastomycosis).

b. Sporotrichosis. A chronic fungal infection caused by Sporothrix schenckii. It is found worldwide in soil, plants, and decaying wood. Organism is introduced by skin trauma, usually on hand, arm, or foot.

S. and O. Commonly begins with a hard, nontender subcutaneous module that later becomes adherent to the overlying skin, ulcerates (chancriform), and may persist for a long time. Within a few days to weeks, similar modules usually develop along the lymphatics draining this area, and these may ulcerate. The lymphatic vessels become indurated and are easily palpable. Infection usually ceases to spread before the regional lymph modes are invaded, and blood-bone dissemination is rare.

Skin infection may not spread through the lymphatics but may appear only as warty or papular scaly lesions that may become pustular. Disseminated sporotrichosis presents as multiple, hard subcutaneous modules scattered over the body. These become soft but rarely rupture spontaneously. Lesions may also develop in bones, joints, muscles, and viscera.

Laboratory findings: Cultures are needed to establish diagnosis.

A. Sporotrichosis.

P. Saturated solution of potassium iodine (S.S.K.I.) 5 drops in a glass of water t.i.d., after meals, orally, increasing by 1 drop per dose until 40 drops t.i.d. are being given. Continue until signs of active disease have disappeared. Then decrease the dosage by 1 drop per dose until 5 drops per dose are being given, then discontinue. Although S.S.K.I. is not fungicidal, it does promote rapid healing. Care must be taken to reduce the dosage if signs of iodism appear.

Amphotericin B IV and miconazole have been effective in systemic infections.

c. Chromomycosis. Mainly a tropical chronic cutaneous infection caused by several species of closely related molds having a dark mycelium. Found in soil and on decaying vegetation. In humans the disease progresses slowly, occurring most frequently on the lower extremities, but it may occur on hands, arms, and elsewhere.

S. and O. Lesions begin as a papule or ulcer. Over a period of months to years, the lesions enlarge to become vegetating, papillomatous, verrucous, elevated nodules with a cauliflowerlike appearance or widespread dry verrucous plaques. The latter spread peripherally with a raised, verrucous border, leaving central atrophic scarring. The surface of the border contains minute abscesses. Satellite lesions may appear along the lymphatics. There may be a foul odor due to secondary bacterial infection. Some patients complain of itching. Elephantiasis may result if marked fibrosis and lymph stasis exist in the limb.

Lab findings: The fungus is seen as brown, thick-walled, spherical, sometimes septate cells in pus.

A. Chromomycosis.

P. Flucytosine - 150 mg./kg./d. orally or thiabendazole 25 mg./kg./d. orally. Surgical excision and skin grafting may prove useful.

d. Dermatophyte infections (Ringworm). Superficial infections caused by fungi that invade only dead tissues of the skin or its appendages (stratum corneum, nails, hair).

S. Microsporum, Trichophyton, and Epidermophyton are the genera most commonly involved.

O. Some dermatophytes produce only mild or no inflammation. In such cases, the organism may persist indefinitely, causing intermittent remissions and exacerbations of a gradually extending lesion with a scaling, slightly raised border. In other cases, an acute infection may occur typically causing a sudden vesicular and bullous disease of the feet, or an inflamed boggy lesion of the scalp (Kerion) may occur that is due to a strong immunologic reaction to the fungus; it is usually followed by remission or cure.

A. Tinea corporis - (Ringworm of the body).

Tinea pedis - (Ringworm of the feet) - athlete's foot.

Tinea unguium - (Ringworm of the nails).

Tinea capitis - (Ringworm of the scalp) - dandruff.

Tinea cruris - (Ringworm of the groin) - jock itch.

Tinea barbae - (Ringworm of the beard area).

Tinea manuum - (Ringworm of the palms and soles of the feet).

Differential diagnosis: Includes pityriasis rosea, discoid eczema, and psoriasis.

Confirmation can be made with Wood's light or KOH preparation.

P. Griseofulvin is effective against true dermatophyte infections, but not against candidiasis or tinea versicolor. Adult dosage is 500 mg. b.i.d. with meals. Duration varies from 2 weeks for tinea corporis to 6-12 months for tinea unguium. Tinactin/Mycostatin are effective against most fungal infections where applied b.i.d. to t.i.d. to affected areas and washed off before reapplication.

1-6. PARASITIC SKIN INFECTIONS.

a. Scabies. A transmissible parasitic skin infection characterized by superficial burrows, intense pruritus, and secondary infections.

S. Caused by the itch mite (Sarcoptes scabiei). The female mite tunnels into the epidermis layer and deposits her eggs along the burrow. Scabies is transmitted by skin-to-skin contact with an infected person. It is <u>not</u> transmitted by clothing or bedding.

O. Nocturnal itching, pruritic vesicles and pustules in "runs" or "galleries" especially on the sides of the fingers and the heel of the palms. Mites, ova, and black clots of feces may be visible microscopically.

A. Scabies. Confirm by demonstrating the parasite in scrapings taken from a burrow, mix with any clear fluid, and examine microscopically.

P. Disinfestation with gamma Kwell 1% cream base applied from neck down and repeated in one week. (WARNING: there is a potential of neurotoxicity from use on infants and from overuse on adults.) Treatment should be aimed at all infected personnel. In cases of severe secondary infections, treatment should be supplemented with systemic and topical antibiotics.

b. Pediculosis (Lice). A parasitic infestation of the skin-- scalp, trunk, or pubic areas--that usually occurs in overcrowded dwellings.

S. Head and pubic lice can be found on the head and in the pubic area. Body lice are seldom found on the body as the insects only come to the skin to feed; you must look for them in the seams of clothing.

O. Pruritis with excoriation, nits (ova) on hair shafts, lice on skin or clothing, occasionally sky-blue macules (maculae caeruleae) on the inner thighs or on the lower abdomen in pubic lice infestations. You may also see secondary infections.

A. Pediculosis pubis (Crabs - Phthirus pubis). Infestation of anogenital region. Pediculosis humanus-var corporis (body louse). Differential diagnosis seborrheic dermatitis, scabies, anogenital pruritis, and eczema.

P. Cure is rapid with gamma Kwell 1% q.d. x 2 days. Repeat after 10 days to destroy the nits; practice good personal hygiene. If the infestation is widespread, wash all clothing and bedding in hot water with a strong detergent and dust the area with lindane powder.

c. See Chapter 2, Section 1, Parasitic, for African trypanosomiasis (sleeping sickness), American trypanosomiasis (Chagas' disease), and cutaneous and mucocutaneous leishmaniasis.

1-7. VIRAL INFECTIONS OF THE SKIN.

a. Herpes simplex (cold/fever sore). An acute viral infection.

S. Clinical outbreaks, which may be recurrent in the same location for years, are provoked by fever, sunburn, indigestion, fatigue, windburn, menstruation, or nervous tension.

O. Recurrent, small, grouped vesicles on an erythematous base, especially around the oral and genital area, lasting approximately 1-2 weeks. Regional lymph nodes may be swollen and tender. Burning and stinging; neuralgia may precede and accompany attacks. The lesions consist of small, grouped vesicles that may occur anywhere, but most often occur on the lips, mouth, and genitals.

A. Herpes simplex. Differential diagnosis: Distinguish from other vesicular lesions, especially herpes zoster and impetigo, in the genital area, syphilis, lymphogranuloma venereum, and chancroid.

COMPLICATIONS: Kaposi's varicelliform eruptions (eczema herpeticum or disseminated herpes simplex), encephalitis, keratitis, and perhaps cervical cancer and other neoplastic diseases.

P. Eliminate precipitating agents when possible. Apply a moistened styptic pencil several times daily to abort lesions. Dust vesicles twice daily with bismuth formic iodide or use shake lotions or camphor spirit. Epinephrine 1:1,000 applied locally b.i.d. may also be used. If there is associated cellulitis and lymphadenitis, apply cool compresses. Treat stomatitis with mild saline mouthwash.

b. Herpes zoster (Shingles). An acute vesicular eruption due to a virus that is morphologically identical with the varicella virus.

S. Usually occurs in adults with or without a history of chickenpox during childhood and is probably a reactivation of a varicella virus infection that has been occult for many years. Persons in anergic states (Hodgkin's disease, lymphomas, or those taking immunosuppressive drugs) are at greater risk, and life-threatening dissemination (varicella) may occur.

O. Pain along the course of a nerve followed by painful groups of vesicular lesions. Involvement is unilateral and persists for approximately 2-3 weeks. Lesions are usually on the face and trunk. Swelling of regional lymph nodes may occur. Pain usually precedes eruptions by 48 hours or more and may persist and actually increase in intensity after the lesions have disappeared.

A. Herpes zoster. Differential diagnosis: Poison ivy, poison oak dermatitis, and herpes simplex, which is usually less painful. COMPLICATIONS: Persistent neuralgia, anesthesia of the affected area following healing, facial or other nerve paralysis, and encephalitis may occur.

P. Barbiturates may help control tension and nervousness associated with neuralgia. Aspirin with or without codeine (30 mg.) usually controls the pain. A single injection of triamcinolone acetonide (Kenalog) suspension (40 mg. intragluteally) may give prompt relief. Prednisone 40 mg. daily for 4 days and then continued in declining doses may also be used. Calamine lotion or other shake lotions are often of value; apply liberally and cover with a protective layer of cotton. DO NOT USE GREASES.

c. See Chapter 2, Section IV, Viral, for measles, smallpox, dengue, Colorado tick fever, and herpes genitalis.

d. See Chapter 6, Pediatrics, for chickenpox.

1-8. RICKETTSIAL DISEASES. See Chapter 2, Section V, Rickettsial and Spirochetal, for epidemic louse-borne typhus, endemic flea-borne typhus, and spotted fevers (Rocky Mountain spotted fever, Rickettsialpox, scrub typhus, trench fever, Q fever).

1-9. SPIROCHETAL DISEASES.

a. See Chapter 2, Section VI, Venereal for syphilis.

b. See Chapter 2, Section V, Rickettsial and Spirochetal, for treponemal infections (yaws, endemic syphilis, pinta).

Section II - Musculoskeletal System

1-10. GENERAL.

a. The history of a musculoskeletal disorder is much like any other history. A concise story of specific complaints will help the medic best determine the extent of the disorder. Questions should include chronological sequence, manner of onset, duration of symptoms, previous history, progress of the complaint, extent of disability, specific complaint of weight bearing, motion of the part, weather changes, what aggravates the complaint, what relieves it, whether it has ever been treated, and if so, what were the effects of treatment.

b. The physical examination should include the general posture and alignment of the body as a whole. Evaluate the patient's body attitude while standing and walking. The relationship of the feet to the legs and of the hips to the pelvis should be noted; also the relationship of the arms to the shoulder girdle and to the upper trunk. Next the general contour of the spine and its relation to the shoulder girdle, thorax, and pelvis should be noted. The local physical examination should include:

(1) Inspection. Contour, appearance, color, deformity, and its general relationship to the body.

(2) Palpation. Tenderness, swelling, muscle spasm, local temperature changes, and gross alterations.

(3) Range of motion. Motion is measured in degrees of a circle as illustrated below. Medic should compare affected area with uninvolved opposites or with his own joints.

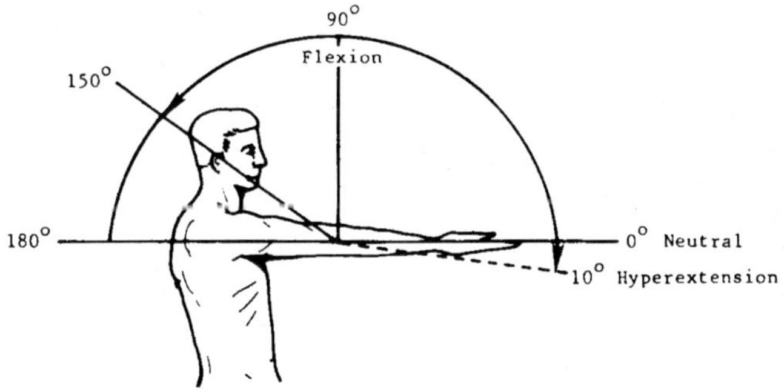

(4) Joint position. Position of function is the position that gives the joint its maximum strength and efficiency. Position of comfort is the position in which the joint feels the most comfortable. Patients will always try to assume the position of comfort. It is up to the medic to insure that the affected joints are always supported in a position of function.

(5) Measurement. Atrophy or hypertrophy may be determined by measuring and comparing with uninvolved opposite.

(6) Neurologic. The strength of the affected muscles and the quality of the superficial and deep tendon reflexes should be noted. Also the integrity of cutaneous sensation should be determined when indicated.

1-11. RHEUMATOID ARTHRITIS. Chronic systemic disease of unknown etiology usually involving the synovial membranes of multiple joints, tendons, or bursae.

S. and O. Common in ages 25-50; women are affected three times as often as men. Abrupt onset with symmetrical swelling of joints in the hands and feet, regional atrophy of bone and muscle, limited joint motion, the skin of the extremities may be smooth, glossy, and atrophic. Other signs and symptoms include elevated temperature, tachycardia, generalized lymphadenopathy, malnutrition, body wasting, morning stiffness, and depression. Synovial fluid is cloudy and sterile, reduced viscosity. Polymorphonuclear leukocytes typically predominate. History should rule out other types of arthritis.

A. Rheumatoid arthritis.

P. Rest, aspirin in high doses (look out for ulcer), corticosteroids, either systemically and/or intra-articular injection. Severe rebound may follow steroid withdrawal. Heat and physical therapy to maintain joint function.

1-12. OSTEOARTHRITIS. A degenerative joint disease usually affecting large weight-bearing joints of older individuals, causing deterioration of articular cartilage.

S. and O. Onset is gradual and localized to a few joints; 60-70-year age bracket; women affected 10 times as often as men; distal interphalangeal joints of the fingers frequently show modulation, obesity; pain is made worse by exercise. The cervical and lumbar spine, hip, and knee are most often involved. History, physical, laboratory findings will show minimal abnormalities.

A. Osteoarthritis.

P. Rest, weight reduction, heat, occasional brace support, aspirin, analgesics, and physical therapy.

1-13. SEPTIC ARTHRITIS. Acute disease process involving a single joint and is secondary to a bacterial infection.

S. and O. Previously healthy, case of gonorrhea usually in women, concurrent bacterial infection, fever, rash possibly, acute joint pain and stiffness, joint is warm, tender, swollen. Leukocytosis, arthrocentesis will show color to be variable, viscosity variable, clarity opaque, culture often positive, Gram's stain, W.B.C. greater than 10,000.

A. Septic arthritis.

P. Evacuate if possible; the joint may be destroyed if not promptly treated. Treat with antibiotics according to infectious organism.

1-14. GOUTY ARTHRITIS. Recurrent metabolic disease usually causing arthritis in peripheral joints due to hyperuricemia that leaves urate crystals within the joint space.

S. and O. Minor trauma may start; overindulgence in pork or alcohol; classically the joint of the big toe is affected; inflammation, pain, swelling, fever, chills, tachycardia; urate salts may precipitate in a collection called a tophus that may be mistakenly reported as calcification. These tophi may be found in the muscle surrounding the joint, the tendons, or the walls of the bursae. Usually made by history and physical. Synovial fluid will have needle-shaped urate crystals that are free in the fluid.

A. Gouty arthritis.

P. Terminate the acute attacks by the use of an anti-inflammatory drug, prophylaxis by daily use of colchicine, and prevention of further deposits of urate crystals by lowering uric acid levels with Benemid or allopurinol. Codeine may be needed to control pain.

1-15. OSTEOMYELITIS. An infection of the bone and bone marrow due to septicemia or bacteremia.

S. and O. Infected tonsils, boils, abscessed teeth, or upper respiratory infections may cause the septicemia. Direct contamination may result from open fracture or war wound. General symptoms are those of an acute toxic illness with sharp rise in temperature. Locally the involved area may be swollen, warm, and very tender to touch. There may be a severe, constant, pulsating pain, usually aggravated by motion. The diagnosis of acute osteomyelitis ideally requires the identification of the causative agent. Staphylococcus aureus is the most common, accounting for 65-70 percent of the cases. Proteus, pseudomonas, salmonella, streptococcus, acid-fast bacilli, fungi, and rickettsiae can also be the cause. Blood test will usually show an elevated leukocyte count and blood culture may be positive.

A. Osteomyelitis.

P. The successful treatment is completely dependent upon establishing an early clinical and bacterial diagnosis. Antibiotics are started as soon as diagnosis is suspected and may be altered after the results of the culture and sensitivity are known. Penicillin G with doses of 12-20 million units daily and 1-8 grams of methicillin daily, depending on patient's age. For patients that are allergic to penicillin, cephalosporin, erythromycin, or lincomycin may be given. Antibiotics should be continued for 8-12 weeks after all signs and symptoms disappear. The affected bone should be immobilized until all signs of active infection have disappeared. Aspiration of abscess may also be necessary. Chronic osteomyelitis requires surgery with radical debridement of the bone with excision of all sinuses, dead bone, scar tissue, and necrotic tissue.

1-16. BURSITIS. Inflammation of the bursa. Bursae are lubricating devices that diminish the friction of movement. They are found beneath the skin, beneath tendons, and overlying joints. Inflammation may be due to trauma, extensive use, infection, gout, or rheumatoid arthritis. Due to the stimulus of inflammation, the lining membrane produces excess fluid causing distension of the bursa sac. The fluid may be bloody or in the case of gout, there may be urate crystals. Treatment consists of local injections of corticosteroids into the inflamed bursa. Treatment of choice is 20-40 mg. hydrocortisone following infiltration of 1% procaine. Phenylbutazone 300 mg. for 2-3 days followed by 100 mg. for 10 days is also effective. Early active movement inhibits development of limiting adhesions.

1-17. ARTHROCENTESIS. Find the effusion. Mark the site for entry. Scrub with Betadine or iodine. Anesthetize the skin 1% lidocaine. Aspirate with 20-gage needle; insure needle is long enough. Record the volume, viscosity, color, and clarity of synovial fluid. Immediately place 0.5 ml. in sterile tube for culture with Thayes-Martin medium. Place 0.5 ml. of synovial fluid in a heparinized tube for leukocyte count. Use 0.3% saline solution as diluent for W.B.C. Prepare smears for Wright's and Gram's stain. Prepare wet smear by placing drop of synovial fluid on slide, cover with cover slip, and seal edges with nail polish.

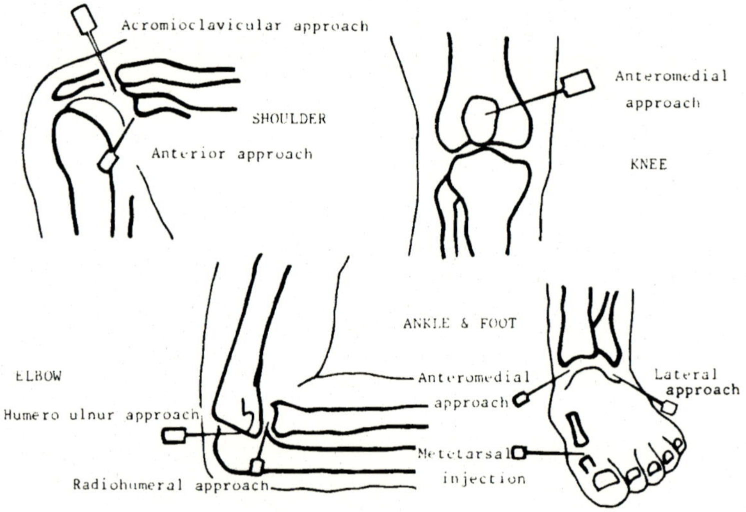

1-18. THE SHOULDER. Shoulder pain may arise from a problem primarily in the joint or it may be referred pain. Referred pain may be due to cervical spine disorders, cardiac disorders, gallbladder diseases, or diseases involving the mediastinum or diaphragm. Referred pain will less likely have local tenderness, inflammation, and limited range of motion.

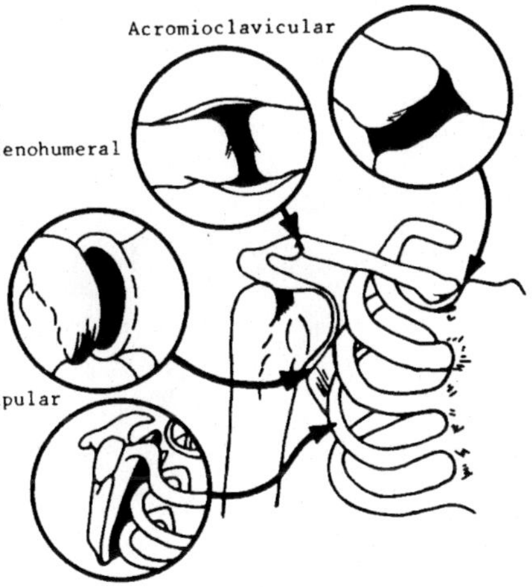

1-19. THE KNEE.

a. Collateral ligament rupture test. With the knee partially flexed, an abnormal opening of the medial aspect of the knee indicates damage to the medial collateral ligament. If the lateral collateral ligament has been injured there will be an opening on the lateral aspect of the knee.

b. Cruciate ligament rupture test. With both knees flexed, the medic grasps the leg just below the knee with both hands and pulls the tibia forward. For best results the medic should place his hip on the patient's foot. Abnormal forward motion of the tibia suggest damage to the anterior cruciate ligaments. Abnormal backward motion of the tibia suggests damage to the posterior cruciate ligaments.

c. McMurray's test for torn meniscus. The patient should be lying in the supine position with the knee fully flexed. The foot is forcibly rotated outward to its full capacity. While the foot is held outward in the rotated position, the knee is slowly extended. If a painful click is felt, this indicates a tear of the medial meniscus. If the painful click is felt when the foot is rotated inward, the tear is in the lateral meniscus.

1-20. LOW BACK PAIN. A thorough knowledge of the anatomy of the spine, particularly of the lumbosacral area, is essential to the diagnosis and treatment of low back pain. Low back pain may be due to congenital disorders, tumors, trauma, metabolic disorders, inflammatory diseases, degenerative diseases, infections, mechanical causes, or psychoneurotic disorders. This does not end the list. Trauma is the most common cause of back pain. A study of the presented disorders will help the medic in his differential diagnosis. General treatment consists of bed rest, heating pads, firm mattress, massage, and possibly a local anesthetic infiltration to trigger points.

a. The malingerer. Malingerers exist, but every patient should be treated as a true patient until other evidence exists.

b. The tests.

(1) Have the patient sit in a chair and try to touch the floor; a patient with a severe disc herniation can usually perform while the malingerer cannot.

(2) Place the patient in the supine position. Put one hand under the heel and raise the opposite leg. A malingerer will usually lift his heel out of the medic's hand while the legitimate patient will press further into the hand.

(3) The malingering patient usually exhibits a marked withdrawal response when the medic palpates any part of his body. Squeezing the sacroiliac joints by compression from both sides usually elicits pain from the patient who is faking and not from the true patient.

(4) Muscle weakness in the injured side is usually too obvious and disproportionate to the neurological findings in the malingerer. The best course of action is to tell the patient that no organic cause can be found for the patient's symptoms.

Section III - Respiratory System

The respiratory system includes the nasal pharynx, sinuses, trachea, bronchial tree, lungs, pleura, diaphram, and the chest wall.

The upper portion of the respiratory system is covered in Chapter 1, Section IX, EENT.

1-21. PNEUMOTHORAX: The presence of air in the pleural cavity resulting in partial or total collapse of the lung.

S. Closed pneumothorax: No direct communication between pleural cavity and the atmosphere.

(1) Spontaneous pneumothorax: Due to rupture of a bleb at the surface of the lung lining. Most common in otherwise healthy males between 20-30 years of age. Sudden onset of progressive dyspnea is the most common complaint. Chest pain of variable quality (but usually pleuritic) is frequently associated. The rupture often occurs during exercise, coughing, sneezing, or straining, and the patient can usually pinpoint the onset of dyspnea to the second. The progression is usually rapid, and the patient may find himself in severe respiratory distress in minutes. The course, however, may be less acute and the patient may note only slowly increasing dyspnea on exertion for days prior to onset of frank dyspnea at rest. The chest pain is usually localized to the affected side.

(2) Tension pneumothorax: Due to rupture of a small bronchus, bronchiole, or alveolus. This results in the formation of a one-way valve that allows inspired air to enter but prevents its escape. The progressive increase in pressure from the trapped air buildup pushes the heart to the opposite side and compresses the univalved lung and great veins resulting in a decreased cardiac output. The symptoms are the same as spontaneous pneumothorax but far more rapid in progression. The chest pain usually localizes well to the affected side, initially, but may become more diffuse as the contralateral lung is involved.

O. General: The patient is usually anxious and tachypneic. Signs of varying degrees of shock may be present depending on the type and extent of the pneumothorax. The same can be said for cyanosis.

Vital Signs: Temperature is usually normal but may be subnormal if severe degree of shock is present. Pulse is usually increased and feeble. Respiration is tachypneic.

B.P.: A postural drop may be noted with significant cardiovascular compromise; a persistently low or falling supine B.P. will be seen as shock becomes more developed.

Chest Exam:	Spontaneous	Tension or Open
Chest expansion	or absent on affected side.	or absent on affected side greater than uninvolved side (which may also demonstrate poor expansion)
Resonance to percussion	Involved side>uninvolved side	Involved side> uninvolved side
Breath sounds & voice sounds	or absent on involved side	or absent on involved side
Fremitus	Absent	Absent
Tracheal deviation	Usually none	When present, is away from affected side.
P.M.I. shift	Usually none	When present, is away from affected side.
Tracheal & P.M.I. "swing" (a pendulum type motion of the heart & trachea during expiration and inspiration is often seen in pneumothorax).	Insp: Toward involved side Expir: Away from involved side	Insp: Away from involved side Exp: Toward involved side

Subcutaneous emphysema: Air in the subcutaneous tissues about the neck and chest usually indicates an underlying pneumothorax.

A. Pneumothorax. Differential diagnosis: May mimic many acute thoraxic events including pulmonary embolus and MI. The specific features of demonstrable hyperresonance with associated poor expansion of one side of the chest will usually differentiate a pneumothorax. Nonetheless, a quick rule of other possible causes should be done.

P. Closed pneumothorax:

(1) Spontaneous - Tube thoracostomy with drainage:

(a) At the 3rd or 4th intercostal space just medial to the anterior axillary line, make a short skin incision just above and roughly parallel to the inferior rib of the interspace.

(b) Use large hemostats to separate the muscles and puncture the pleura.

(c) With the hemostats, introduce a large bore Foley catheter into the pleural space with the tip pointing superiorly (if a chest tube is available, use it).

(d) The tube should be inserted 1/2 to 3/4 of its length and the balloon inflated. The catheter is then slowly pulled outward until the inflated balloon "catches" on the inner chest wall. During this time the patient should be urged to cough and strain to allow removal of pleural fluid. Once the catheter catches, it is secured with sutures. A vertical mattress suture wrapped around the tube is preferred.

The wound, too, is "tightened" with sutures, and petroleum gauze overlaid with dry dressing is placed over the entrance. Secure the edges of the dressing out to 6 inches with tape, tightly. DO NOT secure with circumferential wraps around the chest.

(e) If the tube does not have a one-way valve, one can be improvised by tying a finger cot, a finger cut out of a rubber glove, or a condom over the end of the tube and cutting a small hole in it. A rubber Penrose drain slipped over the end (with a few centimeters "left dangling") will accomplish the same (i.e., prevent air reflux into the chest). The water bowl seal can be used for the same purpose. See illustrations below.

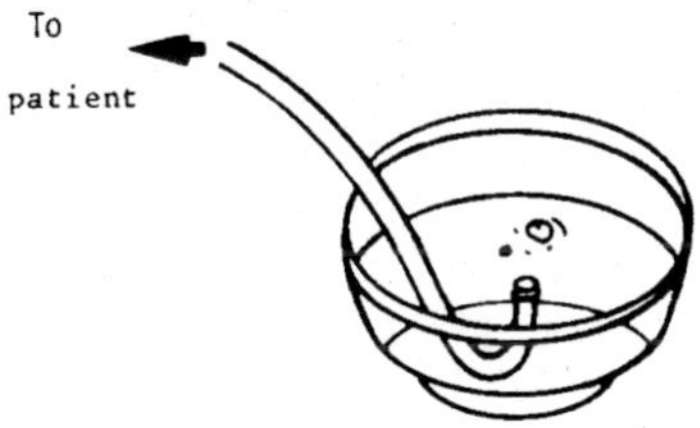

Water bowl seal bowl must be kept below level of patient.

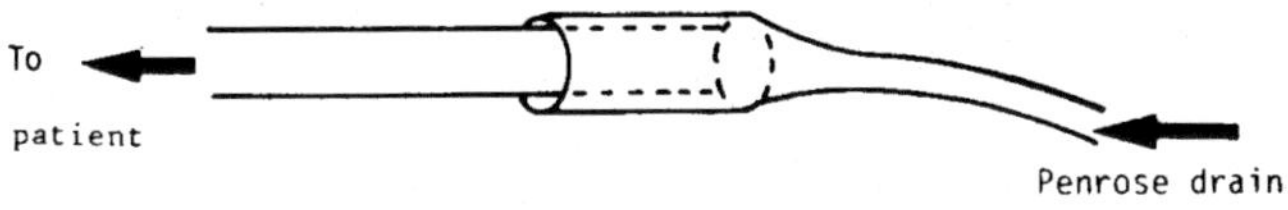

Improvised one-way valve.

(f) If a water seal device is available or can be improvised, it is preferable. A simple 2-bottle water trap suction system is illustrated below.

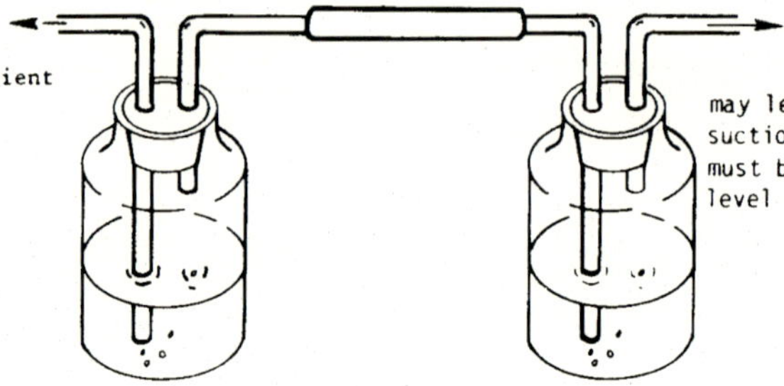

Two-bottle water seal trap for pneumothorax.

(2) Tension Pneumothorax: Because of the rapid progression of derangements and their consequences (i.e., shock), heroic steps may have to be taken to buy time for tube placement and definitive management.

(a) If a tension pneumothorax is suspected and the patient is cyanotic or manifests any signs of cardiovascular compromise (e. g., postural drop in B.P., frank hypotension; cold, clammy skin, etc.), a #18 or #16 needle should be introduced into the chest to decompress the pleural space. The needle should be introduced slowly in the 2d or 3rd intercostal space MCL until the "hiss" of air can be heard (...get your ear down there and listen!!) escaping. Avoid the underside of the superior rib (see 1-27, Pleural Effusions).

(b) When the initial blast of air ceases, remove the needle and institute tube thoracostomy and drainage as outlined above.

(3) General care after closed thoracostomy - tube drainage:

(a) Monitor patient for signs of continued improvement (or deterioration). Have the patient cough occasionally, and check for signs of air movement in the tube or water trap system. If patient exam is consistent with sustained expansion and no air leak is noted for 24 hours, the tube may be clamped. In an uncomplicated spontaneous pneumothorax, the tube may be withdrawn after another 24 hours of continued stability. The mattress suture is drawn tight and closure effected as the tube is pulled clear. Pulling the tube in the field is, however, strongly discouraged in spontaneous pneumothorax and absolutely contraindicated in open or tension pneumothorax.

(b) If the pneumothorax persists with evidence of good air drainage (large leak into the pleural space) or without evidence of good air drainage (obstructed or poorly positioned tube) a second tube should be placed nearby to facilitate drainage. If a significant hemothorax is present (open chest trauma, etc.) a second tube should be placed in the 6th or 7th intercostal space in the mid or posterior axillary line. The presence of fluid there should first be confirmed by needle aspiration.

(c) Tetanus prophylaxis is given and all drainage routinely Gram-stained for evidence of infection.

1-22. ASPIRATION.

a. Definition: Inspiratory sucking into the airways of fluid or other foreign material. Two types:

(1) Active aspiration: The patient's airway defense mechanisms (cough, gag, etc.) are overwhelmed by the sudden collection of matter in the posterior pharynx. This usually happens as a result of vomiting but can happen with rapid hemorrhage that drains into the area (i.e., maxillo facial trauma, severe nose bleeds). Drowning is also a type of active aspiration.

(2) Passive aspiration: Oropharyngeal secretions pool in the posterior pharynx and passively "leak" into the trachea. Almost always occurs in the presence of sluggish or absent airway defense mechanisms (obtundation, coma, etc.).

b. Pathology. Three major events may occur:

(1) Asphyxiation ("strangling"): Occurs when large volumes are aspirated resulting in extensive airway obstruction.

(2) Aspiration pneumonia: Occurs as a result of aspirating oropharyngeal secretions that contain numerous potentially pathological organisms.

(3) Chemical pneumonitis: May result from aspiration of highly acid stomach secretions. It is a type of noncardiac pulmonary edema.

S. The actual event (vomiting, choking, etc.) may have been witnessed, but it is likely that the victim of active aspiration will be found cyanotic and in severe respiratory distress. The usual history of passive aspiration is the onset of fever and progressive respiratory distress after or during a bout of obtundation.

Any recent Hx of obtundation in a patient with respiratory distress should alert the examiner for aspiration. Any Hx of conditions that may produce unconciousness (alcoholism, seizure disorder) has the same significance.

O. General appearance: With massive aspiration, vomitus or other matter may be seen about the nose and mouth. The patient may be cyanotic with varying states of conciousness (ranging from alert to frank coma) depending on degree of obstruction, time obstruction present, and nature of associated injuries.

VS: Temperature may be elevated if pneumonia or chemical pneumonitis has developed. Pulse is usually increased. R. is usually increased and labored. B.P. may be decreased or may exhibit postural drop if shock is present or imminent.

	Asphyxiation	Pneumonia	Pneumonitis
Neck	Use of accessory muscles may be prominent until near the end.	Use of accessory muscles unusual or until advanced stages.	Use of accessory muscles.
Lungs	Poor breath sound over large areas may be noted; coarse rhonchi.	Resembles findings in other pneumonias (i.e., signs of consol-idation).	The findings of pulmonary edema (rales, rhonchi, wheezing, etc.).

Lab: W.B.C.: May have leukocytosis with left shift, especially if pneumonia is present.

Sputum exam: Many W.B.C.; mixed flora.

A. The most important clue to diagnosis is the presence in the Hx of a suspect setting.

P. (1) Clear the airway by manual extraction of foreign matter. Use suction if available. The Heimlich maneuver may be necessary to clear the airway.

(2) If patient is conscious and can cough, administer regular chest percussion and drainage. If the patient is unconscious, he should be intubated and secretions removed by suction.

(3) Med: Oxygen, if available, should be administered. Antibiotics are the preferred methods: Tobramycin or gentamycin 80 mg. IV or IM b.i.d.; Penicillin G two million units IV q.6h. Bronchodilators may be of benefit. Aminophylline (as per asthma).

c. General considerations. The best treatment is prevention. Severely debilitated or obtunded patients should not have food or liquids "forced" upon them. Their heads should be kept at a 30-45° angle. If a patient has no gag reflex, cannot cough or gargle a small amount of water without choking, he should be considered a high risk for aspiration. Wet, gurgling noises on inspiration and expiration may represent impending passive aspiration in the obtunded patient. He should be immediately suctioned or his airway evacuated by postural methods.

1-23. HEMOPTYSIS. Spitting or coughing up blood of respiratory tract origin. Massive hemoptysis: hemorrhage exceeds 200 cc. in 24-hr period.

a. Pathology: The bleeding may come from a lesion anywhere in the respiratory tract. Hemoptysis can be deadly. Few patients "bleed to death;" rather death is almost always due to aspiration asphyxiation (i.e., they "drown" in their own blood).

b. Causes: Lung abscess/TB/some heart diseases (mitral stenosis)/crushing, penetrating or concussive chest trauma/penetrating neck injuries.

S. Question for evidence of disease states outlined above. Trauma should be obvious.

O. General appearance: Search for signs of possible respiratory collapse (cyanosis, lethargy, etc.). In severe states, use of neck accessory muscles and retractions of the chest may be seen. Dullness and poor expansion may be noted on the side where bleeding is originating (if coming from a lung). Rhonchi, rales, and wheezes may be heard. Decreased or absent breath sounds may be heard over the side most involved.

A. Hemoptysis should be obvious, but take care to distinguish from G.I. bleeding.

P. (1) Clear the airway. Chest percussion and drainage. If the bleeding is too brisk or the patient is in severe respiratory distress, intubation should be carried out with vigorous suction. Do not intubate if suction not available unless the patient is unconscious.

(2) Massive hemoptysis or any hemoptysis associated with severe respiratory distress is an emergency that cannot be adequately managed in the field. Evacuate ASAP!! The measures outlined above are temporary supportive measures only.

1-24. PNEUMONIA. An inflammation of the lung parenchyma to include the aveoli and smaller airways. Though the inflammation may be secondary to any number of processes, the term as used in this discussion will apply to infectious processes.

a. Bacterial pneumonia. An acute infection of the alveolar spaces of the lung. Organisms causing pneumonia include pneumococci, staphylococci, Group A hemolytic streptococci, Klebsiella pneumonia, Haemophilus influenzae, and Francisella tularensis.

(1) Pneumococcal pneumonia. The pneumococcus accounts for 60-80 percent of primary bacterial pneumonia. Among conditions which predispose to pneumonia are viral respiratory diseases, malnutrition, exposure to cold, noxious gases, alcohol, drugs, and cardiac failure.

S. Sudden onset of shaking chills, fever, "stabbing" chest pain, high fever (101-105°F.), productive cough with "rusty" sputum, and occasionally vomiting. A history of recent respiratory illness can often be elicited.

O. The patient appears acutely ill with marked tachypnea (30-40/minute), but no orthopnea. Respirations are grunting, nares flaring, and the patient often lies on the affected side in an attempt to splint the chest. Signs of consolidation may be lacking during the first few hours, but fine rales and suppressed breath sounds are soon heard over the involved area. Frank consolidation, involving part of a lobe or several lobes, is found later. A pleural friction rub is often heard in the early stages. Leukocytosis of 20-35 thousand/cu. mm. is the rule. Gram-stained sputum shows many R.B.C., W.B.C., and pneumococci.

A. Pneumococcal pneumonia. Differential diagnosis: Other bacterial pneumonias.

P. Penicillin G is the drug of choice. Give 600,000 units q. 12 h. IM for moderate cases. Severe cases will require up to 10 million units/24 hrs by IV infusion. An adequate airway must be maintained, if necessary, by tracheal suction, endotracheal tube, or tracheostomy. O_2 must be supplied to any patient with severe pneumonia, cyanosis, or marked dyspnea. Treat shock p.r.n. as outlined in chapter 15. Toxic delirium occurs in any severe pneumonia and may be especially difficult to manage in alcoholics. It is best controlled by promazine 50-100 mg. IM q. 4h. p.r.n. Anxiety and restlessness may be treated with phenobarbital 51-30 mg. q. 4h. One-tenth gram phenobarbital h.s. helps insure adequate rest. Force fluid to maintain a daily urinary output of at least 1,500 cc. Liquid diet intially then normal diet when patient can tolerate it. ETH with codeine, 1 tsp q. 3-4h. p.r.n. Mild pleuritic pain may be controlled by spraying the area of greatest pain with ethylchloride x 1 min, then along the long axis of the body through the entire area of pain, so that a line of frost about 1 inch wide is formed. Codeine 15-30 mg. or meperidine 50-100 mg. may be used for severe pain.

(2) Klebsiella pneumonia. Occurs primarily in person 40-60 years of age with a history of alcoholism or debilitating diseases. The causative organism is Klebsiella pneumoniae, which occurs as normal bacterial flora in the respiratory tract or gut.

S. Sudden onset of chills, fever dyspnea, cyanosis, and profound toxicity. The sputum is often red ("currant jelly"), mucoid, sticky, and difficult to expectorate.

O. Physical findings and W.B.C. are variable. Diagnosis is based on finding short, encapsulated gram-negative bacteria as the predominate organism in sputum smears.

A. Klebsiella pneumonia. Differential diagnosis: Pneumococcal pneumonia (you must have a good, well stained smear).

P. Kanamycin 0.5 gm IM q. 6-8h. (15 mg./kg./day); cephalothin 6-10 gm IV. Antibiotic therapy must be continued for at least three weeks. General supportive care is the same as for pneumococcal pneumonia.

(3) Staphylococcal pneumonia. Pneumonia caused by Staphylococcus aureus occurs as a sequel to viral infections of the respiratory tract (e.g., influenza) and in debilitated (e.g., postsurgical) patients or hospitalized infants, especially after antimicrobial drug administration.

S. There is often a history of a mild illness with headache, cough, and generalized aches that abruptly changes to a very severe illness with high fever, chills, and exaggerated cough with purulent or blood-streaked sputum and deep cyanosis.

O. There may be early signs of pleural effusion, empyema, or tension pneumothorax W.B.C. usually 20,000 cu. mm. Gram-staied sputum reveals masses of W.B.C.'s and gram-positive cocci, many of which are intracellular.

A. Staphylococcal pneumonia.

P. Initial therapy (based on sputum smear) consists of full systemic doses of a cephalosporin, a penicillinase-resistant penicillin, or vancomycin. The doses are as follows: cephalotin, 8-14 gm/day IV; methicillin, 8-16 gm/day IV; vancomycin, 2 gm/day IV; nafcillin, 6-12 gm/day IV. If empyema develops, drainage must be established. If pneumothorax develops, treat as described in chapter 16, Emergency War Surgery.

(4) Streptococcal pneumonia. Usually occurs as a sequel to viral infection of the respiratory tract, especially influenza or measles or in persons with underlying pulmonary disease.

S. The patients are usually severaly toxic and cyanotic.

O. Pleural effusion develops frequently and early and progresses to empyema in one-third of untreated patients. Diagnosis rests in finding large number of streptococci in Gram-stained sputum smears.

A. Streptococcal pneumonia.

P. Treat same as penumococcal pneumonia.

b. Viral pneumonia.

S. Relatively slow progressive symptoms. Cough may be hacking and dry or produce small amounts of nonpurulent mucoid or watery sputum. Rarely dyspneic. Usually associated signs of viral syndrome (e.g., myalgias, sore throat, rashes, runny nose, conjuctivitis, etc.). Pleuritic pain may be present but is usually much less severe than in bacterial pneumonia (splinting is rare).

O. Usually only mildly febrile if at all. Does not appear "toxic" as a rule. No chest findings of consolidation. Coarse breath sounds and sometimes sparse rales may be heard. W.B.C. is usually normal but may reach 12,000 or above with slight left shift (early) or right shift (late in course). Gram-stained sputum: No organisms or few mixed organisms.

A. Viral.

P. Therapy: Symptomatic treatment.

c. Mycoplasmal pneumonia.

S. Resembles viral pneumonia in symptomology but with slightly more acute onset and more severe expression of symptoms. Cough is usually more productive but sputum is similar in character. Malaise and myalgias may be more prominent. May occur in limited, small group epidemics (camps, schools, etc.).

O. Patient may appear mildly toxic. Fever may be high but is usually low grade. Signs of consolidation in the chest. Leukocytosis (up to 15,000) seen in only 25 percent of cases. Sputum appears similar to viral sputum.

A. Mycoplasma. Differential diagnosis: Chlamydia and rickettsia.

P. Therapy: Tetracycline P.O. 500 mg. q.4h. or erythromycin 500 mg. +10. Treatment is same for chlamydia and rickettsia.

1-25. CHRONIC BRONCHITIS AND EMPHYSEMA.

a. Chronic bronchitis: A chronic airway disorder characterized by production of thickened secretions, recurrent bouts of infection, and mucosal edema-bronchospasm. Airway obstruction develops as the disease worsens.

b. Emphysema: The term applied to distention and distortion of the alveoli or terminal bronchioles.

S. Chronic bronchitis is characterized by a cough that is persistent or recurs daily for at least 3 months a year for at least 2 successive years. The typical cough is usually worse in the morning; the patient continues to cough until the urge is relieved by coughing up the pool of mucous that has collected during the night. A variable degree of chest tightness and occasionally some wheezing may be noted in the morning, but this too is relieved somewhat once the chest has been "coughed clear." As the disease becomes more advanced, the cough worsens in severity and duration, and sputum production increases. A significant smoking history is almost always present. In the majority of cases it is a superimposed bout of respiratory infection that brings the patient to see you. During this time he usually notes a change in the color (green, brown or grey), character (thickened) or volume (increased) of sputum production. The cough may have become painful. Though a fever (usually low grade) may be present, significant degrees of dyspnea at rest are rare unless chronic obstructive pulmonary disease (COPD) was present.

With the history of chronic cough and the morning distress, the patient may also note a decrease in exercise tolerance secondary to shortness of breath. The greater the exercise intolerance the more advanced the disease.

Emphysema: In the majority of cases, it will be associated with chronic bronchitis, its signs and symptoms. The rare case of pure emphysema usually presents with dyspnea on exertion. Cough is usually not prominent until COPD develops and, when present, is productive of only small amounts of watery mucoid sputum. Likewise, repeated respiratory infections are uncommon.

Evidence of right-sided heart failure is important. In emphysema its appearance represents the onset of the terminal phase whereas in chronic bronchitics right-sided heart failure may be tolerated for some time.

O. In the early stages the findings on physical exam are nonspecific. Indeed, many exams will reveal no abnormalities to explain the respiratory abnormalities.

Chronic Bronchitis: Scattered airway coarseness (rhonchi) clearing with cough is the most consistent finding. Occasionally, wheezes may be heard, but they are very mild and also clear somewhat with cough. As the disease progresses in severity, some hyperexpansion of the chest and prolongation of the expiratory phase may be noted.

Emphysema: Airway coarseness usually not as prominent.

Otherwise the findings are similar.

Lab: The only lab study of any potential benefit in the field will be Gram-stained sputum. This should be done to support a diagnosis of infection. Though pneumonia tends to occur more frequently in these patients, the most common infection in this group is bouts of acute bronchitis. Gram's stain usually shows mod. W.B.C. (15,000-30,000), many epithelial cells, and mixed flora.

A. Differentiating chronic bronchitis from asthma may prove difficult but certain differences are helpful.

	Chronic Bronchitis	Asthma
Cough	Dominant feature, occurs chronically.	Occurs usually in association with attack (e.g. wheezing, dyspnea, etc.).
Wheezing	Mild, most notable in A.M. or during infection; clears somewhat with cough.	Dominant feature.
Dyspnea	Usually on exertion. Subacute in onset.	At rest. Usually acute in onset.
Hx of smoking	Almost always present.	Rare.

As both disorders progress through the years, the clinical pictures become less distinguishable. Both, however, terminate in a chronic obstructive lung disease with right heart problems. The differences at this point, however, are academic because treatment and long-term management will be the same regardless of the courses.

P. Management of less advanced cases of chronic bronchitis and emphysema should be carried out as outlined.

(1) Halt progression of the disease process.

(a) Stop smoking; by far, the single most important factor.

(b) Avoid areas where noxious fumes or high concentrations of particulate matter (e.g., smoke, dust, fibers, etc.) are present.

(c) Chest percussion and postural drainage in the morning and as needed through the day. The patient should be encouraged to maintain hydration (2-3 liters of water per day).

(2) Functional rehabilitation. Progressive exercise programs increase tolerance. Some patients respond to bronchodilators so this therapy is probably worth a try. Aminophylline 200-400 mg. t.i.d.-q.i.d. or theophylline 100-200 mg. t.i.d.-q.i.d. may be given. Terbutaline 2.5-5 mg. t.i.d.-q.i.d. may be administered with either aminophylline or theophylline. Some inhalants (e.g., Isuprel) may also be of some benefit especially when administered prior to a chest percussion and drainage session.

(3) Infection management.

(a) Influenza vaccine should be received yearly.

(b) Pneumococcal vaccination should be received.

(c) Acute bronchitis: Sputum gram stain +5 nonspecific (i.e., mixed flora); ampicillin or tetracycline 500 mg. P.O. q.6h. x 10 days. Sputum shows predominate organism: Treat as indicated (see pneumonia).

(4) Severe bronchitis or emphysema.

(a) Stable: The same general therapeutic program as outlined above is initiated but with more urgency. Exercise programs, as such, should not be attempted; rather the patient should be encouraged to do as much for himself as possible.

(b) "Breakdown" is marked by a sudden worsening in respiratory status (i.e., increased dyspnea, fatigue, etc.). To prevent progression to respiratory failure, some of the measures must be executed rapidly and simultaneously.

1. An IV should be started and IV aminophylline administered as described in the asthma section. Rate should not exceed 125 cc./min.

2. Terbutaline 2.5-5 mg. may be given SQ.

3. Antibiotics should be given. Treat with ampicillin or tetracycline as described.

4. Oxygen may be given CAREFULLY if available. Only Low Flow oxygen should be administered (2 liters/min). High oxygen concentrations can cause sudden respiratory arrest in the patient.

5. During the therapy the patient must be encouraged to cough and clear as much secretion as possible.

6. Right-sided heart failure that is secondary to the lung disease will only respond to improvement in pulmonary status. Digoxin will not help. Diuretics may precipitate shock, hence, should be avoided in the field.

7. Never give narcotics or sedatives that might decrease respiratory drive.

1-26. PULMONARY EMBOLISM

a. Pulmonary embolism occurs when a thrombus (blood clot) or foreign matter lodges in the pulmonary vascular bed (the pulmonary arteries or their branches).

b. Etiology. The most common type of embolus is a blood clot formed in some part of the systemic venous circulation (usually deep leg veins), that breaks loose to travel to and subsequently lodge in the pulmonary circulation. Fat globules and amniotic fluid may also embolize to the lung. Death is usually the result of shock.

S. Chief complaint: Sudden onset of unexplained dyspnea is the most common complaint. This may or may not be associated with chest pain; usually pleuritic (i.e., sharp, localized, aggravated by deep inspiration or coughing) but may resemble that of MI. Hemoptysis may be a feature and is usually seen when pulmonary infarction has resulted. Syncope may sometimes be the presenting symptom. By far the most consistent of these symptoms is dyspnea. This complaint also has some prognostic value, as severe prolonged dyspnea is usually associated with very large emboli and a poor prognosis.

Present Hx: Since 80-90 percent of pulmonary emboli are blood clots, the patient should be questioned about any predisposing conditions. These conditions are usually marked by stasis of venous blood flow with subsequent clot formation. Question carefully for symptoms of deep vein thrombophlebitis in the legs (by far the most common source of emboli). Pre-existing congestive heart failure; shock states (traumatic, cardiac, and septic); prolonged immobilization, either general (i.e., paralysis, bed confinement, etc.) or of an extremity (i.e., paralysis, cast, traction); and post-op states are all associated with sluggish venous blood flow. In pregnant women clots may form in the pelvic veins. Severe cellulitis or gangrene of an extremity may cause clot formation in large veins if these veins are involved in the process.

Past Hx: A tendency toward recurrence has been noted in many cases of pulmonary embolism. A past Hx of pulmonary embolism or unexplained signs and symptoms suspicious of pulmonary embolism are helpful.

Occupational Hx: A high incidence has been noted in civilian occupations with long periods of immobilization (e.g., cab & truck drivers). It is likely that similar military occupations might carry with them some predisposition toward clot formation and subsequent embolization.

O. Physical findings are inconsistent and often absent with small emboli. Generally the larger the embolus, the greater the pulmonary and hemodynamic consequences, hence the more prominent the P.E. findings. The patient is usually very anxious and in moderate to serve respiratory distress. He may grimace on inspiration (secondary to pleuritic pain) and have one or both hands placed over the area where pain is greatest as if wounded there. He may be pale and clammy if obstruction is great enough to produce some degree of shock.

Vital Signs: Temperature is often slightly to moderately elevated (38-39°C.) but may be subnormal if shock is present. Tachycardia is the most consistent P.E. finding of the syndrome and has the same prognostic implications of dyspnea. Note also postural changes (see B.P.). Respirations are usually rapid and often somewhat shallow (secondary to splinting because of pain). B.P. may be normal. The presence of significant postural drop in systolic B.P. may indicate a high degree of obstruction with poor cardiac output. A low systolic B.P. may be seen when frank shock has developed. Use of accessory muscles of respiration is usually seen only when the embolus has triggered diffuse severe bronchospasm (rare). Jugular venous distention may be noted (see cardiovascular below). Asymmetrical expansion between the two sides of the thorax may be seen secondary to pain (i.e, "splinting"). In the lungs a patchy area of e>a change or bronchovesicular (tubular) breath sounds and rales may be discovered if some lung collapse (atelectasis) has occurred. Wheezing may be detected if the embolus has triggered brochospasm. A pleural friction rub may be heard if pulmonary infarction has resulted.

Dullness, e>a change with decreased breath sound may be present if a pleural effusion is present.

Cardiovascular. Kussmaul's sign (failure of the jugular veins to collapse on inspiration) may be noted. With large emboli, signs of acute right ventricular failure (see cardiovascular section) may be seen. Search for signs of venous insufficiency or thrombophlebitis in the lower extremities (the chief source of emboli).

A. Even with the aid of X rays and lab facilities, the diagnosis of pulmonary embolization may be elusive; pulmonary embolism may mimic myocardial infarction, pneumonia, asthma, spontaneous pneumothorax, cardiac tamponade, or virtually any acute or subacute cardiac or pulmonary event. The most consistent finding (tachycardia) is nonspecific and the other findings are so inconsistent as to make formulation of any type of reliable symptom-sign complex impossible. The so-called "classic triad" of dyspnea, pleuritic chest pain, and tachycardia is neither specific nor regular in occurrence. Pulmonary embolism must first be thought of before it can be diagnosed and it should be considered in any patient that develops sudden, unexplained respiratory distress in a suspect setting. In the field, the diagnosis will be a function of three factors: (1) historical and physical findings; (2) the setting in which the event occurred (e.g., thrombophlebitis, prolonged immobilization, etc.); and (3) the exclusion of other possible reasons for the distress (e.g., sudden onset of dyspnea and tachycardia in a 22-year-old trooper who has had a fractured leg immobilized for 3 days is unlikely to be having a myocardial infarction) as rapidly and practical as possible.

P. Therapy: In the field, once embolization is suspected, very little short of general supportive measures (e.g., oxygen, ventilatory assistance, etc.) can be done to remedy the effects of the embolus. Large or extensive embolization producing more than 70-80 percent of the pulmonary circulation (depending on previous respiratory status and overall health) will usually kill regardless of supportive measures. Smaller embolization (the majority) will begin to resolve within the first few days, though significant improvement in the patient's state may be noted within the first hours. Since even small emboli may produce very prominent signs and symptoms initially, it is impossible to preict the severity of the obstruction in the first hours after embolization. Vigorous supportive measures must be instituted to give the patient's body as much time as possible for resolution.

Heparin therapy is instituted to prevent further clot formation. It does not "melt" the clot already lodged in the pulmonary circulation (though it does assist resolution somewhat). Heparin may cause fatal bleeding if the dosages given are too high or the patient has another disease process or injury (e.g., active peptic ulcer, hemorrhagic or inflammatory pericarditis, internal injuries, etc.) from which uncontrollable bleeding may occur.

Given Heparin: An initial bolus of 15,000 to 20,000 units IV followed by 7,500 units SQ q.6h. or 10,000 units SQ q.8h. Heparin therapy must be monitored; in the field, clotting time is the only practical method.

Clotting Time: A stopwatch is started when 5 cc. of venous blood is drawn into a glass syringe. One ml. of blood is placed in each of three dry glass test tubes. After 3 minutes the tubes are tilted every 30 sec until the tubes can be inverted without blood spilling out. The elapsed times are noted in the 3 tubes and averaged to give the clotting time (CT). The test must be done as close to 37° C. as possible. This may be accomplished by taping the tubes to the abdomen of a volunteer. Have him sit erect on the ground with outstretched legs and recline, gradually, back on his elbows every 30 sec to check blood movement in the tubes. In warm weather the tubes may be hand warmed. Normal CT is between 4-10 minutes, but your monitoring should be based on a baseline measurement (e.g., a CT done prior to heparin Rx). Subsequent levels should be drawn just prior to administration of each intermittent dose. The goal should be to maintain a CT of approximately twice the baseline measurement. Heparin doses should be raised or lowered accordingly. If on a given dose the CT seems to stabilize where you want it (for three consecutive readings), you need only obtain this measurement once or twice daily.

Heparin therapy should be continued until the patient's cardiopulmonary status has improved. Once this occurs, the heparin may be tapered over 48 hours to 5,000 units SQ every 12 hours.

Progressive ambulation, before tapering the heparin, should be encouraged. Ace wraps should be employed on the legs during this time.

The patient should be maintained on 5,000 units SQ every 12 hours for 4-6 weeks. This dose (often referred to as "mini-dose" heparin) will not affect clotting times, so none need be done. This low dose does, however, afford some resistance to future possible clot formation.

Fat embolization: Should be suspected if sudden unexplained dyspnea, tachypnea, tachycardia, and neurological deterioration (e.g., delirium, coma, etc.) develop 12-36 hours after bone fracture (especially a major long bone or pelvic fracture). Treatment is supportive.

1-27. PLEURAL EFFUSIONS. The presence of fluid (including blood and pus) in the pleural cavity.

Pathology: The presence of fluid displaces and restricts the lung on the involved side, hindering respiration. The more fluid, the more restriction. Fluid can arise from several processes (see below).

S. and O. Progressive or worsening dyspnea is the most consistent finding. The rapidity of fluid accumulation as well as the amount of fluid present will contribute to the prominence of this symptom. Slowly developing effusions may not produce significant dyspnea until large volumes have accumulated where a rapidly developing effusion will produce dyspnea at smaller volumes. Other symptoms of pleural effusion will be related to the specific causes. Deviation of the trachea away from the affected side may be seen. Poor movement of the involved side of the chest may be noted. Dullness to percussion will be noted in the upright position. The extent of dullness (measured to the intercostal space where dullness disappears) should be marked off. Sometimes an area of hyperresonance will be noted just above the fluid level. Fremitus is absent. Decreased to absent breath sound is the rule, but loud tubular breath sounds may often be present. Also whispered sounds may be absent or less commonly increase.

Lab: Pleural fluid should be examined and the following tests performed:

(1) W.B.C. count and differential: R.B.C. count.
(2) Gram's stain.
(3) Glucose measurement (dextrostix) of fluid and blood.

Other findings related to the specific causes of the effusion may be present.

Congestive heart failure	Usually right-side; may be bilateral. W.B.C. <1,000/mm.3/glucose equals serum glucose R.B.C.<10,000/mm.3. Other evidence of CHF.
Cirrhosis	As above but with evidence of liver disease.
Bacterial or viral pneumonia	Same side as infection. May precede other evidence of pneumonia. W.B.C.>1000/mm.3 with >50%P.M.N.s/glucose<serum glucose organisms (bacteria) may be seen on Gram's stain (rare).
Tuberculosis	Same side as infection. Other evidence of PTB W.B.C.>1,000/mm.3 with >50% lymphocytes.
Pulmonary infarction	May be bloody. R.B.C.>10,000/mm.3 W.B.C.>1,000/mm.3
Subphrenic abscess	W.B.C.>1,000/mm.3 (usually) evidence of intra-abdominal infection.
Chest trauma	Frequently blood. Hx of trauma usually obtainable.
Leakage through a subclavian line	Fluid has characteristic of IV fluid used glucose>serum glucose (if D_5 was component of fluids).
Pneumothorax	Usually unremarkable but may have W.B.C. increase.

P. Thoracentesis: Because of the danger of inducing a pneumothorax, evacuation of the fluid (therapeutic thoracentesis) should be reserved for conditions where severe respiratory distress is present. A small sampling of fluid may be obtained for studies (diagnostic thoracentesis) relatively safely.

The major therapeutic effort should be directed at resolving the process responsible for the effusion. Most effusion will resorb once this is done.

1-28. ASTHMA. A disease of the airways characterized by recurrent bouts of dyspnea usually associated with wheezing and coughing.

S. Chief complaint: Dyspnea is the most outstanding complaint. Onset is usually abrupt (seconds to minutes) though there may occur, prior to the onset of frank dyspnea, a period of vague chest discomfort not always clearly defined upon questioning the patient, but often described as a "rightness" by some. Many asthmatics have learned to recognize this "aura" as a warning of impending attack. The dyspnea, when it does become recognized, is usually progressive. Because the sensation of shortness of breath is subject to modification by factors not directly the result of the pathophysiology (i.e., anxiety, intoxication), the degree of apparent dyspnea does not correlate well with the severity of airway obstruction; hence it should not be used as a concrete clinical guide to therapy or the patient's response to therapy. Cough is usually present and may be productive of a thick, tenacious, grey-white sputum. This sputum mostly consists of bronchial secretions that have "dried out" somewhat (i.e., the water is evaporated off by air flow leaving behind the thick mucous component of the secretions) and can reach the consistency of gelatin. This inspissated mucous can plug airways, thus increasing airway obstruction. Hence a dry cough in an asthmatic during an attack may indicate a severe degree of obstruction due to the "mucous plugging" phenomena. Wheezing may or may not be perceptible to the patient and is defined further below. The duration between onset of symptoms and presentation should be obtained as the rapidity with which a patient approaches a given amount of distress (as obtained from history and physical) may prove a valuable index to the severity of the episode.

Past history: Most asthmatics are very familiar with their state and may tell you both what usually triggers an attack and what therapy they usually respond to.

Medications: Many attacks probably result from loss of medical control. Determine what medications, if any, the patient uses for asthma. If he discontinued them, determine when generally; the more medications and the higher the dosages, the more severe his disease. Steroids are the "big guns" of asthma therapy and the asthmatic requiring them for control has severe disease.

Allergies: Some asthmatics give a history of various and sundry allergic responses (hives, rhinitis, etc.) to specific substances. These patients are especially prone to anaphylactic reactions, so special attention should be given to this segment of questioning. Note here that certain drugs can precipitate or worsen an asthma attack. The most notable being salycilates and other nonsteroidol anti-inflammatory agents (e.g. Indocin, Motrin, etc.) as well as propranolol (Inderal).

O. General appearance. Asthmatics appear anxious during an attack, and the expression of fear on their faces is evident across a room. They inhale through open mouths often throwing their heads back as they do. Exhalation may be through pursed lips and the patient may lean forward as if straining to defecate. Asthmatics in moderate to severe distress prefer to sit as maximal mechanical advantage of the respiratory muscles are obtained in this position. When an asthmatic in this type of distress "lays down" on you, it may indicate he is tiring; hence, you must move quickly.

Vital signs: Should be obtained prior to any therapy.

Temperature, if elevated, may indicate presence of a concomitant infection.

Pulse is usually rapid and regular; slow or irregular pulse may indicate severe hypoxia acidosis. Pulsus paradoxus should be searched for (see B.P.).

Respirations are very important. Both the rate and character of the respirations should be noted. Because inspiration has more muscular assist than expiration, air can be forced through partially obstructed airways, but has considerably more difficulty getting out. This results in a prolonged expiratory phase, the length of which parallels roughly the degree of obstruction. Further, as the patient breaths faster (because of hypoxia) his inspirations begin before the slower expirations are completed, hence air is trapped and the chest becomes progressively hyperexpanded. As hyperexpansion increases, the amount of air the patient is able to forcefully inspire decreases. He compensates by breathing still faster. More air is trapped and a vicious cycle ensues. For these reasons a low respiratory rate with markedly prolonged expiratory phase (exhaustion) or a rapid shallow rate in the presence of marked hyperinflation are preterminal events in the asthmatic...seconds count.

B.P.: When the B.P. is markedly elevated (>160/>100) caution should be used in the administration of epinephrine. The drugs should probably be withheld altogether in the older patient with elevated B.P. especially if there is a history of heart disease or stroke. The severity of the elevation and the patient's overall state must be weighed together. There are no hard and fast rules. An abnormal degree of pulsus paradoxus (PP) should be searched for. When the cuff is inflated, SLOWLY deflate it (1mm. Hg every 2 secs) and note at what point the systolic tones begin. If pulsus paradoxus is present, these tones will disappear during inspiration and reappear on expiration. Continue to deflate the cuff slowly and note the range over which this finding persists. If the finding persists over a range greater than 12mm./Hg, there is an abnormal degree of paradox present. This sign correlates well with the degree of obstruction (the greater the range, the more severe the obstruction) and usually reflects trends in the patient's status before they can be fully appreciated in other aspects of the physical.

The degree of pulsus paradoxus should be noted through the treatment until normal and recorded with frequently collected vital signs. In more severe degrees, the pulsus paradoxus may be noted in the peripheral pulses where it manifests as an inspiratory disappearance or weakening of the pulse. This finding is an invaluable aid to estimating the severity of obstruction and the adequacy (or inadequacy) of therapy when arterial blood gases and other labs are not available or not practicable. A note of caution here: A decrease in PP may be noted as the patient begins to succumb to exhaustion or approaches the state of maximal hyperinflation. Like any other physical sign, PP must be interpreted in light of the general clinical picture; yet here, any change is of significance.

HEENT - Dry mucous membranes should be interpreted (as an indication of possible dehydration) with caution as there is invariably some drying secondary to the prominent mouth breathing.

Neck - Use of the accessory muscles of respiration, specifically the anterior and anterolateral neck muscles, have been shown to correlate roughly with the degree of obstruction. Straining of these muscles on inspiration is seen in moderate to severe degrees of obstruction and their use will decrease and eventually disappear as obstruction is relieved. Remember, however, that use of these muscles will also become less prominent as the patient becomes exhausted...monitor the WHOLE patient!

Chest - In the field, probably the most valuable indications of the adequacy of ventilation are the magnitude and nature of chest movements.

For all practicable purposes if there is no chest expansion, the patient is not moving air. All the other parameters used to monitor the asthmatic in the field (e.g., changes in PP; presence or absence of wheezes; use of accessory muscles, etc.) should be interpreted in light of chest expansion (and to a lesser extent on the presence or absence of breath sounds).

By the mechanism previously outlined, the chest may become "locked in" a progressively increasing state of expansion by air trapping and be unable to relax to its preinspiratory position. Since the chest wall can only expand so far, the amount of air that can be forced in progressively decreases. Signs of hyperexpansion include increased or increasing anterior-posterior chest diameter (best noted at the end of expiration); decreasing respiratory excursions; increasing chest hyperresonance to percussion with loss of cardiac area dullness and widened intercostal spaces. In severe instances (approaching maximal hyperinflation) air movement decreases to the point that breath sounds and wheezes begin to fade and disappear. Expiratory movement: As stated previously, the degree of expiratory phase prolongation should be noted.

Lungs - Breath sounds may be heard in mild to moderate states, but usually become obscured by wheezing in more severe cases. Wheezing is a hallmark of partial airways obstruction. The sound is produced by air "whistling" through partially obstructed channels. Both inspiratory and expiratory wheezes are heard in asthma though expiratory wheezes are more prominent and may be the only type present in mild episodes. As obstruction is relieved, wheezing will diminish and clear breath sounds with improved respiratory excursions will be noted. Since the production of wheezes depends also on air flow, they will also diminish or vanish when ventilation falls (e.g., high degrees of hyperexpansion or patient exhaustion). Here no breath sounds will be heard, and chest expansion will be minimal to nonexistent.

Egophony ('e>a' changes) may be noted in patchy areas over all lung fields. In this case, the finding is probably secondary to collapse of small areas of lung because their airways have been completely obstructed. If the finding is very prominent over a fairly large, well demarcated area, then an associated pneumonia or collapse of a lung segment, lobe, or entire lung (depending on extent of the area) secondary to obstruction of a bronchus by a large mucous plug must be considered.

Lab: An elevated W.B.C. count and/or leftward shift in the differentiation may indicate an associated infection. If this test is to be performed, it should be done before administration of epinephrine as this agent will itself increase W.B.C. count in the leftward direction. This effect may persist for 24 hours. Exam of the sputum may reveal tiny mucous plugs that have been dislodged from the smaller airways (called Curschmann's spirals). Eosinophils may also be present in large numbers. The presence of many non-eosinophilic polymorphonuclear cells should raise suspicion of a possible associated pneumonia or bronchitis. In general, however, most of the above provide merely supportive evidence, and since more sophisticated labs will not be available, the diagnosis and management of the asthmatic in the field will depend on your abilities to obtain and interpret clinical findings.

A. Asthma.

P. Management: Therapy is aimed at reversing the pathophysiologic factors while correcting the derangements (e.g., hypoxia, dehydration, etc.) they have produced. The treatment is staged to correspond to the classes of severity previously outlined.

	Mild	Severe
Bronchospasm:	.3-.5cc. 1:100 solution of epinephrine SQ repeat q.20min x 3 or until wheezes cleared	Administer epinephrine as scheduled but immediately after first injection administer aminophylline as follows:
	If no improvement noted or patient worsens during Tx	Aminophylline 400 mg. in 250 cc. D5 /1/2 NS run in IV over 15 min. Followed by an IV administered solution of aminophylline 200 mg. in 500 cc. D5 /1/2 NS at rate of 150-200 cc./hr until cleared. If no improvement noted at 2 hrs or patient worsens, continue infusion and, Give terbutaline 0.25-0.5 mg. SQ. If no improvement in 1 hr or patient worsens continue infusion and... Give Solu-Medrol (methylprednisolone) 1 gm IV push followed by 1 gm IV push q.6h. until clear. Solu-Cortef (hydrocortisone) may be substituted. An initial 10 gm is given IV push and subsequently q.6h. thereafter until clear.
Dehydration:	P.O. hydration (force fluids) is usually adequate	Hydration is accomplished with the aminophylline solution. D5 /1/2 is preferred but NS or Ringer's solution will suffice. ($D5^W$ in extreme emergency).
Hypoxia:	O_2 not required	O_2, if at all attainable, must be employed preferably by mask (because of mouth breathing)

Inspissated secretions: Are thinned by hydration and released by relief of bronchospasm to be effectively coughed up and cleared.

General therapeutic considerations: Many would view this outlined plan of management as aggressive. However, in the field, removed from sophisticated diagnostic-monitoring facilities, mechanical ventilatory assistance, and most probably oxygen, the only hope the asthmatic has is an approach that relieves his obstruction ASAP! The old adage of "push it (aminophylline) till they puke" may be quite necessary in field practice to assure adequate blood levels. It must be remembered that it is impossible to reliably predict which episodes will respond to lower dosages or less vigorous management and that as the attack progresses your chances of retrieval diminish by large factors. In these instances, you can expect mortality rates approaching 20 times those of a hospital emergency room.

Special Considerations:

Exhaustion: Close monitoring is necessary to head off complete respiratory collapse. If the patient shows signs of "giving it up" (i.e., weakened respiratory effort manifested by a decreased or erratic respiratory rate or decreased inspiratory excursions associated with a progressive decrease in breath sounds--or wheezes in the absence of breath sounds-- and a lethargic fatigued overall appearance), therapy should be stepped up by progressing directly to steroid administration. Talk to the patient and encourage him to hang in there! Slap him or pinch him if you have to but try to buy any additional time you can. If he does not answer coherently and continues to "slip away," you must intubate and bag him until therapy begins to take effect and he can breath on his own.

Cyanosis: Slight discoloration may be noted at the nail beds and should be managed by oxygen and continued bronchodilation therapy. When it occurs in the setting of impending exhaustion (above), it is an indication for immediate intubation and ventilatory assistance.

Hyperinflation: High degrees of hyperinflation associated with decreasing excursions are an indication to step up therapy as outlined above. Once the chest becomes "fixed" at a high level of expansion, however, ventilatory assistance can usually force no more air in than the patient could. It should nonetheless be attempted since some degree of exhaustion is usually active.

Large mucous plugs: May be relieved with hydration, bronchodilators, and chest percussion. To perform percussion, the patient is placed in a manner to position the affected side up and in a head-down tilt of approximately 30º. The area is briskly slapped with cupped palms and the patient is asked to increase expiratory effort, if possible, or cough.

Intubation: Once intubated the patient's own effective mechanisms for clearing secretions (cough) are removed. Frequent suctioning is a must. Never leave a tube in place in an asthmatic unless you are ventilating him.

Immediate follow-up therapy:

Once the patient has cleared, he should be placed on theophylline 100-300 mg. t.i.d.-q.i.d. depending on severity of the episode. Terbutaline 2.5-5 mg. P.O. t.i.d.-q.i.d. may also be given with this. Those patients that require steroid therapy should be placed on prednisone 40 mg. P.O. the first day after the episode and the dose reduced by 5 mg. each day thereafter (e.g., 35 mg. the 2nd day; 30 mg. the 3rd, etc.) until they have been tapered to 5-10 mg. day. These patients and indeed all severe cases should be evacuated as soon as possible for further evaluation.

Section IV - The Circulatory System.

1-29. The circulatory system is composed of the heart, blood vessels, lymphactic system and their contained fluids, blood, and lymph.

a. Arterial hypertension. Elevation of systolic and/or diastolic blood pressure, either primary (essential hypertension) or secondary. Although the etiology of essential hypertension is unknown, the family history is usually suggestive of hypertension (stroke, sudden death, heart failure). Secondary hypertension is associated with kidney disease (e.g., chronic glomerulonephritis or pyelonephritis), or occlusion of one or more of the renal arteries or their branches (renovascular hypertension). An untreated hypertensive patient is at great risk of developing fatal heart failure, brain hemorrhage, or kidney failure.

S. Primary hypertension is asymptomatic until complications arise. Complications include left ventricular failure; atherosclerotic heart disease; retinal hemorrhages, exudates, and vascular accidents; cerebral vascular insufficiency; and renal failure. Hypertensive encephalopathy due to cerebral vasospasm and edema is characteristic of hypertension.

O. Consistent diastolic pressure >100 mm. Hg in patients >60 years of age; diastolic pressure >90 mm. Hg in patients <50 years of age; or systolic pressure >140 mm. Hg regardless of age. Retinal changes will range from minimal arteriolar narrowing and irregularity to frank hemorrhages and papilledema, i.e., elevation of the optic disk or blurring of the disk margins.

A. A Dx of hypertension is not warranted in a patient under 50 years of age unless the B.P. exceeds 140/90 mm. Hg on at least three separate occasions after the patient has rested for 20 minutes or more in quiet and familiar surroundings. Secondary complications will present symptomatology of the "target organs" involved:

(1) Cardiac involvement often leads to nocturnal dyspnea or cardiac asthma (inspiratory and expiratory wheezing). Angina pectoris or myocardial infarction may develop.

(2) Renal involvement may produce nocturia and hematuria. The patient may have a uremic odor. Kidneys may be enlarged and palpable.

(3) Cerebral involvement will demonstrate neurological signs ranging from a positive Babinkşi or Hoffman reflex to paralysis.

(4) Peripheral arterial disease causes intermittent claudication (limping). If the terminal aorta is involved, pain in the buttocks and low back pain appear on walking and men become impotent.

P. Treat mild hypertension (diastolic pressure 90 to 110 mm. Hg) with an oral diuretic such as chlorothiazide (Diuril) 500 mg. b.i.d. If the diuretic does not control the hypertension, methyldopa (Aldomet) 250 mg. b.i.d. to 500 mg. q.i.d., or clonidine (Catepres) or reserpine 0.25 to 0.5 mg./day should be added. Methyldopa is preferred because its side effects are better tolerated. For moderate hypertension (diastolic pressure between 111 and 125 mm. Hg) start therapy with an oral diuretic and a sympathetic depressant (e.g., methyldopa, clonidine, reserpine, or propranolol). For severe hypertension (diastolic pressure >125 mm. Hg) therapy should be started with an oral diuretic and guanethidine (10 mg. to 150 mg./day in a single dose) simultaneously. Methyldopa should be added if needed. Patients with acute severe hypertension (diastolic pressure >150 mm. Hg) or with pressures somewhat lower but with commanding symptoms of headache, visual disturbances, somnolence or other signs of cerebral, cardiac, or renal involvement or acute pulmonary edema should be placed on strict bed rest (semi-Fowler position) and parenteral therapy instituted immediately. Diazoxide (Hyperstat) is the drug of choice; 300 mg. IV push will reduce B.P. to normal values within 5 minutes. The drug should be used only for short periods and combined with a potent diuretic such as furosemide (Lasix) 40 to 80 mg. IV. Vital signs must be monitored continuously. Be prepared to treat hypotension (see Chapter 5, Shock). Discontinue if any sign of hearing impairment develops. When B.P. has been brought under control, combinations of oral antihypertensive agents can be added as parenteral drugs are tapered off over a period of 2-3 days.

b. Thrombophlebitis. Partial or complete occlusion of a vein by a thrombus with a secondary inflammatory reaction in the wall of a vein. It occurs most frequently in the deep veins of the legs and pelvis in postoperative and postpartum patients during the fourth to fourteenth day, and in patients with fractures or other trauma, cardiac disease, or stroke, especially if prolonged bed rest is involved. Deep venous thrombosis is usually benign but occasionally terminates in lethal pulmonary embolism or chronic venous insufficiency. Superficial phlebitis alone is usually self-limiting and without serious complications; aging, malignancy, shock, dehydration, anemia, obesity, and chronic infection are predisposing factors.

S. Approximately half of patients with thrombophlebitis are asymptomatic: Others may complain of a dull ache, tightness, or frank pain in the calf or the whole leg, especially when walking. A feeling of anxiety is not uncommon.

O. Slight swelling in the involved calf (measure); bluish discoloration or prominence of the superficial veins; warmth of affected leg when both legs are exposed to room temperature; tenderness and induration or spasm in the calf muscles, with or without pain in the calf produced by dorsiflexion of the foot (Homans' sign). With deep thrombophlebitis involving the popliteal, femoral, and iliac segments, there may be tenderness and a hard cord may be palpable over the involved vein in the femoral triangle in the groin, the medial thigh, or popliteal space; slight fever and tachycardia may be present. The skin may be cyanotic if venous obstruction is severe, or pale and cool if a reflex arterial spasm is superimposed.

A. Thrombophlebitis. Differential diagnosis: Calf muscle strain or contusion. NOTE: Pain due to muscular causes is absent or minimal on dorsiflexion of the ankle with the knee flexed and maximal on dorsiflexion of the ankle with the knee extended or during SLRs (Homans' sign); cellulitis; lymphatic obstruction; acute arterial occlusion (distal pulses are absent and there is no swelling); bilateral leg edema due to heart, kidney, or liver disease.

P. Treatment: Strict bed rest; elevate legs 15-20 degrees. Ace bandage from toes to just below the knees; moist heat. Anticoagulation therapy with heparin should be initiated if there are no contraindications to its use (contraindications are peptic ulcer, significant kidney or liver disease; Hx of cerebrovascular hemorrhage, recent head trauma, or known clotting defect). Prior to initiation of heparin therapy, a baseline clotting time must be established. (Normal Lee-White clotting time is 6-15 minutes). The dose should be adjusted to provide 2-3 times the baseline pretreatment value. Continuous IV infusion is the preferred route. Give a loading dose as an IV bolus (2,000 units) prior to starting constant infusion at a rate of approximately 1,500 units/hour for the average-sized adult. Remember that the ultimate rate must be established on the basis of clotting times obtained q.2-3h. from an arm not being infused and verified by at least 2 successive clotting times in the therapeutic range. Subsequent clotting times are repeated q.6-10h. The required dosage will usually decrease with time. If an infusion pump is not available, give deep SQ q.6h. (use small needle and inject slowly). Start dose in the range of 7,000-9,000 units for an average-sized adult. Obtain clotting time 30 minutes before each planned dose and adjust to maintain therapeutic range. The required dose should drop to 4,000-6,000 units after a day or two of therapy. Therapy should be continued until the patient is asymptomatic and the danger of embolism has passed (normally 2-3 weeks). The diagnosis of thrombophlebitis is difficult without the use of sophisticated diagnostic aids that normally are not available (phlebography isotopic scan, etc.); therefore, maximum use must be made of past and current history and the most thorough P.E. possible. The dangers of lethal pulmonary embolism must be carefully weighed against the dangers of uncontrolled hemorrhage, and each decision is made on a sound assessment of all factors involved.

Prevention: The best cure for postoperative thrombophlebitis is its prevention. Assure that circulation is maintained by active and passive exercise while patients are bedridden. Avoid tight clothing. Elevate legs or foot of bed 15-30 degrees. Flex knees. Encourage deep breathing exercise. Ambulate patient as soon as possible (walking, not standing). Dextran, 500 ml. IV during surgery and repeated on first postoperative day, appears to have a prophylactic effect, as does ASA 1 gm daily P.O. NOTE: ASA is contraindicated once anticoagulation therapy has begun.

c. Hemorrhoids. Varicosities of the veins of the hemorrhoidal plexus, often complicated by inflammation, thrombosis, and bleeding. May be external (distal to anorectal line) or internal (proximal to anorectal line).

S. Rectal bleeding, pain (may be severe), itching, protrusion, mucoid discharge from rectum.

O. Small, rounded, purplish skin-covered masses that are soft and seldom painful unless thrombosed. When thrombosed, they are hard and often extremely painful when palpitated.

A. Hemorrhoids (internal or external). Differential diagnosis: Perianal abcess, rectal neoplasms, or colitis.

P. Use stool softners or nonirritating laxatives, such as mineral oil, and soft diet to prevent hard stools and straining. Small uncomplicated hemorrhoids are usually self-limiting and respond well to conservative or minimal treatment. Manage local pain and infection with warm sitz baths and insertion of a soothing anal suppository b.i.d.-t.i.d. Avoid the use of benzocaine and other types of similar ointments as much as possible to preclude sensitizing the patient. Use hot sitz baths t.i.d.-q.i.d. to reduce thrombosed hemorrhoids. If this is unsuccessful or patient is in extreme discomfort, excise the thrombus under 1% lidocaine local; pack lightly with iodoform gauze initially and cover with dry sterile dressing. Change dressing daily. Continue warm sitz baths. Instruct patient to avoid trauma when cleansing the anal area after bowel movements by patting with damp tissue rather than rubbing. Instruct patient not to attempt to defecate unless there is a real urge and to avoid straining at stools.

1-30. DISEASES OF THE HEART.

a. Myocardial infarction (MI). Ischemic myocardial necrosis usually resulting from a sudden reduction in blood flow to a section of the myocardium due to occlusion of a coronary artery.

S. Sudden onset of intense, crushing substernal or precordial pain, often radiating to the left shoulder, arm, or jaw. Patients break out in a cold sweat, feel weak and apprehensive, and move about seeking a position of comfort. They prefer not to lie quietly. Lightheadedness, syncope, dyspnea, orthopnea, cough, wheezing, nausea and vomiting, or abdominal bloating may also be present, singly or in combination. The pain is not relieved by nitroglycerin.

O. Patient may be cyanotic and the skin is usually cool. The pulse may be thready and the blood pressure variable. Most show some degree of hypertension unless cardiogenic shock is developing (incidence about 8-14 percent). In a severe attack, the first and second heart sounds are faint and often indistinguishable. Arrhythmia is common. Rales may be heard on auscultation and the neck veins are often distended. Fever is absent at the onset but usually rises to 100-103° F. within 24 hours. W.B.C. will be elevated with a shift to the left by the second day. The sedimentation rate is normal at onset and will rise on the second or third day.

A. Acute myocardial infarction. Differential diagnosis: Angina pectoris, acute pericarditis, acute pulmonary embolism, reflux esophagitis, acute pancreatitis, acute cholecystitis, spontaneous pneumothorax, pneumonia.

P. Be alert for cardiac arrest, particularly during the first few hours after onset (50 percent of all MI deaths occur during this period). Be prepared to initiate CPR immediately if patient does arrest (see Chapter 3, Emergency Resuscitation). Morphine SO_4 2-5 mg. slow IV, stat. repeat q. 15 min p.r.n. unless respiration falls below 12/min. Shock position, O_2 (do not use positive pressure). Lidocaine initial bolus 50-100 mg. (1 mg./kg.) IV, then IV drip at 1-4 mg. per minute. Hospitalize with strict bed rest and complete nursing care for at least 6 weeks. Sedate with 1/2 gm phenobarbital t.i.d. Low sodium, low fat, low protein diet. Monitor vital signs constantly. Be alert for signs of left-sided heart failure (see para e, Congestive heart failure), hypotension, and cardiogenic shock (see Chapter 15, Shock); evacuate when feasible.

b. Acute myocarditis. A focal or diffuse inflammation of the myocardium occurring during or after many viral, rickettsial, spirochetal, fungal, and parasitic diseases or administration of various drugs. Severe myocarditis occurs most commonly in acute rheumatic fever, diphtheria, scrub typhus, and Chagas' disease.

S. Fever, malaise, arthralgias, chest pain, dyspnea, and

palpitations. The patient may have associated pericarditis, with chest pain characteristic of pericardial involvement (see para f, Acute pericarditis). The chest pain is frequently vague and nondiagnostic.

O. Tachycardia out of proportion to the amount of fever. The B.P. is usually normal. Ausculation may reveal a tic-tac rhythm and systolic murmur. Acute circulatory collapse, emboli, and sudden death may occur.

A. Acute myocarditis. Differential diagnosis: Viral, protozoan, or bacterial infections must be distinguished from acute toxic myocarditis due to drugs or diphtheria and from myocarditis associated with acute rheumatic fever and acute glomerulonephritis by a careful analysis of each history and clinical picture as it presents.

P. Direct treatment toward underlying cause if known. In all cases when myocarditis is suspected or apparent, complete bed rest and sedation plus continued therapy of the underlying disease are needed. Oxygen is indicated when cyanosis or dyspnea occurs. Continue bed rest until all evidence of cardiac involvement disappears.

c. Bacterial endocarditis. Bacterial infection of the lining membrane of the heart. Acute bacterial endocarditis (ABE) begins abruptly and progresses rapidly. The usual cause is staphylococci and occasionally pneumococci. It may follow postabortal pelvic infection, surgery on infected tissue, or unsterile intravenous techniques. Subacute bacterial endocarditis (SBE) is usually due to alpha-hemoliticus streptococci and frequently follows a dental procedure. The disease is fatal if untreated.

S. Fever is usually present but afebrile periods may occur. Night sweats, chills, malaise, fatigue, anorexia, weight loss; myalgia; arthralgia, or redness and swelling of joints; sudden visual disturbances; paralysis; pain in the abdomen, chest, or flanks; nose bleeds; easy bruisability; and symptoms of heart failure may also occur.

O. Findings in SBE include tachycardia; splenomegaly; petechiae of the skin, mucous membranes, and ocular fundi, or beneath the nails as splinter hemorrhages; clubbing of the fingers and toes; pallor or a yellowish-brown tint of the skin; neurologic residual effects of cerebral emboli; and tender finger and toe pads. In ABE symptoms and signs are similar to those of SBE, but the course is more rapid. Suspect ABE if an otherwise healthy individual with a focal infection suddenly develops chills, high fever, and prostration. An unexplained fever in patient with a heart murmur is indicative of endocarditis. Anemia, markedly elevated sedimentation rate, variable leukocytosis, microscopic hematuria, proteinuria, and casts are commonly present in SBE and ABE.

A. Infective endocarditis due to _________. Differential diagnosis: Lymphomas, thrombocytopenic purpura, leukemia, acute rheumatic fever, lupus erythematosus, septicemia (may be the forerunner), URIs.

P. Endocarditis due to streptococcus: Penicillin G 20-40 M.U. daily, or ampicillin 6-12 gm daily in divided doses as bolus injections q.2-4h. into an IV infusion. Probenecid 0.5 gm P.O. t.i.d. x 4-5 weeks. Streptomycin, 1 gm day; kanamycin 15 mg./kg./day; or gentamicin 5 mg./kg./per day b.i.d.-t.i.d. in divided doses. Endocarditis due to staphlococcus (penicillin resistant), nafcillin, 8-12 gm daily as a bolus q.2h. in an IV infusion. If patient is hypersensitive to penicillin, desensitize or use vancomycin 2-3 gm IV daily in divided doses q.4h. continue Tx x 5-6 weeks. Complete nursing care. Monitor for signs of neurotoxicity and thrombophlebitis. Change injection site q.48h. and keep scrupulously clean. Evacuate if at all feasible.

d. Angina pectoris. A clinical syndrome due to myocardial ischemia producing a sensation of precordial discomfort, pressure, or a strangling sensation, characteristically precipitated by exertion and relieved by rest or nitroglycerin.

S. Squeezing or pressurelike pain, retrosternal or slightly to the left, that appears quickly during exertion and increases rapidly in intensity until the patient is compelled to stop and rest. The distribution of the distress may vary widely in different patients, but is always the same for each individual patient. The attacks usually last less than 3 minutes unless following a heavy meal or precipitated by anger, in which case they may last 15-20 minutes. The distress of angina is never a sharply localized darting pain that can be pointed to with one finger. If the patient points with one finger to the area of the apical impulse as the only site of pain, angina may almost certainly be ruled out.

O. The diagnosis of angina pectoris depends almost entirely upon the history, and it is of utmost importance that the patient be allowed to describe his symptoms to the examiner. The diagnosis is strongly supported (1) if 0.4 mg. nitroglycerin invariably shortens an attack and (2) if that amount taken immediately before hand invariably permits greater exertion before onset of an attack or prevents it entirely. Examination during an attack frequently reveals elevated B.P.; occasionally, gallop rhythm is present during pain only.

A. Angina pectoris. Differential diagnosis: Musculosketal disorders, cholecystitis, reflux esophagitis, peptic ulcer, myocardial infarction.

P. Nitroglycerin 0.3 mg. sublingually is the drug of choice. Increase dose to 0.4-0.6 mg. if smaller dose is ineffective. One amyl nitrite ampule crushed and inhaled will act in about 10 seconds. The patient should stand still or lie down as soon as the pain begins and remain quiet until the attack is over. Patients should be warned not to try to work the attack off.

e. Congestive heart failure. A clinical syndrome in which the heart fails to maintain an adequate output, resulting in diminished blood flow to the tissues and in congestion in the pulmonary and/or systemic circulation. The left or right ventricle alone may fail initially (usually the former), but ultimately combined failure is the rule. The basic causes of ventricular failure are: (1) Myocardial weakness or inflammation (e.g., myocarditis, ischemia), (2) Excess workload (e.g., hypertension, aortic insufficiency anemia, pregnancy, etc.).

S. Early manifestations of left ventricular failure include undue tachycardia, fatigue with exertion, dsypnea with mild exercise, and intolerance to cold; paroxysmal nocturnal dyspnea and cough. In advanced failure severe cough is prominent. The sputum may be tinged rusty or brown. Frank hemoptysis is rare but can occur. Acute pulmonary edema is a serious life threatening manifestation of left ventricular failure. The patient presents with extreme dyspnea, cyanosis, tachypnea, hyperpnea, restlessness, and anxiety with a sense of suffocation. Right ventricular failure presents with increasing fatigue, awareness of fullness in the neck and abdomen, anorexia, bloating, or exertional RUQ pain. Oliguria is present in the day time; polyuria at night.

O. Signs of left ventricular failure include reduced carotid pulsation, diffuse apical impulse, palpable and audible third and fourth heart sounds, inspiratory rales, and pleural effusion. With acute pulmonary edema the pulse may be thready and the B.P. difficult to obtain. Respirations are grunting and labored with inspiration, and expiration is prolonged. Expiratory rales can be heard over both lungs. There may be marked bronchospasm or wheezing. Hypoxia is severe and cyanosis deep. Patients with right ventricular failure show signs of venous hypertension, an enlarged and tender liver, murmurs, and pitting edema of the lower extremities. CBC and sed. rate are normal in uncomplicated left heart failure. Urinalysis often shows significant proteinuria and granular casts.

A. Congestive heart failure due to__________. Differential diagnosis: Pericardial effusion, constrictive pericarditis, pulmonary disease, carcinoma of the lung, anemias, and rebound edema following the use of diuretics.

P. Bed rest (Fowler or semi-Fowler position), sedation with morphine or phenobarbital; frequent (4-6) small, bland, low calorie, low residue, sodium restricted meals with vitamin supplements. Diuretics such as hydrochlorothiazide 50 mg./day or chlorothiazide 500 mg. daily or b.i.d. are essential to management of chronic heart failure. Increase daily ingestion of foods with a high potassium content (bananas, orange juice) for potassium replacement. Administer O_2 p.r.n. for respiratory distress and hypoxia. Acute pulmonary edema is grave medical emergency demanding prompt and effective Tx. Unless in shock, the patient should sit upright with legs dangling. Give high concentrations of O_2 by mask or nasal cannula. Morphine SO_4 5-10 mg. IV or IM. Sublingual nitroglycerin 0.4-0.6 mg. q.10 min for several doses may be immediately effective. If severe, apply B.P. cuffs (or soft rubber tourniquets) to three limbs and inflate or tighten sufficiently to obstruct venous return (midway between systolic and diastolic pressure) but not arterial flow. Rotate q.15 min. NOTE: Do not apply to a limb in which an IV is running. If IV is running, deflate q.15-20 min but do not rotate. Give a rapid acting diuretic, e.g., Lasix (furosemide) 40-80 mg. IV or Edecrin 25-50 mg. IV. Aminophylline, 0.25-0.5 gm slow IV or aminophylline suppositories, 0.25-0.5 gm may be of help. Rapid digitalization is of value; however, it must be remembered that all digitalis preparations are toxic and the difference between the theraputic and toxic level is small. Do not use digitalis if there is any indication of renal failure. If renal function is normal, the following schedule may be used: Digoxin 0.25 mg. IV or P.O. stat., then 0.25 mg. q.6h. x 2 days and 0.25 mg. daily thereafter. NOTE: Digitalis maintenance may be required for the remainder of the patient's life. When stable, the patient should be carefully monitored for: (1) Status of original symptoms, (2) new symptoms or signs, (3) weight changes, (4) vital signs, (5) evidence of phlebothrombosis. Evacuate as soon as feasible.

f. Acute pericarditis. Inflammation of the pericardium. It may result from trauma, infection, or neoplasm or secondary to systemic diseases such as rheumatic fever, rheumatoid arthritis, or uremia.

S. Pleuritic or persisting substernal or precordial pain

radiating to the neck, shoulder, or back. Pain may be aggravated by thoracic motion, cough, and respiration. It is relieved by sitting up and leaning forward and may be accentuated by swallowing. Tachypnea, nonproductive cough, fever, chills, weakness, and anxiety are common.

O. Auscultation reveals to and fro friction sounds (friction rub) over 4th (L) intercostal space near sternum. Inspection and palpation sometimes reveal a diffuse apex beat. With purulent effusion may present with high, irregular fever, sweats, chills, and progressive pallor. Bulging of the precordium, increased dullness to percussion, and edema of the precordium may also be present. Leukocytosis and elevated sed. rate will be present at the onset.

A. Acute pericarditis due to ____________. Differential diagnosis: Acute MI, pleurisy.

P. (1) Treat underlying condition.

(2) ASA 600 mg. P.O., codeine 15-60 mg. P.O., meperidine 50-100 mg. P.O. or IM, or morphine 10-15 mg. SQ q.4h. for pain. Sedate with phenobarbital 15-30 mg. P.O. t.i.d.-q.i.d.; 100-200 mg. phenobarbital may be given h.s. for insomnia. Prednisone 20 to 60 mg. daily in divided doses t.i.d.-q.i.d. may be required to control pain, fever, and effusion. The dose should be reduced gradually and discontinued over a period of 7-14 days. If the pericarditis is due a pyogenic infection, surgical drainage of the pericardial sac may be indicated.

1-31. DISEASES OF THE BLOOD.

a. Anemia (general). A condition in which there is a reduction in the number of circulating R.B.C.s and/or Hb in the blood. Fundamentally, all anemias are caused by one of the following conditions:

(1) Increased loss of R.B.C. due to:

(a) Hemorrhage.
(b) Increased rate of R.B.C. destruction (hemolytic anemias).

(2) Decreased production of R.B.C. due to:

(a) Deficiencies.
(b) Bone marrow suppression.

b. Iron-deficiency anemia. Chronic anemia characterized by small, pale R.B.C. and depletion of iron stores. In adults it is almost always due to occult blood loss (G.I. bleeding, excessive menstrual, excessive salicylate intake, etc.).

S. Easy fatigability, dyspnea, palpitation, angina, and tachycardia. Inability to swallow or difficulty in swallowing may exist in advanced cases. There often exists a craving for strange foodstuffs (dirt, chalk, paint, etc.).

O. Skin and mucous membranes are usually pale. In advanced cases the skin may have a waxy appearance; the hair and nails are brittle, longitudinal ridging with progressive concavity (spooning) may appear on the fingernails. The tongue may be smooth, and the lips inflamed and cracked. Hb may be as low as 3 Mg% but R.B.C. is rarely below 2.5 m. W.B.C. is normal.

A. Iron deficiency anemia due to __________. Differential diagnosis: Other hypochromic anemias (anemias of infection, thalassemia, etc.) pernicious anemia, aplastic anemia.

P. (1) Treat underlying cause.

(2) Oral $FeSO_4$ 0.2 gm t.i.d. p.c. Continue for 3 months after Hb returns to normal. If there is bleeding in excess of 500 ml./wk over a sustained period, iron therapy will not work until the cause of bleeding is corrected. NOTE: Iron causes a color change in the stool (dark green or black). Advise patient not to be alarmed if this occurs.

c. Pernicious anemia. Anemia due to impaired absorption of vitamin B_{12}.

S. Same as iron deficiency. In addition the patient may complain of a "burning of the tongue"; constant, symmetric numbness of the feet; various G.I. disturbances (anorexia, constipation, diarrhea, vague abdominal pain); transient paresthesias of the upper extremities; and severe weight loss. There may be mental disturbances ranging from mild depression to delirium and paranoia.

O. Pallor with a trace of jaundice; loss of vibratory sensation in the lower extremities, loss of positional sense, loss of coordination; hyperactive deep tendon reflexes and positive Babinski. Occasional splenomegaly and hepatomegaly may be present. Differential smear will demonstrate large oval R.B.C. with a few small misshapen R.B.C. W.B.C. is usually less than 5,000. The granulocytes tend to be hypersegmented.

A. Pernicious anemia. Differential diagnosis: Anemia due to folic acid deficiency. NOTE: The oval shape of the R.B.C. and hypersegmentation of the W.B.C. are not characteristic of folic acid deficiency anemia.

P. Give 100 mg. vitamin B_{12} IM stat., then 100 mg. 3 times per week until blood picture returns to normal. If anemia is severe, give transfusion (after type and X-match) of packed red cells slowly.

d. Hemolytic transfusion reactions. Hemolysis of the recipient's or donor's R.B.C. (usually the latter) during or following the administration of solutions, plasma, blood, or blood components. Hemolytic reactions vary in severity depending on the degree of incompatibility, the amount of blood given, and the rate of administration. The most severe reaction occurs when donor R.B.C. are hemolized instantaneously by antibody in the recipient's plasma. These reactions constitute a grave medical emergency.

S. Sudden onset of chills and fever and pain in the vein at the local injection site or in the back, chest, or abdomen. Anxiety, apprehension, and headache are common. Under general anesthesia, spontaneous bleeding may be the only sign of a transfusion reaction.

O. Evidence of shock (see Chapter 15, Shock). Oliguria, anuria, progressing to uremia. If a hemolytic reaction is suspected, immediately take a blood sample from the patient and centrifuge it. Hemolysis will be clearly visible as a pink to dark red color in the serum.

A. Hemolytic transfusion reaction. Differential diagnosis: Minor allergic reactions. (Serum will remain clear.)

P. (1) STOP TRANSFUSION STAT.

(2) Treat for shock.

(3) To prevent renal failure, give 10% mannitol solution IV infusion at a rate of 10-15 ml./min until 1,000 ml. have been given. If diuresis occurs, continue the mannitol infusion until serum and urine are clear.

1-32. DISEASES OF THE LYMPHATIC SYSTEM.

a. Lymphadenitis. Inflammation of one or more lymph nodes. Usually secondary to a primary infection elsewhere involving the skin or subcutaneous tissue.

S. Enlarged, tender, often acutely painful lymph nodes. Systemic symptoms may be minimal or severe.

O. Primary focus of infection in the region of the affected node(s). Cellulitis, suppuration with abcess formation may occur. Low grade or chronic infections may produce firm, nontender nodes that persist indefinitely (e.g., TB and fungal infections). They may form cold abcesses or erode through the surface to create draining sinuses.

A. Lymphadenitis secondary to ___________. Differential diagnosis: Lymphedema secondary to blockage of the lymph channels.

P. Treat primary infection. Apply moist heat to localize infection. Analgesics for pain. I&D abcesses.

b. Lymphangitis. Acute or chronic inflammation of the superficial or deep lymphatic channels, usually caused by streptococci or staphylococci.

S. Fever (102 to 105° F.), chills, malaise, generalized aching, and headache.

O. Patchy areas of inflammation along the path of a lymphatic channel resembling cellulitis. Lymphangitis occurring as the result of hand or foot infection presents as irregular pink, tender, linear streaks extending toward the regional lymph nodes. Lymphadenitis usually follows. Leukocytosis (W.B.C. 15,000-30,000) with shift to the left.

A. Acute lympangitis due to ___________. Differential diagnosis: Acute thrompophlebitis, cellulitis.

P. Treat the original infection, but avoid all undue surgical manipulation of the wound. Use same antibiotic therapy as for acute cellulitis (Chap 1, Sec I). Antibiotics should be continued until the temperature has been normal for 72 hours and inflammation has subsided.

Section V - Digestive System

1-33. GENERAL. The digestive system covers the entire alimentary tract (mouth, esophagus, stomach, intestines, colon, and rectum) and all organs that aid in digestion (liver, gallbladder, and pancreas). Diseases of the mouth are covered in the dental section. Diseases of the esophagus are either minor or of such a nature that we can only treat them symptomatically.

1-34. ACUTE ABDOMEN. Usually manifested by pain, anorexia, nausea, vomiting, and fever. Physical exam shows tenderness, muscle spasm, and changes in peristalsis. Correct diagnosis depends on the precision and care in taking history and doing physical exams.

a. History.

(1) Mode of onset of abdominal pain.

(a) Patient is well one moment and seized with agonizing (explosive) pain the next; most probable diagnosis is free rupture of a hollow viscus or vascular accident. Renal and biliary colic may be very sudden in onset but are not likely to cause severe and prostrating pain.

(b) If pain is rapid in onset--moderately severe at first and becoming rapidly worse--consider acute pancreatitis, mesenteric thrombosis, or strangulation of the small bowel.

(c) Gradual onset of slowly progressive pain is characteristic of peritoneal infection or inflammation. Appendicitis and diverticulitis often start this way.

(2) Character of the pain.

(a) Excruciating pain not relieved by narcotics indicates a vascular lesion such as massive infarction of the intestine or rupture of an abdominal aneurysm.

(b) Very severe pain readily controlled by medication more typical of acute pancreatitis or the peritonitis associated with a ruptured viscus. Obstructive appendicitis and incarcerated small bowel without extensive infarction occasionally produce the same type of pain. Biliary or renal colic is usually promptly alleviated by medication.

(c) Dull, vague, and poorly localized pain usually gradual in onset strongly suggests an inflammatory process or low grade infection, e.g., appendicitis.

(d) No abdominal pain but complains of feeling of fullness that might be relieved by a bowel movement, enema provides no relief ("gas stoppage sign"). This may be present when any inflammatory lesion is walled off from free peritoneal cavity.

(e) Intermittent pain with cramps and rushes commonly seen in gastroenteritis. The peristaltic rushes have little or no relation to abdominal cramps in gastroenteritis. If the pain comes in regular cycles, rising in crescendo fashion, synchronous with the pain and then subsiding to a pain-free interval, small bowel obstruction is very likely.

(f) Radiation or a shift in localization of pain. Pain in the shoulder follows diaphragmatic irritation due to air, peritoneal fluid, or blood. Biliary pain is often referred to the right scapula and rarely to the left epigastrium and left shoulder, simulating angina pectoris. Classically, appendicitis begins in the epigastrium and settles in the right lower quadrant. A shift or spread of abdominal pain often indicates spreading peritonitis.

(g) Anorexia, nausea, and vomiting. The time of onset of these symptoms is important; if they precede the onset of pain, gastroenteritis or some systemic illness is much more likely the diagnosis than acute abdominal disorder requiring an emergency operation. The most likely possibilities are gastroenteritis, acute gastritis, acute pancreatitis, common duct stone, and high intestinal obstruction. In most other acute surgical emergencies, nausea and vomiting are not dominant symptoms though they may be present.

(h) Diarrhea, constipation, and obstipation. Some alteration of bowel function is common in most cases of acute abdominal emergencies. Diarrhea is the classic manifestation of gastroenteritis, but it may also be a dominant symptom of pelvic appendicitis. Bloody and repetitive diarrhea indicates ulceration of the colon, but you should consider bacillary or amebic dysentery first.

(i) Chills and fever. Repeated bouts of chills and fever are characteristic signs of pylephlebitis and bacteremia. Chills and fever are common in infections of the biliary or renal tract. Acute cholangitis and pyelitis present with intermittent chills and fever. In appendicitis, fever is not usually very high and there are usually no chills unless you have a perforation. In a woman with no apparent general systemic illness, a very high fever with peritoneal signs is characteristic of acute pelvic inflammatory disease (PID).

b. Routine for physical exam of the acute abdomen.

(1) General inspection (patient standing).

(2) Cough tenderness. Examine hernial rings and male genitals.

(3) Feel for spasm.

(4) One-finger palpation.

(5) Costovertebral check for tenderness.

(6) Deep palpation.

(7) Rebound tenderness.

(8) Auscultation.

(9) Rectal and pelvic examination.

1-35. DISEASES OF THE STOMACH.

a. Acute simple gastritis. This is probably the most common disturbance of the stomach and is frequently accompanied by generalized enteritis. Causes are chemical irritants (e.g., alcohol, salicylates), bacterial infection or toxins (e.g., staphylococcal food poisoning, scarlet fever, pneumonia), viral infections (e.g., viral gastroenteritis, measles, hepatitis, influenza), and allergy (e.g., shellfish).

S. Anorexia is always present and may be the only symptom. Usually, patient complains of epigastric fullness and pressure and nausea and vomiting. Diarrhea, colic, malaise, fever, chills, headache, and muscle cramps are common with toxins or infections.

O. The patient may be prostrated and dehydrated. Examination shows mild epigastric tenderness. Hemorrhage is frequent with chemical irritants (e.g., salicylates). This may be found using a guaiac test. CBC may show a leukocytosis or in viral infections, a leukopenia.

A. Acute simple gastritis caused by ________________. Differential diagnosis: Includes peptic ulcers and appendicitis.

P. Treat the specific infection or problem. Correct fluid and electrolyte disturbance. Place patient N.P.O. until acute symptoms of pain and nausea have subided, then start giving clear liquids and progress to a soft diet as tolerated. Sedatives, Compazine, or opiates may be used as indicated. Symptoms last from 1-7 days.

b. Food poisoning and acute gastroenteritis. Food poisoning is a general term applied to the syndrome of acute anorexia, nausea, vomiting, and/or diarrhea that is attributed to food intake, especially if it affects a group of people who ate the same foods. There are numerous causative agents and organisms that have similar signs and symptoms to a greater or lesser degree. The only positive way of differentiating between these agents or organisms is by culturing the suspected food and stools of the affected individuals. Most forms of food poisoning are self-limiting and require symptomatic treatment, such as replacement of fluids and electrolytes, control of diarrhea with Lomotil, and control of nausea and vomiting with Compazine. Very rarely patients may develop hypovolemic shock and respiratory embarrassment, and this will have to be managed. Antimicrobial drugs should not be given unless the specific organism can be identified as they may aggravate the anorexia and diarrhea and prolong the course of the illness. <u>The exception to the rule is if you suspect BOTULISM; then polyvalent antitoxin must be administered.</u> The following chart will help in identifying the various types of food poisoning and their specific treatments.

Organism	Incubation Period (Hours)	Epidemiology	Clinical Features
Staphylococcus	1-18	Staphylococci grow in meats, dairy, and bakery products and produce enterotoxin.	Abrupt onset, intense vomiting for up to 24 hours, regular recovery in 24-48 hours. Occurs in persons eating the same food. No treatment usually necessary except to restore fluids and electrolytes.

Clostridium perfringens	8-16	Clostridia grow in rewarmed meat dishes and produce enterotoxin.	Abrupt onset of profuse diarrhea; vomiting occasionally. Recovery usual without treatment in 1-4 days. Many clostridia in cultures of food and feces of patients.
Clostridium botulinum	24-96	Clostridia grow in anaerobic foods and produce toxin.	Diplopia, dysphagia, dysphonia, respiratory embarrassment. Treatment requires clear airway, ventilation, and intravenous polyvalent antitoxin. Toxin present in food and serum. Mortality rate high.
Escherichia coli (some strains)	24-72	Organisms grow in gut and produce toxin. May also invade superficial epithelium.	Usually abrupt onset of diarrhea; vomiting rare. A serious infection in neonates. In adults, "traveler's diarrhea" is usually self-limited in 1-3 days. Use diphenoxylate (Lomotil) but no antimicrobials.
Vibrio parahaemolyticus	6-96	Organisms grow in seafood and in gut and produce toxin.	Abrupt onset of diarrhea in groups consuming the same food, especially crabs and other seafood. Recovery is usually complete in 1-3 days. Food and stool cultures are positive.
Vibrio cholerae (mild cases)	24-72	Organisms grow in gut and produce toxin.	Abrupt onset of liquid diarrhea in endemic area. Needs prompt replacement of fluids and electrolytes IV or orally. Tetracyclines shorten excretion of vibrios. Stool cultures positive.

Shigella spp. (mild cases)	24-72	Organisms grow in superficial gut epithelium and gut lumen and produce toxin.	Abrupt onset of diarrhea, often with blood and pus in stools; cramps; tenesmus; and lethargy. Stool cultures are positive. Give ampicillin, chloramphenicol, or sulfamethoxazole with trimethoprim (co-trimoxazole) in severe cases. Often mild and self-limited. Restore fluids.
Salmonella spp.	8-48	Organisms grow in gut. Do not produce toxin.	Gradual or abrupt onset of diarrhea and low-grade fever. No antimicrobials unless systemic dissemination is suspected. Stool cultures are positive. Prolonged carriage is frequent.
Clostridium difficile	?	Drug intake, e.g., clindamycin.	Especially after abdominal surgery, abrupt bloody diarrhea and fever. Toxin in stool. Oral vancomycin useful in therapy.
Campylobacter fetus	?	Organism grows in jejunum and ileum.	Fever, diarrhea; P.M.N.'s and fresh blood in stool, especially in children. Usually self-limited. Special media needed for culture. Erythromycin in severe cases with invasion.
Yersinia enterocolitica	?	Fecal-oral transmission. Food-borne.? In pets.	Severe abdominal pain, diarrhea, fever; P.M.N.'s and blood in stool; polyarthritis, erythema nodosum, especially in children. If severe, tetracycline or

gentamicin.

c. Bacillary dysentery (shigellosis). Shigellosis is a common, often mild and self-limiting disease that occasionally is serious. It is usually found in conjunction with poor sanitary conditions.

S. Abrupt onset of diarrhea (often with blood and mucus), lower abdominal cramps, and tenesmus. This is usually accompanied by fever, chills, anorexia, malaise, headache, lethargy, clouded mental condition, and in the most severe cases meningismus (S and S of meningeal irritation without actual infection), coma, and convulsions. As the illness progresses, the patient becomes weaker and more dehydrated.

O. Temperature up to 104o F., tender abdomen, and blood, mucus, and pus in the stool. Stool culture is positive for shigellae.

A. Bacillary dysentery (shigellosis). Differential diagnosis: Amebic dysentery, salmonella, gastroenteritis, E. coli, viral diarrhea, and ulcerative colitis.

P. IV fluid and electrolyte replacement, place patient N.P.O.; antispasmodics (e.g., tincture of belladonna) are helpful when cramps are severe. Avoid Lomotil or paregoric; they may improve the general symptoms but prolong fever, diarrhea, and excretion of shigella in feces. Effective stool isolation and disposal should be initiated. Drug of choice is ampicillin 250 mg. q.6h. x 5-7 days; second choice is tetracycline 250 mg. q.6h. x 5-7 days. After bowel has been at rest for a short time, start patient on clear fluids for 2-3 days, then soft diet and gradually build.

d. Amebic dysentery (see Chapter 2, Section I, Parasitic Diseases).

e. Typhoid fever (see Chapter 2, Section III, Bacterial Diseases).

f. Cholera (see Chapter 2, Section III, Bacterial Diseases).

g. Infectious hepatitis (see Chapter 2, Section IV, Viral Diseases).

h. Peptic ulcer disease. An acute or chronic benign ulceration in a portion of the digestive tract exposed to gastric secretions.

(1) Duodenal ulcer. Most common type of ulcer, four to five times more prevalent than gastric ulcer.

S. Symptoms may be vague or absent. In a typical case pain is described as gnawing, burning, cramplike, aching, or as heartburn; it is usually mild to moderate, located near the midline and near the xiphoid process. Pain may radiate below the ribs into the back or occasionally to the right shoulder. Patient may have nausea and may vomit small quantities of highly acid gastric juices with little or no food. Usually occurs 45-60 minutes after meals; absent in the morning before breakfast and gets progressively worse as the day passes. May be most severe between midnight and 0200. Pain is relieved by food, milk, antacids, and vomiting within 5-30 minutes. Ulcers can spontaneously get better or worse. Causative factors may be unknown but may include physical or emotional distress, trauma, or infections.

O. Examination shows superficial and deep epigastric tenderness, voluntary muscle guarding, and unilaterial spasm over duodenal bulb. Lab work will show occult blood in the stool and anemia in chronic ulcers. Definite diagnosis depends on X ray and endoscopic examination.

NOTE: Complications include severe hemorrhage due to ulceration into a vein or artery or even bleeding from granulation tissue; perforation into the peritoneal cavity causing peritonitis; puretration into surrounding organs, usually into the pancreas, but the liver, biliary tract or gastrohepatic omentum may be involved. In 20 to 25 percent of untreated patients, minor degrees of pyloric valve obstruction occur, but major or complete obstructions are rare.

A. Peptic ulcer disease duodenal ulcer. Differential diagnosis: functional gastrointestinal disease, gastritis, gastric carcinoma, and irritable colon syndrome.

P. 2-3 weeks rest from work if possible. Relieve or avoid anxiety whenever possible. Forbid alcohol. Discontinue or avoid drugs that aggravate ulcers (e.g., phenylbutazone, indomethacin, and large amounts of salicylates). Place patient on a dietary management program.

(a) In the acute phase, start full liquid diet with hourly antacids liberalized rapidly to a regular diet.

(b) Avoid milk as therapy.

(c) Avoid interval feeding (eating small meals every few hours).

(d) Nutritious diet.

(e) Regular meals.

(f) Restrict coffee, tea, and cola beverages.

(g) Avoid foods that are known to produce unpleasant symptoms in a given individual.

Antacids, in order to be effective, must be taken frequently. In the acute phase, antacids should be given hourly. The schedule may then be changed to a full dose 1 and 3 hours after meals and at bedtime.

(2) Gastric ulcer. In many respects it is similar to duodenal ulcer.

S. There may be no symptoms or vague and atypical symptoms. Pain is epigastric and described as gnawing, burning, aching, or hunger pangs referred at times to left subcostal area. Usually occurs 45-60 minutes after meals and is relieved by food, antacids, or vomiting. Weight loss, constipation, and fatigue are common.

O. Epigastric tenderness or voluntary muscle guarding is usually the only finding. If there has been bleeding, a guaiac test will show occult blood.

NOTE: Complications are the same as with duodenal ulcers.

A. Peptic ulcer disease, gastric ulcer. Differential diagnosis: Duodenal ulcer, irritable colon, functional gastrointestinal distress, and gastritis.

P. Treatment is the same as for duodenal ulcer. Failure to respond in 3-4 weeks is indication for surgery.

Gastric ulcers tend to be recurrent. Recurrent uncomplicated ulcers usually heal faster than the previous ulcer.

i. Acute organic intestinal obstruction. Usually involves the small intestines, particularly the ileum. Major causes are external hernia and postoperative adhesions. Less common causes are gallstones, neoplasms, foreign bodies, intussusception, granulomatous processes, internal hernia, and vovulus.

S. Colicky abdominal pain in periumbilical area becoming more constant and diffuse as distention develops. Vomiting associated with waves of pain. If obstruction is of the distal bowel, vomiting becomes fecal in nature. Loud stomach growling, unmanageable constipation, weakness, sweating, and anxiety are often present.

O. Patient is restless, often in shocklike state with tachycardia and dehydration, tender distended abdomen (can be localized but usually generalized) without peritoneal irritation. Audible and visible peristalsis, high pitched tinkles, and pain related to peristaltic rushes may be present. Temperature is normal or slightly elevated. A tender hernia may be present. W.B.C. is normal or slightly elevated.

A. Acute organic intestinal obstruction. Differential diagnosis: Renal colic, gallbladder colic, or mesenteric vascular disease.

P. Place patient N.P.O. Decompress intestinal tract by nasogastric suction (see illustration on next page). Replace fluids and electrolytes by IV. Treat the cause of the obstruction. Start broad-spectrum antibiotic therapy if needed.

j. Appendicitis. One of the most frequent causes of acute abdomen. Signs and symptoms usually follow a fairly stereotyped pattern, but it can display many different manifestations that should be considered in the differential diagnosis of every case of abdominal sepsis and pain.

S. Appendicitis usually begins with generalized periumbilical or epigastric pain and 1 or 2 episodes of vomiting Within 2-12 hours, the pain shifts to right lower quadrant where it persists as a steady soreness aggravated by walking or coughing. Patient can usually place a finger on a specific point. Anorexia, malaise, slight fever, and constipation are usual, but diarrhea occurs occasionally.

O. Rebound tenderness and spasm of the overlying abdominal muscles. Rectal tenderness is common; peristalsis is diminished or absent. Slight to moderate fever. Pain localized in right lower quadrant. W.B.C. 10-20,000 with an increase in neutrophils.

NOTE: Complications include perforation leading to generalized peritonitis, appendiceal abscess, pylephlebitis, and intestinal obstruction.

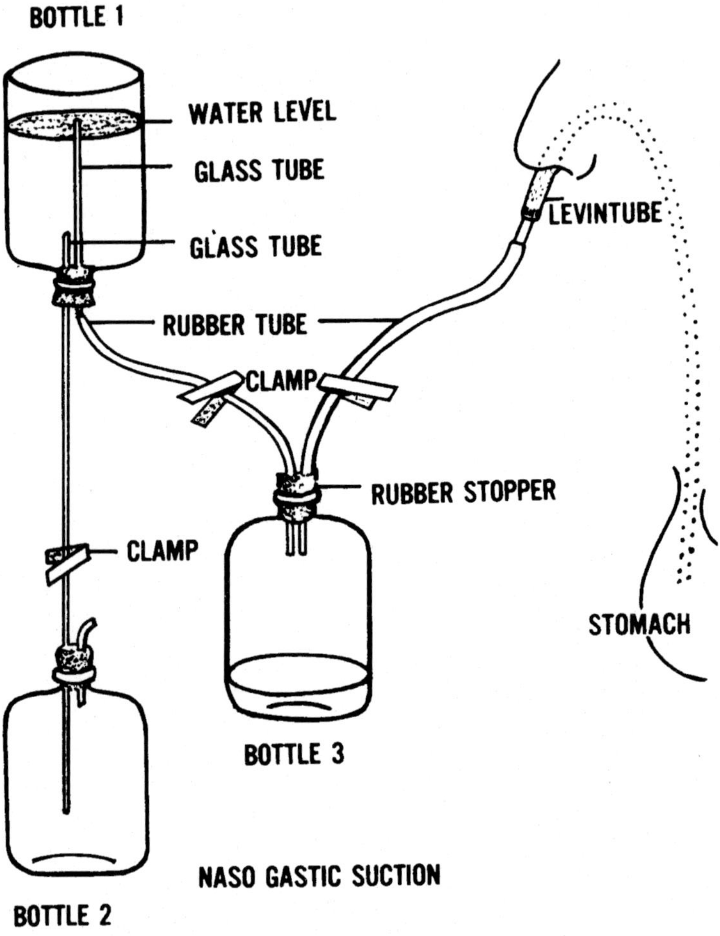

NASO GASTIC SUCTION

A. Appendicitis. Differential diagnosis: Acute gastroenteritis, mesenteric adenitis, Meckel's diverticulitis, regional enteritis, amebiasis, perforated duodenal ulcer, ureteral colic, ruptured ectopic pregnancy, and twisted ovarian cyst may at times mimic appendicitis.

P. Place patient under observation for diagnosis within the first 8-12 hours. Bed rest, N.P.O., start maintaining IV, avoid narcotic medication as it might mask symptoms necessary for proper diagnosis. Abdominal and rectal exam, white blood count, and differential count are repeated periodically.

(1) Once diagnosis is made, an appendectomy should be performed as soon as fluid imbalances and other systemic disturbances are controlled.

(2) Antibiotics should be administered in the presence of marked systemic reaction with severe toxicity and high fever.

(3) Emergency nonsurgical treatment when surgical facilities are not available; treat as for acute peritonitis. Acute appendicitis may subside and complications will be minimized.

k. Acute peritonitis. Localized or generalized peritonitis is the most important complication of numerous acute abdominal disorders. May be caused by infection or chemical irritation.

S. Malaise, prostration, nausea, vomiting, fever, depending on extent of involvement localized or generalized pain and tenderness, abdominal pain on coughing.

O. Elevated W.B.C., rebound tenderness referred to area of peritonitis, and tenderness to light percussion over the area. Pelvic peritonitis is associated with rectal and vaginal tenderness. Spastic muscles over area of inflammation. When peritonitis is generalized, there will be marked rigidity of the entire abdominal wall. This rigidity is frequently diminished or absent in the late stages of peritonitis, in severe toxemia, and when the abdominal wall is weak, flabby, or obese. Diminished to absent peristalsis and progressive abdominal distention is found. Vomiting occurs due to pooling of gastrointestinal secretions and gas. W.B.C. will increase to 10-20,000.

A. Acute peritonitis. Differential diagnosis: Peritonitis may present a highly variable clinical picture and must be differentiated from acute intestinal obstruction, acute cholecystitis, renal colic, gastrointestinal hemorrhage, lower labor pneumonia, porphyria, periodic fever, hysteria, and central nervous system disorders.

P. Treatment is generally applicable as supportive treatment in most acute abdominal disorders. The objectives are: Control infection; minimize the effects of paralytic ileus; correct fluid, electrolyte, and nutritional disorders.

(1) Specific measures: Identify and treat the cause; this usually entails surgery to remove sources of infection such as appendicitis, gangrenous bowel, abscesses, or perforated ulcers.

(2) General: Bed rest in medium Fowler position (semi-sitting). Nasogastric (NG) suction to prevent abdominal distention and continued

until peristalsis returns and patient begins passing flatus. Place patient N.P.O. until after NG suction is discontinued, then slowly resume oral intake. IV for fluid electrolyte therapy and parenteral feeding are required. Narcotics and sedatives used liberally to insure rest and comfort. Broad-spectrum antibiotic therapy to prevent and control infections should be initiated. Blood transfusions as needed. Watch patient for signs of toxic shock and treat as required.

1. Acute Pancreatitis. A severe abdominal disease produced by acute inflammation in the pancreas and associated "escape" of pancreatic enzymes into the surrounding tissues. The exact cause is not known, but more than 80 clinical causes have been related to acute pancreatitis, everything from alcoholism to drugs.

S. Epigastric pain generally abrupt in onset is steady and severe, made worse by lying down and better by sitting up leaning forward. Pain usually radiates to the back but may radiate right or left. Nausea, vomiting, and constipation are present, and severe prostration, sweating, and anxiety are usually found. There may be a history of alcohol intake or a heavy meal immediately before the attack.

O. Tender abdomen mainly in upper abdomen, usually without guarding, rigidity, or rebound. Abdomen may be distended and bowel sounds may be absent. Temperature of 101.1-102.2°F., tachycardia, pallor, hypotension, and a cool clammy skin are often present.

Mild jaundice is common. Upper abdominal mass may be present. Acute renal failure may occur early in the course of the disease. W.B.C. 10-30,000. Urinalysis shows proteinuria, casts in 25 percent of the cases, and glucosuria in 10-20 percent of the cases.

A. Acute pancreatitis. Differential diagnosis: Pancreatitis is hard to tell from common duct stone or perforated peptic ulcer. It must also be differentiated from acute mesenteric thrombosis, renal colic, acute cholecystitis, and acute intestinal obstruction.

P. Emergency measures for impending shock: Place patient N.P.O. If bowel sounds are absent, initiate nasogastric suction. Patient should be placed at bed rest and given 100-150 mg. demerol SQ as necessary for relief of pain. Atropine may be given as an antispasmodic 0.4-0.6 mg. SQ. Start IV to replace fluids and monitor urinary output. Use shock drugs if necessary; calcium gluconate must be given IV if there is evidence of hypocalcemia with tetany. Initiate prophylactic antibiotic therapy only if fever exceeds 102°F. Patient should be constantly attended and vital signs checked every 15-30 miunutes. CBC and urinalysis should be done frequently and monitored.

(1) Follow-up care: Patient should be kept N.P.O. for 48-72 hours. Examine frequently and closely for evidence of continued inflammation of the pancreas or related structures. Conduct periodic CBC and urinalysis. Hyperfeed the patient parenterally for first 48-72 hours, then gradually introduce oral feeding. When clinical evidence of pancreatitis has cleared, place the patient on a low fat diet.

(2) Prognosis: Recurrence is common. Surgery is indicated only when diagnosis is in doubt, if conservative treatment is not working, or in the presence of an associated disorder such as stones in biliary tract.

m. Acute Cholecystitis. Cholecystitis is associated with gallstones in over 90 percent of cases. It is caused by a partial or complete cystic duct obstruction. If the obstruction is not relieved, pressure builds up within the gallbladder. Primarily as a result of ischemic changes secondary to distention, gangrene may develop with resulting perforation. This may cause generalized peritonitis but usually remains localized and forms a chronic well-circumscribed abscess cavity.

S. Usually follows a large or fatty meal. Relatively sudden onset of severe, minimally fluctuating pain localized in the epigastrium or right upper quadrant frequently radiating to infrascapular area. In the uncomplicated case, the pain may gradually subside over a 12-18 hour period. Vomiting occurs in 75 percent of cases and 50 percent of these get variable relief.

O. Right upper quadrant abdominal tenderness, guarding and rebound pain. About 15 percent of cases have a palpable gallbladder and 25 percent of cases have jaundice. Fever is usually present. W.B.C. is usually 12-15,000.

A. Acute cholecystitis. Differential diagnosis: Perforated peptic ulcer, acute pancreatitis, appendicitis, hepatitis, and pneumonia with pleurisy on the right side.

P. Place patient N.P.O. Initiate IV for maintenance and feeding. Start prophylactic antibiotic therapy. Give analgesics as needed (morphine or meperidine). Smooth muscle relaxants, such as IM atropine or probanthine, should be used. Patient should be watched closely. W.B.C. should be done several times a day. Treatment is continued until symptoms subside. Cholecystectomy is usually required but not as emergency surgery unless there is evidence of gangrene or perforation.

Section VI - Genitourinary System

1-36. The genitourinary system is made up of the male and female sexual organs, the urethra, the bladder, the ureters, and the kidneys.

1-37. GENITOURINARY TRAUMA.

a. Kidney trauma. Most commonly caused by blunt external force such as blows, kicks, falls, etc., in the flank area. Other causes are wounds such as gunshot, stabs, etc.; it is very rarely caused by spontaneous rupture of a diseased kidney.

S. Pain at site of injury with a boring or tearing sensation felt in loin or upper abdomen.

O. Swelling and progressive rigidity of affected side. If there is a tear in the renal capsule, there is usually a rapidly expanding mass in the flank. From mild to gross hematuria is present in 90 percent of the cases. Shock occurs in varying degrees. W.B.C. elevates rapidly to 20,000 and higher.

A. Kidney trauma.

P. Conservervative treatment will usually provide satisfactory results in most cases where there is no penetrating wound. Bed rest for at least 2 weeks, until urine is clear. Shock and pain measures as required. Monitor urinary output closely. Patient must force fluids to insure urinary output of 25-40 ml./hr. In serious cases, an indwelling catheter should be installed and through IV therapy provide a urinary output of 25-40 ml./hr. Antibiotic therapy should be initiated in all cases as a prophylaxis. If an infection is allowed to develop, it will cause scar tissue and further complications. If at all possible, med evac all penetrating wounds and serious cases.

b. Bladder trauma. Causes include crushing injury from blows, seatbelts, etc., particularly if the injury occurs when the bladder is full; gunshot or stab wounds; or bony fragments from fractured pelvis.

S. Severe pain in lower abdomen. Slow and painful urination due to muscle spasm after injury.

O. Hematuria, often only a few drops of blood. Progressive symptoms of peritonitis depending on the extent of bladder rupture.

A. Bladder trauma.

P. Flat in bed. Treat for shock; install indwelling catheter. Prophylactic antibiotic treatment. Treat related problems (fracture, wound, etc.).

c. External genitalia trauma. Usual causes are heavy blows, cuts, direct injury, pelvic fracture, or straddle injury.

S. Intense to excruciating pain, swelling, and rapid development of a large hematoma.

O. Vary with the severity of the condition but will consist of hematuria, spasmodic contractions of the vesicle sphincter with pain, and persistent desire to empty the bladder with involuntary ineffectual straining efforts and shock.

A. External genital trauma.

P. Indwelling catheter, cold packs, scrotal support, pain medication, and treat related problems (shock, wound, etc).

1-38. GENITOURINARY TRACT INFLAMMATION.

a. Renal calculi. Caused by a concentration of mineral salts and crystals that are formed in the calyx of the kidney. These kidney stones vary from small sandlike particles to large oval or branching (staghorn) stones that may fill the entire renal pelvis. Many factors are contributory such as infection, obstructions, dehydration, and hereditary tendency.

S. Severe intermittent colicky pain, radiating to pelvis, testicle, and/or inner aspect of the thigh. While the stone is in the kidney, the pain is dull and intensified by motion. When the stone enters the ureter, a sudden stab of excruciating pain is felt. If stone is in the bladder, the patient may be able to void only in the horizontal position.

O. Usually accompanied by chills, fever, violent movements, sweating, and shock as the stone moves through the ureter. Frequency, urgency, oliguria (diminished amount of urine formation), dysuria (painful or difficult urination), hematuria, and possibly pyuria (pus in the urine) are contributory findings. If anuria (complete urinary suppression) develops, it is indicative of renal failure.

A. Renal calculi.

P. Relieve pain (morphine 1/4 gr. q.2-3hr). Relax ureteral spasms with Pro-Banthine, 1/100-1/150 gr. atropine, or 1/100 gr. nitroglycerin. Force fluids and keep close record of intake and output. Strain all urine for stones; these should pass within 24-36 hours. At the first sign of anuria this becomes an acute emergency and patient should be evacuated to a definitive treatment facility.

b. Acute pyelonephritis. An acute infection of the kidney usually due to an ascending infection (from bladder through ureters to kidney) but may start from a systemic bacterial infection.

S. Sudden onset with chills, fever, some muscular rigidity, frequency, urgency, and dysuria.

O. Pain on percussion of the back with radiation to costovertebral angles and along the course of the ureters. Urinalysis shows albumen, pus cells, casts, R.B.C.'s, W.B.C.'s, and bacteria. W.B.C. in excess of 20,000.

A. Acute pyelonephritis. Differential diagnosis: Cystitis.

P. Bed rest, force fluids, and soft diet. Eliminate irritants such as alcohol or cocoa. Antibiotic therapy using Gantrisin, tetracycline, or penicillin/streptomycin. Symptomatic treatment.

c. Cystitis. Bladder infection usually due to bacteria.

S. Sudden or more gradual onset of burning pain on urination, often with turbid, foul-smelling, or dark urine; frequency; difficult or painful urination; and occasionally blood in the urine. Chills and fever are rare and if temperature is over 100° F., consider possibility of other causes than cystitis.

O. Usually no positive physical findings unless the upper tract is involved. Urinalysis shows pus, bacteria, and occasional hematuria. W.B.C.'s are rare unless upper tract is involved.

A. Cystitis. Differential diagnosis: Urethritis, pyelonephritis.

P. Gantrisin (sulfisoxazole) 1 gm q.i.d. x 10 days, alternate tetracycline 1-2 250 mg. tablets q.i.d. or ampicillin 1-2 250 mg. tablets q.i.d. Give Pyridium or methenamine urinary analgesic. NOTE: This may stain urine red to deep orange. Follow up in 2 weeks.

d. Urethritis. Caused by a wide range of agents that include gonococcus, Trichomonas, E. coli, and staphylococcus.

S. Burning on urination with pyuria. Discharge from urethra with a consistency from mucoid to purulent.

O. Discharge elicited by milking the penis. Gram's stain of discharge will usually show causative agent.

A. Urethritis. Differential diagnosis: Cystitis, prostatitis.

P. Ensure correct diagnosis with Gram's stain or culture. Treat causative organism with appropriate antibiotic.

e. Epididymitis. Frequent history of infection elsewhere in the general area such as urethritis, etc. Strenuous activity may precipitate spread of the bacteria.

S. Fever, malaise, nausea, tenderness, and pain that may radiate to the groin.

O. Inflammation of scrotal skin that may flake or crack. Scrotum dusky red and warm to the touch. Slight mass in the epididymis.

A. Epididymitis. Differential diagnosis: Orchitis.

P. Bed rest with scrotal elevation. Analgesics for pain, antibiotic therapy. DO NOT massage the prostate. If swelling persists, surgery will be required.

f. Orchitis. Usually results from a complication of mumps or other acute infections.

S. Fever; pain in the groin region.

O. Swelling of the affected testicle (may be bilateral).

A. Orchitis. Differential diagnosis: Epididymitis.

P. Bed rest; suspend the scrotum in suspensory or toweling

"bridge" and apply ice bags. Give codeine or morphine as necessary for pain. Inflammatory reaction can be reduced with hydrocortisone sodium succinate, 100 mg. IV followed by 20 mg. orally q.6h. x 2-3 days. Orchitis often makes the patient very uncomfortable but very rarely results in sterility.

g. Prostatitis. Caused by bacterial infection from systemic or urethral infections. Prostatitis may be acute or chronic; overmanipulation (a lot of sex) of chronic prostatitis gives rise to acute stage symptoms.

S. Acute symptoms: Perineal pain, fever, dysuria, frequency, and urethral discharge. Chronic symptoms: Lumbosacral backache, perineal pain, mild dysuria and frequency, and scanty urethral discharge.

O. Acute stage: Palpation of the prostate shows it is enlarged, boggy, and very tender. Even gentle palpation of the prostate gland results in a copious purulent urethral discharge. Chronic stage palpation of the prostate reveals an irregularly enlarged, firm, and slightly tender prostate. CBC will often show leukocytosis. Expressed prostatic fluid shows pus cells and bacteria on microscopy.

A. Prostatitis. Differential diagnosis: Urethritis. Lower urinary tract infections.

P. Bed rest, force fluids, sitz baths t.i.d. for 15 min, analgesics, and stool softeners. For acute prostatitis initial treatment may consist of sulfamethoxazole 400 mg., plus trimethoprim 80 mg. (co-trimoxazole), 6-8 tablets daily, or tetracycline 500 mg. q.i.d. x 2 weeks or ampicillin 500 mg. q.4h. x 2 weeks; two-week treatment usually results in subsidence of the acute inflammation, but chronic prostatitis may continue because most drugs fail to reach the prostatic acini. Chronic prostatitis should be treated with prolonged antibiotic therapy accompanied by vigorous prostatic massage once weekly to promote drainage.

h. Benign prostatic hyperplasia. Caused by hyperplasia (abnormal multiplication or increase in the number of normal cells in a tissue) of the prostatic lateral and subcervical lobes resulting in enlargement of the prostate and urethral obstruction.

S. Hesitancy and straining to urinate; reduced force and caliber of the urinary stream, and nocturia. Symptoms may be overlooked until the problem is well developed when the progression of the obstruction is slow.

O. Prostate is usually enlarged on palpation. The bladder may be seen and palpated as urine retention increases. Infections commonly occur as retention increases. Hematuria may occur.

A. Benign prostatic hyperplasia. Differential diagnosis: Urethral strictures, renal calculi, bladder tumor, or carcinoma of the prostate.

P. Relieve acute urinary retention by catheterization. Maintain catheter drainage if degree of obstruction is severe. Surgery is usually necessary. Treat infections that develop.

i. Carcinoma of the prostate. Rare before age 60. It metastasizes early to the bones of the pelvis and locally may produce urethral obstruction with subsequent renal damage.

S. Obstructive symptoms similar to those of benign prostatic hyperplasia are common. Low back pain occurs with metastases to the bones of the pelvis and spine.

O. Rectal exam reveals a stone-hard prostate that is often modular and fixed. Obstructions may produce renal damage and the symptoms and signs of renal insufficiency. Urine may show evidence of infection.

A. Carcinoma of the prostate. Differential diagnosis: Benign prostatic hyperplasia, urethral strictures, renal calculi, and bladder tumor.

P. Evac to a definitive care center.

j. Acute glomerulonephritis. Glomerulonephritis is a disease affecting both kidneys. It is most common in children 3-10 years old. Most common cause is a preceding infection of the pharynx or of the skin with group AB-hemolytic streptococci.

S. Malaise, headache, anorexia, low-grade fever, puffiness around the eyes and face, flank pain, and oliguria (diminished amount of urine output in relation to fluid intake). Hematuria is usually noted as "bloody" or if the urine is acid as "brown" or "coffee-colored." Respiratory difficulty with shortness of breath may occur as a result of salt and water retention and circulatory congestion. Tenderness in the costovertebral angle is common.

O. Mild generalized edema, mild hypertension, and retinal hemorrhages may be noted. There may be moderate tachycardia and moderate to marked elevation of B.P. The diagnosis is confirmed by urine examination that may be grossly bloody or coffee-colored or may only show microscopic hematuria. In addition, the urine contains protein (1-3+), red cell casts, granular and hyaline casts, white cells, and renal epithelial cells.

A. Acute glomerulonephritis. Differential diagnosis: Other diseases in which glomerular inflammation and tubule damage are present.

P. There is no specific treatment, but eradication of B-hemolytic strep is desirable. In uncomplicated cases, treatment is symptomatic and designed to prevent overhydration and hypertension. Bed rest until clinical signs abate. Blood pressure should be normal for 1-2 weeks before resuming normal activity. When protein excretion has disminished to near normal and when white and epithelial cells excretion has decreased and stabilized, activity may be resumed on a graded basis. Excretion of protein and formed elements in the urine will increase with resumption of activity, but such increases should not be great. Fluids should be restricted in keeping with the ability of the kidney to excrete urine. If edema becomes severe, a trial using an oral diuretic should be tried.

k. Phimosis.

(1) Cause and symptoms: Foreskin not pliable enough to retract over the glans penis. This causes pain on erection and may be complicated with paraphimosis.

(2) Treatment: Cut a dorsal slit in foreskin and schedule for

circumcision.

1. Paraphimosis.

(1) Cause and symptoms: Foreskin is constricted around the glans penis and cannot be reduced.

(2) Treatment: Cut a dorsal slit in the foreskin and schedule for circumcision.

Section VII - Nervous System

1-39. This section is not intended to cover all neurological problems because most neurological problems are beyond your scope for definitive treatment. It should, however, provide you with enough information to make you aware of the neurological problems you may face and enable you to make a tentative diagnosis.

1-40. COMPOSITION OF THE NERVOUS SYSTEM.

a. The nervous system is composed of (1) Central Nervous System (C.N.S) - Cerebrum, Cerebellum, Brain Stem, Spinal Cord; (2) Peripheral Nervous System (P.N.S.) - Peripheral nerves.

b. Review of the twelve cranial nerves.

(1) First: Olfactory. Sense of smell. Injury causes loss of sense of smell.

(2) Second: Optic. Sense of sight. Injury causes optic disturbances to loss of sight in one or both eyes.

(3) Third: Oculomotor. Supplies all the muscles of the orbit except the superior oblique and external rectus; also supplies the sphincter muscle of the iris and the ciliary muscle. Injury causes dilated and fixed pupils, slight prominence of the eyeball, and drooping of the upper eyelid.

(4) Fourth: Trochlear. Supplies the superior oblique muscle (smallest of the cranial nerves). Injury makes patient unable to turn eyes downward and outward. If attempted, affected eye is twisted inward causing double vision.

(5) Fifth: Trigeminal. Innervates facial sensation and motor to muscles of mastication (largest cranial nerve). This nerve also supplies the eye, nose, teeth, gums, palate, etc." Injury can cause numerous problems from dryness of the nose and eyeball to impaired action of the lower jaw.

(6) Sixth: Abducens. Supplies the external rectus muscle. More frequently involved in base of the skull fractures than any other nerve. Injury causes an internal or convergent squint often with a certain amount of contraction of the pupil.

(7) Seventh: Facial nerve. Motor nerve of all the muscles of facial expression: the platysma and buccinator; external ear muscles; posterior belly of the digastric and stylohyoid; nerve of taste for the anterior two-thirds of the tongue; the vasodilator nerve of the submaxillary and sublingual glands; and tympanic branch supplies the stapedius muscle. Most common effect of injury is Bell's facial palsy.

(8) Eighth: Auditory. Sense of hearing. Injury causes deafness.

(9) Ninth: Glossopharyngeal. Nerve of sensation to pharynx, fauces, and tonsil. Also sensation of taste to posterior third of tongue.

(10) Tenth: Vagus. Supplies the organs of voice and

respiration with motor and sensory fibers and the pharynx, esophagus, stomach, and heart with motor fibers.

(11) Eleventh: Spinal accessory. Consists of accessory portion which is motor to larynx and pharynx and spinal portion which is motor to sternocleidomastoid and trapezius muscles.

(12) Twelfth: Hypoglossal. Motor nerve of the tongue.

1-41. RECOGNITION OF NEUROLOGICAL PROBLEMS.

a. Not all problems have neurological origin. Your first task is to recognize the potential neurologic origin of the patient's complaint. There are eight different complaints or problems that point to neurologic disease. Although each of these complaints may be produced by diseases that do not involve the nervous system, differentiating between neurological and non-neurological causes is usually easy (e.g., a patient's leg may not move correctly because it is broken; he can't see properly because he needs glasses; or he has a headache and fever after taking a typhoid immunization). The eight complaints/problems are:

(1) Something doesn't move right.

(2) Something doesn't feel right (including disorders of other sensory modalities).

(3) I can't see properly.

(4) I can't think or communicate properly.

(5) I have spells.

(6) I am dizzy.

(7) My head hurts.

(8) Patient is unconscious, unrousable, or excessively drowsy.

1-42. NEUROLOGIC HISTORY. Most patients with neurologic disease will tell their physician what is wrong with them if he can properly interpret what they are trying to say and expands the history with skillful questioning. The history should give a profile of the disorder. This provides a valuable clue to the basic disease process. A few general principles are worth mentioning.

a. Seizures (convulsions) develop more rapidly than any other form of neurologic disorder. In many cases they develop in less than one second and may disappear as quickly as they come. Neuralgias are the only other group of disorders this abrupt. Vascular disorders including stroke and migraine usually take seconds to minutes to develop. Instead of clearing rapidly they melt away over hours or days. Demyelination seldom develops as rapidly as stroke but may progress over hours to days. Tumors usually develop in weeks to months and degenerative disorders in months to years. Toxic, metabolic, and infectious disorders are variable and more likely to leave their mark on other organ systems.

b. A brief neurologic review of systems should be made. It helps the medic be sure that the neurologic disorder is restricted to the problem area he is evaluating. Possible intellectual defects can be elicited by asking about any difficulty in thinking or remembering, comparing recent job or school performance with past achievements may be helpful, asking whether he has any difficulty understanding what is said to him or expressing himself in oral or written language. Other possible complaints relative to the head are logically explored next. These include a discussion of the patient's headaches. He should be asked about any spells, attacks of dizziness, or alteration of consciousness he may have had. Visual complaints including diplopia, scotomata, and loss of visual acuity should be solicited.

1-43. NEUROLOGICAL EXAMINATION.

a. The following checklist will help you make a neurological examination: See para b, below, for details.

(1) Mental status.

(a) Affect and mood
(b) Orientation
(c) Memory
(d) Calculation and abstraction
(e) Aphasia

(2) Patient standing.

(a) Routine gait - note:

1. Arm swing
2. Width of gait
3. Limp or other abnormality

(b) Toe walking
(c) Heel walking
(d) Tandem walking
(e) Romberg's test

(3) Patient seated on exam table.

(a) Cranial nerve tests:

1. Visual acuity
2. Visual fields to confrontation
3. Ocular fundus
4. Extraocular movements
5. Pupillary reactions
6. Smiling, voluntary and emotional
7. Tongue protrusion
8. Voluntary palate movement
9. Hearing

(b) Arm strength and coordination

1. Strength

a. Shoulder abduction
b. Elbow flexion - extension
c. Thumb adduction

d. Thumb opposition
e. Wrist dorsiflexion
f. Handgrip

2. Reflexes
   a. Biceps
   b. Triceps
   c. Radial - periosteal

3. Coordination
   a. Finger to nose
   b. Rapid alternating movements
   c. Muscle tone

(4) Patient lying down.

(a) Leg strength and coordination

1. Strength

   a. Hip flexion
   b. Knee extension
   c. Dorsiflexion of the foot

2. Reflexes

   a. Abdominal
   b. Knee jerk
   c. Ankle jerk
   d. Babinski

3. Heel to shin test

(b) Sensory examination

1. Pain

   a. Face
   b. Extremities

2. Vibration - extremities
3. Light touch

   a. Cornea
   b. Face
   c. Extremities

4. Position
   a. Fingers
   b. Toes

b. Further details on neurological examination.

(1) Mental status exam. The medic who is evaluating a patient's mental status is usually looking for elements of dementia, aphasia, depression, or anxiety. These can often be observed during history taking.

(a) Affect and mood should be observed and recorded.

Affect is how the patient transmits his feelings and mood is what he is trying to transmit. In most individuals a depressed affect reflects a depressed mood and vice versa. Flattening or dulling of affect is seen in most depressed, schizophrenic, or parkinsonian patients.

(b) Orientation to time, place, and person should be recorded.

(c) Memory can usually be judged from the quality of the history, but should be commented on. Formal memory testing is unnecessary unless there is some reason to suspect difficulty.

(d) Calculation and abstraction should be tested in patients over 50 years of age. Serial 7's and a well-known parable (such as "why shouldn't people who live in glass houses throw stones?") are usually adequate.

(2) Gait and station. Four types of gait are routinely tested: ordinary gait, heel walking, toe walking, and tandem gait. Ordinary gait is observed for gross abnormalities of carriage and width of base. Arm swing may be deficient if there is weakness (especially hemiparesis) or a basal ganglion disease such as Parkinson's disease. Asymmetric heel elevation during toe walking indicates weakness in plantar flexors of foot while asymmetric toe and foot elevation in heel walking suggests weakness of the dorsiflexion of foot and toes. Tandem walking brings out gait ataxia (broad-based gait) seen in midline cerebellar disorders. Romberg's test is an evaluation of position sense. The patient is told to stand with his feet as close together as possible. If, with his eyes open, he can only stand with a wide base, the problem is most likely cerebellar. If he stands firm with eyes open, but tends to fall upon closing his eyes, the problem is position sense (posterior column or peripheral nerve) and Romberg's sign is present. While performing the Romberg test, it is convenient to examine for arm drift, a useful test of mild shoulder weakness or proprioceptive loss. Before the patient closes his eyes, have him extend both arms, palms up and elbows stiff in front of him. If while his eyes are closed he displays a tendency for either hand to pronate or either arm to "drift" downward, you may have discovered a significant defect. About 20 seconds of holding against gravity is sufficient.

(3) Cranial nerves. Now the patient can be seated and cranial nerves tested. Smell and taste need not be routinely evaluated. Vision requires more attention. Acuity should be checked first. With glasses on, the ability to read newsprint at about two feet constitutes 20/30 vision; and at 14 inches 20/50 vision. Each eye should be tested separately. Visual fields should also be tested in each eye separately. Always check all four quadrants. In patients over 50 years, check simultaneous stimulation by quadrants, preferably by superior temporal against the inferior nasal and then inferior temporal against the superior nasal. The optic nerve head is routinely examined as part of the ophthalmoscopic exam. A simple tuning fork test for hearing should be included. Extraocular movements and pupillary reactions should always be tested. Emotional and volitional face movements should be observed. Tongue protrusion, voluntary palate elevation, and voice timbre should be examined, but these are usually included as part of the routine oropharyngeal exam. Corneal reflexes, Myerson's sign, and snouting responses should be tested. Ordinary sensation in the face is best checked later with the rest of the general sensory exam.

(4) Motor strength and coordination in the upper extremities. Acceptable techniques of muscle testing consist of the examiner trying to move a joint against resistance or evaluation of a maximum effort by the patient to overcome the examiner. I generally prefer to have the patient exert a maximum effort against my resistance for internal and external rotation at the shoulder, flexion and extension of the elbow, and flexion and extension of the knee. I usually try to overcome the patient's fixation for shoulder abduction, wrist flexion and extension, hip flexion, and foot dorsiflexion. When a patient is making a maximum effort and the examiner is able to overcome the force of his muscle contraction, gradual movement of the joint will be felt. There should be no sudden "give" or relaxation, suggesting a lack of full cooperation. There are several numerical and descriptive scales for recording weakness. Like describing unconsciousness as coma, semicoma, and lethargy, they suffer from a lack of consensus among physicians as to what the numbers mean. At this stage in the examination, shoulder abduction, elbow flexion and extension, wrist dorsiflexion, and thumb opposition and adduction should be tested bilaterally. Biceps, triceps, and radial-periosteal reflexes may be tested at this time or deferred until the patient is supine. Coordination and muscle tone should be checked. Three maneuvers are essential. The first is the familiar finger to nose test. While this is being done, watch for any tremor or involuntary movement. Rapid alternating movements consisting either of opening and closing the hands or touching the tips of each finger with the tip of the thumb is tested next. Finally, passive circumduction of each wrist should be tried while the patient opens and closes the other hand as fast as he can. This will bring out any latent muscle rigidity.

(5) Completion of the motor and reflex exam. The patient should now be placed in the supine position. Up to this point we have been deliberately sloppy in testing strength. We have been testing it without providing fixation of the limb. As a screening procedure, this is fine. If any weakness has been suspected, shoulder rotation and elbow movements should be retested with the shoulder fixed against the examining table. Wrist and hand movements can similarly be isolated. Extension of the hip, extension of the knee, and dorsiflexion of the foot should be routinely examined. If there is a question of knee weakness, have the patient assume the prone position, fix the thigh against the table, and retest flexion and extension.

Biceps, triceps, and radial-periosteal reflexes in the arm should be tested if they have not been previously. Knee jerks, ankle jerks, and abdominal reflexes should be tested, and Babinski's sign sought. All reflexes require three elements: a sensory limb, some form of central integration, and a motor response. Reflexes will be altered if any of these three elements are disturbed. Any peripheral sensory disturbance or disturbance of the lower motor neuron or muscle can abolish reflexes. The only thing that will exaggerate reflexes is a disorder of the corticospinal system (the upper motor neuron syndrome). Finally, leg coordination should be observed with the heel-to-shin test.

(6) Sensory exam. It is convenient to perform the entire sensory exam at one time with the patient lying supine. During an ordinary screening exam, pain sensation with a sharp pin and fine touch with a wisp of cotton or Kleenex should be checked on both cheeks, both hands, and both feet. Position sense should be tested at least in the toes, and vibration sense in both feet and hands. A tuning fork should be used to test vibratory sensation on bony prominences.

1-44. EPILEPSY. Any recurrent seizure pattern. Violent, involuntary contractions of the muscles, occurring singly or in series, often accompanied by sudden loss of consciousness.

a. Grand mal attacks.

(1) Focal or jacksonian seizures. Initiated by specific focal phenomena (motor or sensory). Seizures are one-sided or localized. Head and eyes may turn to one side (that opposite the lesion). Jerking of the limbs may be one-sided. This is an acquired type of epilepsy. Convulsive movements start in small muscle groups (e.g., the hand) and slowly spread to other areas, it is termed the jacksonian "march." Loss of consciousness results when it becomes a generalized convulsion. Indicates specific portion of the cerebrum where lesion is located. May have an "aura," often referred to as a warning, but in reality it is a part of the seizure. The focal point indicates area of the brain where attack originates. Should be considered the focal trigger for the seizure.

(2) Typical grand mal seizures are characterized by a cry; loss of consciousness; falling; tonic then clonic muscle contractions of the extremities, trunk and head; urinary and fecal incontinence; frothing in the mouth; biting of the tongue. About 50 percent have an aura (auditory, visual, olfactory, visceral, or mental) disturbance. Losing consciousness after crying out, the person falls making no effort to protect himself.

(a) Tonic phase: sustained contraction of all muscles; body is rigid, jaws fixed, hands clenched, legs are extended, dilated pupils, face is red or cyanotic due to spasm of respiratory muscles.

(b) Clonic phase follows tonic phase in less than a minute with jerky movements due to alternating contraction and relaxation of muscles. The attack lasts 2 to 5 minutes usually. These attacks may be followed by deep sleep, headache, or muscle soreness.

b. Petit mal attacks. Fleeting attacks of staring into space without loss of consciousness (absence attack) for 1 to 30 seconds. Can occur with loss of muscular tone. Occurs predominantly in children and can recur as frequently as 100 attacks per day. Petit mal may eventually develop into grand mal later in childhood or adolescence.

c. Status epilepticus (continuous seizures).

(1) A serious condition in which seizures of the grand mal type follow in rapid succession with no intervening period of consciousness.

(2) Treatment of this particular condition: Give sodium phenobarbital (Luminal) 0.4 to 0.8 gm or paraldehyde 3 to 6 ml. intravenously to produce brief anesthesia and to help prevent further attacks.

d. Psychomotor seizures do not conform to the classic criteria of grand mal, petit mal, or jacksonian seizures. These are minor seizures with loss of contact with environment for 1 to 2 minutes. The patient does not fall but may stagger around performing automatically and does not understand what is being said. He may resist aid. Mental confusion continues for 1 to 2 minutes after attack has ended. May develop at any age. Usually associated with brain damage.

e. Treatment of convulsive seizures.

(1) Prevent the patient from injuring himself by placing a tongue depressor, handkerchief, or padded gag between teeth to prevent biting of the tongue. Do not restrain patient. Do not leave him alone. If possible, before seizure, place a gag between the teeth, but do not use a metal object. Do not pry the teeth open. Loosen clothing, especially around the neck. Turn head to the side, allowing mucus to flow from mouth and throat. After the attack, give phenobarbital 15-30 mg. t.i.d.

(2) Patient should be hospitalized. If hospitalization is not possible, you will have to control the seizures using anticonvulsant drugs such as Dilantin 100 mg. t.i.d. to q.i.d. P.O. or IM. If seizures add phenobarbital 15-30 mg. t.i.d. to q.i.d. What you want is the lowest dose possible to prevent seizures. To accomplish this start with a low dosage and if the patient has another seizure add a little to the dosage until seizures disappear completely. Patient must not drink alcohol.

1-45. HYSTERICAL ATTACKS VS. GRAND MAL ATTACKS.

a. May resemble grand mal epilepsy. With hysterical attacks the onset is slower and movements are purposeful, incontinence and cyanosis are absent, pupils do not dilate, patient does not injure himself when he falls, does not bite his tongue, usually has history of emotional upset and neurosis.

b. Treatment is the same as (1) of epilepsy treatment.

1-46. BELL's PALSY. A paralysis of the muscles of one side of the face sometimes precipitated by exposure, chill, or trauma. Can occur at any age but most common from 20-50.

S. and O. One side of the face sags--eyelids, lips, eyebrows, or entire face.

A. Bell's palsy.

P. Keep face warm and avoid further exposure, especially to wind and dust. Protect eye with patch if necessary. Gentle upward massage of the involved muscles 5-10 minutes 2-3 times a day helps maintain muscle tone. Prednisone 40 mg. daily x 4 days, then taper to 8 mg. a day in 8 days may help. In most cases partial or complete recovery occurs usually in 2-8 weeks (1-2 years in older patients).

Section VIII - The Endocrine System

1-47. The endocrine system is made up of glands of internal secretion (ductless glands). The secretions (hormones) enter directly into the blood or lymph circulation. Very small quantities of hormones are produced, only a trace being necessary to produce an effect, and some of them influence the body as a whole. Because of this and the fact that endocrine disorders can mimic a wide variety of primary disease states, the diagnosis of endocrine diseases is extremely difficult to make. The hormone producing glands include the pituitary, thyroid, parathyroids, ardrenals, gonads, and pancreas.

1-48. GOITER (see Chapter 5, Nutritional Diseases and Deficiencies).

1-49. DIABETES MELLITUS. A chronic metabolic disorder, characterized by abnormal insulin secretion and a variety of metabolic and vascular manifestations reflected in a tendency toward abnormally elevated blood glucose levels, large vessel disease, microvascular disease, and neuropathy.

S. Polyuria, increased thirst and hunger, paresthesia, and fatigue. Bed wetting may signal the onset of diabetes in children. Vaginitis and pruritus vulvae are frequent initial complaints of adult females. There may be marked weight loss despite normal or increased appetite. Diabetes should be suspected in obese patients, patients with a positive family Hx of diabetes, and in women who have delivered large babies (over 9 lbs) or who have had unexplained fetal losses.

O. In mild or moderate diabetes there may be no abnormal signs at onset, whereas the patient with severe insulin deficiency may present with loss of SQ fat, dehydration, muscle wasting, anorexia, nausea, vomiting, air hunger, and if untreated, coma and death. The retina may show microaneurysms, intraretinal hemorrhages, and hard exudates. Cardiovascular signs include signs of circulatory embarrassment of the lower extremities and hypertension. Neurological signs are predominantly sensory in nature with dulled perception of vibration, pain, and temperature, particularly in the lower extremities. The ankle jerk is often absent, but the knee jerk may be retained. Urinalysis is positive for glucose and ketones with specific gravity 1.020-1.040. NOTE: Certain common therapeutic agents, e.g., ascorbic acid, salicylates, methyldopa, and levodopa, when taken in large doses, can give a false positive for glucose when using Clintest measurements or false negatives when using glucose oxidase paper strips (Clinistix, Tes-Tape, etc.). Despite the importance of the above signs and symptoms to the diabetic syndrome, none constitute the basis for a conclusive diagnosis. Whenever diabetes is suspected, it should be confirmed by a fasting blood or serum glucose and a glucose tolerance test if indicated.

A. Diabetes mellitus. Differential diagnosis: Nondiabetic (renal) glycosuria, hyperglycemia due to end organ insensivity to insulin.

P. A well balanced (sugar free) 1,000-1,200 calorie diet and weight reduction will manage many cases of mild to moderate diabetes, especially in obese patients who demonstrate symptomatology at age 40 or above. If glycosuria persists, the use of hypoglycemic agents such as insulin or tolbutamide (Oranase) is indicated. The ultimate choice of agents, route, dose, and interval must be determined by a careful analysis of serum glucose levels.

1-50. COMPLICATIONS OF DIABETES.

a. Hypoglycemia (insulin shock). An abnormally low blood sugar level and the most common complication of patients on insulin therapy.

S. Sudden onset (slower with long acting insulins) of mental confusion, bizarre behavior, sweating, palpitations, and tremulousness that may lead to coma, convulsions, and death.

O. Skin is moist, pale, and cool. There may be drooling from the mouth. Respirations are normal or shallow and the breath is usually odorless. B.P. is normal with a full bounding pulse. The urine in negative for glucose and ketones by the second voiding (there may initially be some residue from earlier hyperglycemia.) Serum glucose is <60 mg./100 ml.

A. Hypoglycemia due to insulin reaction. Differential diagnosis: Diabetic ketoacidosis, alcohol or drug induced coma, head injury, and cerebrovascular accidents. NOTE: If serum glucose is <50 mg./100 ml. the Dx is confirmed.

P. If still conscious and able to swallow, give orange juice, glucose, or any beverage containing sugar. If stuporous or unconscious, give 20-50 ml. 50% glucose IV stat. Then continue infusion at a rate of 10 gm/hr. If patient is still hypoglycemic, give a second bolus of 25 ml. 50% glucose. If unable to start IV, give 1 mg. glucagon IM or SQ then sugar by mouth when patient is awake and can swallow. If neither glucose nor glucagon is available, give 30 ml. syrup or honey in 500 ml. warm water rectally. Monitor patient response and plasma glucose level carefully.

b. Diabetic ketoacidosis. Hyperglycemic coma. Usually occurs in insulin dependent and juvenile (age <30) onset diabetics.

S. Gradual onset (1-2 days). Nausea, vomiting, abdominal pain, polyuria, intense thirst, and marked fatigue progressing to mental stupor and finally coma and death, if untreated.

O. Skin is hot, dry, and flushed with a loss of turgor. Mouth is dry. Respirations are deep, rapid, and labored. A fruity (acetone) odor is usually present on the breath. There may be signs of shock (see chapter 15). The eyeballs are soft. Urine glucose and ketones are strongly positive. Plasma glucose is >300 mg./100 ml. and ketones are strongly positive. NOTE: A rapid blood glucose determination can be made using commercially available glucose test strips (Dextrostix) and a rough quantitation of serum or plasma ketone can be made using either Ketostix or Acetest tablets. The presence of ketone may be masked if there is a strong level of lactic acid present.

A. Diabetic ketoacidosis. Differential diagnosis: Hypoglycemia, lactic acidosis due to septic, cardiogenic, or hypovolemic shock. NOTE: With lactic acidosis, the clinical picture will be approximately the same without the acetone breath or ketonuria. Blood glucose is variable.

P. (1) Diabetic ketoacidosis. Start IV .5 N saline at rate of 1 L./hr x 2 hrs, then adjust to 5-8 L. (total) over a period of 24 hours. If patient is already in shock, give N saline. Insulin (regular) 5-10 units/hr slow IV drip or IM. When blood glucose is <250 mg./100 ml., start

IV D5W at a rate of approximately 200 ml./hr with insulin q.2-4h. p.r.n. to maintain glucose level between 200 and 250 mg./100 ml.

(2) Lactic acidosis. Start IV .5 N saline at rate of 1 L./2 hours, then 1 L./2-3 hours. Na bicarbonate 2 ampules (90 mEq.) stat. Repeat with 3-4 ampules if necessary. Stop when breathing returns to normal.

c. Prevention of soft tissue complications. Diabetics are susceptible to bedsores, infection, and gangrene. Because of poor circulation, feet should be kept scrupulously clean and dry. Extreme care should be used when trimming toenails, and corn and callouses should be removed by soaking, not cutting. Use oil or lanolin to keep feet soft and avoid tight shoes. Do not apply local heat to legs and feet. Instruct the patient to brush teeth at least three times a day. Take warm baths daily and seek prompt attention for any bruise or break in the skin.

1-51. ACUTE ADRENAL INSUFFICIENCY. A clinical syndrome caused by marked deprivation or insufficient supply of adrenocortical hormones following trauma, surgery, overwhelming sepsis (principally meningococcemia), or sudden withdrawal of corticosteroid drug therapy. Acute adrenal insufficiency constitutes a grave medical emergency and is rapidly fatal if not treated.

S. Headache, lassitude, nausea, vomiting, abdominal pain, C.V.A. pain, and tenderness. Confusion or coma may be present.

O. Fever 105°F. or more, B.P., cyanosis, petechiae (especially with meningococemia), dehydration, abnormal skin pigmentation, and lymphadenopathy marked eosinophilia. NOTE: A high eosinophil count in the presence of severe stress due to trauma, infection, or other mechanisms is strongly suggestive of adrenal failure.

A. Acute adrenal insufficiency due to ____________. Differential diagnosis: Diabetic coma, cerebrovascular accident, acute poisoning.

P. IF ADRENAL FAILURE IS SUSPECTED, TREAT AT ONCE WITHOUT WAITING FOR CONFIRMATION BY LAB RESULTS. Treat for shock (see chapter 15). Start IV fluids stat., vasopressor drugs and O_2 p.r.n. Do not give narcotics or sedatives. 100 mg. Solu-Cortef IV stat. and continue IV infusion of 50-100 mg. q.6h. x 1 day, then same amount q.8h. x 1 day. Continue to give q.8h. with a gradual reduction in dose until the patient is able to take food by mouth, then give oral cortisone 12.5-25 mg. q.6h. and reduce to maintenance levels p.r.n. Monitor B.P. and observe for signs of edema and hypertension. If signs of cerebral edema (unconsciousness or convulsions) or pulmonary edema occur, withhold sodium and fluids and treat these conditions. If signs of hypokalemia occur, give potassium salts or food high in potassium content (orange juice or bananas). Evacuate when feasible.

(8) Scar. The result of healing after destruction of the dermis.

1-3. SKIN DISORDERS.

a. Pruritus (Itching).

S. Compulsive itching accompanies primary skin disease or may be the only signs and symptoms.

O. Redness, uticarial papules, excoriated papules, fissures, crusting, etc.

A. Pruritus/Pruritus secondary to __________ skin disease.

P. Correct the skin disease, or discontinue using irritating substance, e.g., soap, clothing, chemical, etc. Use of mild tranquilizers: Valium, Vistiral. Use of major tranquilizers: Thorazine. Use of antihistamines: Benadryl 50 mg. t.i.d.

b. Contact dermatitis is divided into two types:

(1) Primary irritant contact dermatitis. Develops within a few hours, reaches peak severity in 24 hours then disappears; caused by contact with a chemical irritant.

(2) Allergic eczematous contact dermatitis. Has a delayed onset of about 18 hours, peaks in 48-72 hours, and often lasts 2-3 weeks after discontinuing exposure to the offending antigen. (Poison ivy, oak, or sumac or allergy to clothing, etc.)

(3) Symptoms vary from minor itching and redness to vesicles, redness, edema, oozing, crusting, and scaling; itching is usually sharply demarcated.

(4) Remove offending agent. Use tap water, soaks, or compresses. Blisters may be drained but leave the tops on. Oral corticosteriods - Prednisone 40-60 mg./day x 10-14 days in severe cases. Topical corticosteriods are not effective in acute phase. Antihistamines - Benadryl 50 mg. t.i.d.

1-4. BACTERIAL SKIN INFECTIONS.

a. Impetigo/Ecthyma. Superficial vesiculopustular skin infection seen chiefly in children. Ecthyma is an ulcerative form of impetigo.

S. Group A B-hemolytic streptococcus is usual cause, but Staphylococcus aureus may be cultured also.

O. Usually affects arms, legs, and face, with the legs being more susceptible to ecthyma than unexposed areas. Both may follow superficial trauma or may be secondary to skin disease or insect bites, but it is not uncommon for it to arise on normal skin.

Lesions vary from pea-sized vesicopustules to large bizarre circinate ringwormlike lesions that progress rapidly from maculopapules to vesicopustules or bullae to exudative and then to heavily crusted circinate lesions. Ecthyma is characterized by small, purulent, shallow ulcers

Section IX - Eye, Ear, Nose, and Throat (EENT)

1-52. EYE DISORDERS.

Conjunctivitis. Conjunctivitis is the most common eye disease. It may be acute or chronic. Most cases are due to bacterial, viral, or chlamydial infections. Other causes are allergy, chemical irritation, and fungal or parasitic infection. The mode of transmission is usually direct contact via fingers, towels, etc.

a. Bacterial conjunctivitis.

S. Copious purulent discharge and redness with no pain or blurring of vision.

O. Gram's stain of discharge usually shows streptococcus or staphylococcus organisms.

A. Bacterial conjunctivitis. Differential diagnosis: Iritis, glaucoma, corneal trauma, keratitis, and other causes of conjunctivitis.

P. Disease is usually self-limiting, lasting 10-14 days if untreated. Sulfonamide or antibiotic ophthalmic ointment applied locally t.i.d. usually clears the infection in 2-3 days.

b. Viral conjunctivitis.

S. Redness, copious watery discharge, and scanty exudate from the eye. Usually associated with systemic symptoms, pharyngitis, fever, malaise, and adenopathy.

O. Children are more often affected. Contaminated swimming pools are a major cause.

A. Viral conjunctivitis. Differential diagnosis: See bacterial conjunctivitis.

P. No specific treatment. Use antibiotic ophthalmic ointment to prevent secondary infections. Usually lasts at least 2 weeks.

c. Chlamydial keratoconjunctivitis (trachoma). Trachoma is a major cause of blindness. In endemic areas it is contracted in childhood. It is usually insidious with minimal symptoms. In adults it is acute.

S. Redness, itching, tearing, and slight discharge.

O. Bilateral follicular conjunctivitis, inflammation of the cornea, and pannus (cloudy, uneven, newly formed vascular tissue over the cornea). In the later stages, scarring of the eyelid margin may cause inversion of the eyelid and the eyelashes causing them to rub against the cornea thereby scratching and scarring the cornea. This decreases the vision, leading to blindness. Giemsa stain scraping from conjunctiva shows typical cytoplasmic inclusions in the epithelial cells. In active trachoma, the smear may also include polymorphonuclear leukocytes, plasma cells, and debris-filled macrophages.

A. Trachoma. Differential diagnosis: Other eye infections.

P. Nasal decongestants to keep eustachian tube open. Antihistamines if there is any suggestion of nasal allergy. Treat cause of blockage, e.g., tonsillitis or sinus infection. If all else fails to relieve the fluid, a myringotomy is necessary to drain the ear. Indwelling plastic tubing for drainage can be used in persistent cases.

c. Diseases of the inner ear.

(1) Meniere's disease. Characterized by recurrent episodes of severe vertigo associated with deafness and tinnitus. Meniere's disease is usually encountered in men 40-60 yrs old. Cause is not known.

S. Intermittent severe vertigo that may cause the patient to fall. Nausea, vomiting, and profuse perspiration are often associated. These attacks may last from minutes to several hours. Frequency of attacks varies. Headache, hearing loss, and tinnitus occur during and persist between attacks. Hearing loss may be progressive and in 90 percent of the cases unilateral. Involuntary eyeball movement may occur during attacks of vertigo.

O. Increased sensitivity to loud sounds and decreased speech discrimination. Marked psychic disturbance is found in many patients.

A. Meniere's disease. Differential diagnosis: Systemic infections, psychiatric disorders, and cerebrospinal injuries or disorders.

P. Reassurance, salt-free diet; antihistamines (Benadryl and Dramamine) 50-150 mg. orally 3-4 times daily may help some patients. Parenteral Dramamine, Benadryl or 0.6 mg. atropine sulfate may stop acute attacks. Meniere's disease is chronic, recurrent, and may persist for years.

(2) Acute nonsuppurative labyrinthitis.

S. Usually follows respiratory tract infections. Manifested by intense vertigo, usually with marked tinnitus, a staggering gait, and involuntary eyeball movement.

O. Hearing loss is often not present.

A. Acute nonsuppurative labyrinthitis. Differential diagnosis: Meniere's disease.

P. Bed rest, preferably in a darkened room until severe symptoms subside. Antibiotics are of little value unless there is an associated infection of the middle ear or mastoid bone. Antihistamine (Benadryl or Dramamine) may be of value. Phenobarbital 15-60 mg. 3-4 times a day is generally helpful. Thorazine HCl 50 mg. IM is useful in the acute early phase. Attacks may last for several days but recovery is usually complete.

1-54. NOSE DISORDERS.

a. Sinus infection.

S. History of an acute upper respiratory infection, swimming or diving, dental abscess or extraction, or nasal allergies. Pain, tenderness, redness, swelling over the involved sinus, fever, chills, malaise, and headache.

O. Nasal congestion and purulent nasal discharge. Lab: Smear of nasal discharge may show causative organism; white count may be elevated.

A. Sinus infection. Differential diagnosis: Acute dental infection.

P. Bed rest, sedatives, analgesics, light diet, force fluids, nasal decongestants (nose spray or drops) 2-3 times a day, local heat, and systemic antibiotics will usually clear up the infection.

b. Common cold. Caused by a wide variety of viruses, all of which exist in multiple antigenic types, and recurrent infection is common.

S. Malaise, fever, headache, nasal discomfort with watery discharge and sneezing followed by mucoid to purulent discharge, and nasal obstruction. Throat symptoms are dryness and soreness rather than actual pain and hoarseness.

O. Nasal mucosa is reddened and swollen. Pharynx and tonsils show mild to moderate infection usually without edema or exudate; cervical lymph modes may be enlarged and slightly tender. Lab: Not remarkable unless there is a secondary bacterial infection.

A. Common cold. Differential diagnosis: Flu or URI.

P. General measures: rest, forced fluid, symptomatic treatment, e.g., asiprin for headache, etc.

c. Allergic rhinitis (hay fever).

S. Nasal congestion; a profuse, watery nasal discharge; itching nose often leading to paroxysms of violent sneezing; nasal mucosa is pale and boggy; itching watery eyes; conjunctiva is often red and swollen.

O. Gram's stain of nasal secretion reveals numerous eosinophils, C.B.C. shows 5-40% eosinophilia.

A. Hay fever. Differential diagnosis: Other common upper respiratory infections.

P. Antihistamines give relief in 60-80 percent of cases but effectiveness wanes as the allergy season progresses. Sympathomimetic drugs such as ephedrine are effective by themselves or in combination with antihistamines. Sedation may be of value for tense or nervous patients.

1-55. THROAT DISEASES.

a. Acute tonsillitis is nearly always a bacterial infection, often due to streptococci.

S. Sudden onset of sore throat, fever, chills, headache, anorexia, and malaise.

O. Swollen and red tonsils with pus or exudate. Cervical nodes are frequently enlarged and tender. White count may be elevated. Gram's stain of pus or exudate may show causative organism; throat culture will.

A. Tonsillitis. Differential diagnosis: Simple pharyngitis, infectious mononucleosis, Vincent's angina, and diphtheria.

P. Bed rest, fluids, light diet, warm salt water gargles, analgesics, and antibiotics as required.

b. Simple pharyngitis. Usually bacterial or viral in nature; may be part of the syndrome of an acute specific infection (e.g., measles, scarlet fever, etc.).

S. In acute pharyngitis the throat is dry and sore; systemic symptoms are fever and malaise. Chronic pharyngitis may produce few symptoms, e.g., throat dryness with thick mucus and cough or recurrent acute episodes of more severe throat pain, dull hyperemia.

O. Acute pharyngitis, red mucosa slightly swollen with a thick sticky mucus. Chronic pharyngitis, mild swelling of the mucosa with a thick tenacious mucus often in hypopharynx.

A. Simple pharyngitis. Differential diagnosis: Other upper respiratory infections and part of the syndrome of an acute specific infection (e.g., measles, whooping cough, etc.).

P. Symptomatic treatment; rest, light diet, analgesics, warm saline gargles, and antibiotics if it is a bacterial infection.

c. Influenza transmitted by respiratory route. Although sporadic cases occur, usually occurs as pandemic or epidemic in the fall or winter. Incubation period is 1-4 days.

S. and O. Abrupt onset of fever, chills, malaise and muscular aching, substernal soreness, headache, sore throat, nonproductive cough, nasal stuffiness, mild pharynged infection, flushed face, conjunctival redness, and occasional nausea. Fever lasts 1-7 days (usually 3-5). If fever persists more than 4 days, cough becomes productive or if W.B.C. rises to about 12,000, secondary bacterial infection should be ruled out or verified and treated. Most fatalities are due to bacterial pneumonia.

Lab findings: Leukopenia is common and proteinuria may be present.

A. Influenza.

P. Symptomatic, bed rest to reduce complications, forced fluids, analgesics, and sedative cough mixture. Do Not Use antibiotics unless secondary bacterial infection develops.

CHAPTER 2

COMMUNICABLE DISEASES

Section I - Parasitic

2-1. GENERAL. Of all the diseases that afflict mankind, many parasites, especially malaria, cause the highest morbidity and mortality worldwide.

2-2. AMEBIASIS. Caused by the one-celled parasite Entamoeba histolytica. It is present throughout the world, but is especially severe in third world countries and in tropical countries. Diarrhea is the most common presentation.

S. Recurrent bouts of diarrhea and abdominal cramps, sometimes alternating with constipation.

O. Tenderness and enlargement of the liver are frequent. Semifluid stools containing no pus and only flecks of blood-stained mucus. Stools 5-10 per day often with fever up to 105° F. Abdominal colic and vomiting. Lab findings: Entamoeba histolytica trophozoites and cysts in stool specimens are difficult to detect. Even with the best lab techniques a minimum of six separate stool specimens are needed to diagnose the disease. Trophozoites are found in liquid stools; cysts are found in formed stools.

A. Amebiasis. Differential diagnosis: Other causes of diarrhea, bacillary dysentery, emotional diarrhea, diarrhea 2° to laxative abuse, diverticulitis, drugs, pernicious anemia.

P. Collect six stool samples to look for trophozoites and cysts. Trophozoites that contain ingested red blood cells are diagnostic for invasive Entamoeba histolytica. Leukocytes and macrophages are relatively rare in the stool sample; whereas in bacillary dysentery many white blood cells are present.

Treatment: Metronidazole (Flagyl) 750 mg. t.i.d. x 10 days followed by diiodohydroxyquin 650 mg. q.i.d. x 21 days.

Follow-up care: The stool should be examined six times over one week after symptoms have disappeared. If any cysts or trophozoites are found in these specimens, initiate the treatment above until symptoms are cleared.

2-3. MALARIA. Malaria is perhaps the most debilitating illness worldwide, especially in the tropics. Four species of Plasmodium are responsible: Plasmodium vivax, falciparum, malariae, and ovale.

S. Acute episodes of chills, fever, and sweating. Occasionally delirium, coma, convulsions, gastrointestinal disorders, and jaundice. The chills last from 15 minutes to an hour; nausea, vomiting, and severe headache are common at this time. Fever that follows the chills will last several hours and will often get to 104° F. or higher. The third stage, or sweating, concludes the cycle. The fever subsides and the patient falls asleep to awaken feeling fairly well. In vivax, ovale, and falciparum infections, the episodes occur every 48 hours (tertian malaria). In malariae infections (quartan malaria) the cycle takes 72 hours.

O. The thick and thin blood film, stained with Giemsa's stain or Romanovsky stain, is the mainstay of malaria diagnosis. The thin film is used primarily for species differentiation after the presence of an infection is detected on a thick film. The level of parasites in the blood varies from hour to hour; therefore the blood should be examined several times a day for 2-3 days. Anemia may be present and is usually more severe with falciparum infections. Jaundice may develop in severe infections.

A. Malaria. Differential diagnosis: Other causes of fever in tropics, urinary tract infections, typhoid fever, infectious hepatitis, dengue, leptospirosis. Examination of the blood film is essential to differentiate the above from malaria.

P. Chloroquine is used to prophylatically suppress symptoms of malaria, but it does not prevent infection. If falciparum malaria does not respond promptly to chloroquine (within 24 hours), parasite resistance to this drug must be considered.

Give chloroquine phosphate, 1 gram as initial dose, 500 mg. in 6 hours, and 500 mg. daily for the next 2 days. If patients cannot absorb the drug rapidly because of vomiting or severe diarrhea, or if they are comatose, give 250 mg. (salt) of chloroquine hydrochloride intramuscularly. Repeat in 6 hours, if necessary, and follow with oral therapy as soon as possible. Do not use chloroquine for severely ill patients whose infections originated in an endemic region for P. falciparum.

Prophylactic (suppressive) dosage: Before leaving home, the patient should take a test dose of the medication to detect possible allergic readings. Starting about 1 week before arrival in the area of malaria risk, the patient should begin chloroquine phosphate 500 mg. (salt) weekly, or the combined tablet of chloroquine 500 mg. (salt) plus primaquine phosphate 78.9 mg. (salt) weekly. After leaving the endemic area, the chloroquine should be continued for 6 weeks or the combined tablet for 8 weeks. For those taking chloroquine dose, a 14-day course of primaquine should be given if there has been significant exposure to P. vivax or P. ovale.

Primaquine phosphate: This drug has been shown to be the most effective agent against the tissue forms of P. vivax and P. ovale. The dosage for primaquine phosphate is 26.3 mg. daily for 14 days.

Treatment of malaria due to P. falciparum strains resistant to chloroquine.

When the patient can take medication orally, give quinine sulfate 650 mg. 3 times daily for 14 days plus pyrimethamine 25 mg. twice daily for 3 days, plus either sulfadiazine 500 mg. 4 times daily for 5 days, or dapsone 25 mg. daily for 28 days.

For prophylaxis, Fansidar for nonimmune individuals (pyrimethamine, 25 mg. and sulfadoxine, 500 mg.) should be given once weekly. The medication should be continued for 6 weeks after leaving the endemic area. Although Fansidar is not available in the USA, it is usually available in countries with chloroquine-resistant malaria under the trade names of Fansidar, Falcidar, or Antemal.

2-4. AFRICAN TRYPANOSOMIASIS (sleeping sickness). Rhodesian and Gambian trypanosomiasis are caused by two morphologically similar parasites

Trypanosoma rhodesiense and Trypanosoma gambiense. Trypanosomiasis occurs throughout tropical Africa from south of the Sahara to about 20 degrees South latitude. Trypanosoma gambiense is limited to West Africa up to the western Rift Valley. Trypanosoma rhodesiense occurs to the east of the Rift Valley. Both trypanosomes are transmitted by the bites of tsetse flies.

S. The patient may complain of a local inflammatory reaction (called a trypanosoma chancre). It occurs within 48 hours after a bite. The lesions may be painful or pruritic for up to 3 weeks. The patient may have personality changes, headache, apathy, somnolence, and tremors. The patient may become severely emaciated and finally become comatose.

O. Irregular fever, tachycardia, painless lymph nodes. Multiple thick wet blood smears should be taken. Other lab findings include anemia and increased sedimentation rate.

A. Trypanosomiasis. Differential diagnosis: May be mistaken for a variety of other diseases including malaria, tuberculosis, kala-azar, and cerebral syphilis.

P. Pentamidine is the drug of choice for prophylaxis of sleeping sickness, but is effective with certainty only against the Gambian type. In Rhodesian infection, pentamidine may lead to suppression of early symptoms resulting in recognition of the disease too late in its course for effective treatment. One intramuscular injection (4 mg./kilogram, maximum 300 mg.) will protect against Gambiense infection for 6 months. The drug is potentially toxic and should be used for persons at high risk. It must be emphasized that the drugs used to treat trypanosomiasis are available only from the Parasitic Disease Drug Service, Center for Disease Control, Atlanta, GA 30333, (404) 329-3670.

Suramin sodium is the drug of choice for treatment of the early stages of trypanosomiasis. Treatment is 1 gm dosages @ 1, 3, and 7 days and then weekly until a total of 7 grams have been given.

Tryparsamide has been used for a long time for Gambiense infections of the central nervous system. It is given intravenously in a 20% solution in water. The dosage is 20-40 mg./kg. (maximum dose 2 gm) given at weekly intervals for a total of 10-12 injections.

General measures: Good nursing care and treatment of anemia, concurrent infections, and malnutrition are essential in the management.

Prognosis: If untreated, most cases of African trypanosomiasis are fatal. If treated properly, the prognosis is excellent.

2-5. AMERICAN TRYPANOSOMIASIS (Chagas' disease). Chagas' disease is caused by Trypanosoma cruzi, a one-celled parasite of the blood and tissues of humans and other animals. T. cruzi is found in wild animals from southern South America to northern Mexico, Texas, and the southwestern USA. Many species of reduviid bugs (cone-nosed or kissing bugs) transmit the infection, which results from rubbing infected bug feces, passed during feeding, into the wound.

S. Intermittent fever, swollen painful lymph nodes, and occasionally convulsions.

O. Hard, edematous, red, and painful cutaneous nodules (chagoma). Unilateral palpebral and facial edema and conjunctivitis.

A. Chagas' disease. Differential diagnosis: Can be confused with kala-azar. The chagoma may be mistaken for a variety of tropical skin diseases.

P. Establish the diagnosis by taking thick and thin blood films and finding the parasite in the smears. Trypanosomes should be looked for in the blood of all patients but will usually be seen only in the acute stage of infection. Treatment of Chagas' disease is symptomatic and supportive. The best plan of action is preventive: Living quarters should be cleaned and pesticides used to eradicate the insects that transmit the disease.

2-6. LEISHMANIASIS. The clinical manifestations of leishmaniasis may be classified as (1) visceral, (2) cutaneous, and (3) mucocutaneous. These distinctions are not rigid because in the course of illness one type may develop into another. The leishmaniases are caused by different species of leishmania transmitted by the bites of sandflies (Phlebotomus).

a. Visceral leishmaniasis (kala-azar). Visceral leishmaniasis is geographically widespread. It is caused mainly by two species: Leishmania donovani in the Indian region and Leishmania infantum in USSR, China, Middle East, Mediterranean basin, and Africa. It also occurs in South America.

S. Irregular fever, insidious and chronic; onset may be acute.

O. Progressive anemia, loss of weight, progressive darkening of the skin especially the forehead and hands, gradual enlargement of the spleen and liver. The fever may be very high and the patient sometimes does not look very ill. There is a marked decrease in the W.B.C., usually less than 3,000/ml. The diagnosis is established by demonstrating Leishman-Donovan bodies in stained blood smears.

A. Leishmaniasis. Differential diagnosis: malaria.

P. Treatment of visceral leishmaniasis is difficult--the best drugs are not available for general use. The drug that is available is highly toxic, but it should be used if necessary. Amphotericin B at a dose of 0.5 mg./kg. per day is dissolved in 500 ml. of 5% dextrose and given over 6 hours on alternate days. Patients must be closely monitored. Without treatment, kala-azar is usually fatal.

b. Cutaneous leishmaniasis. Cutaneous leishmaniasis may present as self-healing ulcers (oriental sore), non-ulcerating nodules that resemble leprosy, and chronic mutilating ulcers. Cutaneous leishmaniasis is seen in the USSR, India, the Middle East, the Mediterranean basin, Africa, and Central and South America.

S and O. Cutaneous swellings appear about 2-8 weeks after bites of sandflies. The swellings may ulcerate and discharge pus, or they may remain dry. Dry and moist sores are caused by distinct leishmanias, with the dry forms having longer incubation periods.

A. Cutaneous leishmaniasis. Differential diagnosis: Syphilis, other forms of skin disease.

P. Metronidazole in the dosage required to treat amebiasis has proven éffective.

c. Mucocutaneous (naso-oral) leishmaniasis. Naso-oral lesions caused by leishmaniasis are seen in South America. There it is referred to as espundia. The anterior cartilage of the nose is involved and sometimes leads to a complete erosion of the bone with disfigurement. Amphotericin B 0.25-1 mg./kg. every other day for up to 8 weeks is required to kill the organism.

2-7. SCHISTOSOMIASIS (bilharziasis). A blood fluke (trematode) infection with adult male and female worms living in veins of the host. Symptoms are related to the location of the parasite in the human host. Schistosoma mansoni and Schistosoma japonicum give rise to intestinal symptoms. Schistosoma haematobium gives rise to urinary tract symptoms.

S. Transient red itching skin rash with fever, malaise. The patient may have diarrhea, abdominal pain, loss of appetite, loss of weight. Urinary frequency, urethral and bladder pain.

O. Diarrhea and abdominal pain are common in the early stages of the disease. Diagnosis depends on finding the eggs in stool specimens. As many as 8-10 stool specimens are needed to detect the eggs.

A. Schistosomiasis should be considered in all unresponsive gastrointestinal disorders in endemic areas. Differential diagnosis: Early schistosomiasis may be confused with amebiasis or bacterial dysentery.

P. Treatment should be given only if live ova are identified. In the USA, the first drug of choice for S. haematobium and S. mansoni infections is niridazole. Outside the USA, in countries where it is available, the drug of choice is oxamniquine for S. mansoni and metrifonate for S. haematobium. Niridazole should be administered in high doses, under close medical supervision. Oral doses are 25 mg./kg. (maximum 1.5 grams) daily in 2 divided doses for 7-10 days. The side effects of the drugs include nausea, vomiting, headache, and brownish discoloration of the urine.

2-8. FASCIOLOPSIASIS. Fasciolopsis buski is a large intestinal fluke found in China, Taiwan, Southeast Asia, and India. The intermediate host is a snail. Humans are infected by eating uncooked water plants that have the parasite encysted in them. After an incubation period of several months in humans, manifestations of gastrointestinal irritation appear in all but light infections. In severe infections:

S. and O. Cramping epigastric and hypogastric pains, diarrhea, intermittent constipation, anorexia, and nausea. Edema, particularly of the face and ascites (accumulation of fluid in the abdominal cavity) may occur later. Death may result from the parasite or secondary infection.

Lab findings: Leukocytosis with moderate eosinophilia. Diagnosis is made by finding the eggs or occasionally flukes in the stools.

A. Fasciolopsiasis. Differential diagnosis: Other intestinal flukes.

P. Crystalline hexylresorcinol is the drug of choice. Adults 1 gm orally on an empty stomach in the morning. Repeat in 3-4 days. Children 0.1 gm/year of age to age 10. Same as with adult. After 2 hours give sodium sulfate or sodium citrate as a purgation to flush the intestinal tract. Two treatments are usually sufficient. Alternate drug piperazine citrate in recommended course of therapy.

2-9. LIVER FLUKES.

a. Fascioliasis. Sheep liver fluke found primarily in Latin America and the Mediterranean area. Man is infested by ingesting the metacercariae on watercrest or other aquatic vegetables.

b. Clonorchiasis. Endemic in areas of Japan, Korea, China, Formosa, and Indochina. Imported cases are seen in USA. Man is infested by eating raw or undercooked freshwater fish.

S. and O. Light infestations may be asymptomatic. Heavy infestations may present as malaise, fever, liver tenderness, and jaundice. These symptoms are transient. Progressive liver enlargement, right upper quadrant pain, and vague abdominal symptoms such as diarrhea, weakness, weight loss, tachycardia, and a variety of other symptoms may occur.

Lab findings: Leukocytosis with eosinophilia sometimes from 10-40%. Diagnosis is made by finding the eggs in the stool.

A. Fascioliasis or clonorchiasis.

P. Bithional 40 mg./kg. P.O. on alternate days over 20-30 days. Alternate drug: Emetine HCl, 1 mg./kg. IM up to 65 mg. daily for 7 days. Recovery is slow even if all the flukes are killed.

2-10. PARAGONIMIASIS. A lung fluke found throughout the Far East, West Africa, South Asia, central and northern South America. Man is infected by eating infected snails, crabs, and crayfish. Ingested immature flukes migrate through the small intestines usually to the lungs, although they can lodge in other tissues of the body or even migrate to the brain or spinal cord, but these usually fail to mature. The flukes that reach the lungs encapsulate, reach maturity, and lay eggs. These capsules swell and usually rupture into a bronchiole.

S. and O. The infection is usually asymptomatic until the flukes mature and begin laying eggs. The onset is insidious with low-grade fever and a cough that is dry at first, then turning to a viscous sputum that is rusty or blood-flecked. Pleuritic chest pain is common. The condition is chronic and progressive with dyspnea, signs of bronchitis and bronchiectasis, weakness, malaise, and weight loss. In heavy infestations, parasites in the abdomen may cause abdominal pain, diarrhea, or dysentery. Parasites in the brain or spinal cord, depending on their location, may cause seizures, palsies, or meningoencephalitis.

Lab findings: Slight leukocytosis with eosinophilia. Eggs can be readily found in the sputum if it is spun down and a smear is made from the bottom of the tube. Eggs can also be found in stool specimens.

A. Paragonimiasis.

P. Drug of choice is bithionol 40 mg./kg. of body weight given on alternate days for 10-15 doses (20-30 days).

2-11. TAPEWORM INFECTIONS. A number of tapeworms can infect humans, but only six are commonly found. Distribution is worldwide. Infestations usually occurs by eating infected and undercooked or raw beef, pork, fresh water fish, and crustaceans. Tapeworms vary in size from 1 cm. or less to 300 cm. or more.

S. and O. Adult tapeworms in human intestines usually cause no symptoms. Heavy infestations may present as weight loss, vague abdominal complaints, diarrhea, anorexia, abdominal pain, and nervous disturbances, particularly in children.

The larva of some tapeworms migrate throughout the body. In muscle or connective tissue they cause no problems, but in the brain they may cause a wide variety of manifestations: epileptic seizures, mental deterioration, personality disturbances, and internal hydrocephalus.

Lab findings: Segments of the tapeworm may be found in stool, clothing, or bedding. The ova often can be found using the scotch tape method (as used to diagnose pinworms). The eggs (ova) are found occasionally in the stool.

A. Tapeworm.

P. Drug of choice: Niclosamide. Give 2 gm orally in the morning before eating for 5 days. If niclosamide is not available, use quinacrine HCl (mepacrine). Place patient on liquid diet 24 hours prior to treatment (no milk). The evening before treatment, give saline or soapsuds enema. On morning of treatment, withhold breakfast and confine patient to bed. Give an antiemetic (Compazine) and wait 1 hour. For children 18-34 kg. give 0.5 gm; for adults or children over 45 kg. give 0.8 gm. Dose may be divided but must be given within 30 minutes. Wait 2 hours after the 30 minutes, then give saline or soapsuds purge.

2-12. TRICHINOSIS. Worldwide distribution, but it is a greater problem in the temperate areas than in the tropics. Infection occurs from eating raw or undercooked pork, but bear and walrus meat has also been implicated. Symptoms may appear in a few hours, but usual incubation period is 5-15 days.

S. and O. Symptoms vary considerably depending on the number of larva and the tissue invaded. Initial symptoms occur when mature female roundworms burrow into the small intestinal mucosa and may persist until the adults die at about 5 weeks. Diarrhea, abdominal cramps, malaise, nausea, vomiting, and occasionally constipation. The larva migrate through the bloodstream to most tissues of the body beginning at the end of the first week. This brings fever, low-grade to marked; muscle pain, especially on movement; muscle tenderness; edema; spasms; periorbital and facial edema; sweating; headaches; photophobia; weakness or exhaustion; pain on swallowing; dyspnea; coughing; hoarseness; conjunctival, retinal and nail hemorrhages; and rashes. Inflammatory reactions may produce meningitis, encephalitis, myocarditis, pneumonitis, nephritis, and peripheral and cranial nerve disorders. Death can occur in 4-6 weeks.

Lab findings: Eosinophilia 20-75% in the third or fourth week, slowly declining to normal. Adult worms are rarely found in the feces. Larva may occasionally be found in the blood in the second week. Definitive diagnosis is possible by biopsy of skeletal muscle in the third or fourth week.

A. Trichinosis.

P. Symptomatic treatment is normally all that is required. If it is known a patient has eaten infected meat within the last few days (not over 1 week), give thiabendazole 25 mg./kg. (maximum of 1.5 gm) b.i.d. after meals for 2-4 days. Severe infections, when the larva invade muscle tissue, require hospitalization and high doses of corticosteroids for 24-48 hours followed by lower doses for several days or weeks to control symptoms.

2-13. TRICHURIASIS (whipworms). Small slender worms, 30-50 mm. in length, found worldwide, particularly in the subtropics and tropics.

S. and O. Light to moderate infections rarely cause symptoms. Severe infections (10,000 or more ova per gram of feces) may present with a variety of symptoms that include abdominal pain, tenesmus (spasmodic contraction of anal sphincter with pain and persistent, involuntary, ineffectual straining effort to empty the bowel), diarrhea, distention, flatulence, nausea, vomiting, and weight loss. Blood loss may be significant and rectal prolapse may occur.

Lab findings: Characteristic barrel-shaped eggs in the stool. Eosinophilia of 5-20% in all but light infections and hypochromic anemia may be present in heavy infections.

A. Trichuriasis.

P. Mebendazole, 100 mg. b.i.d. before or after meals x 3 days. Tablets should be chewed before swallowing. No alcohol 24 hours before and after treatment. Alternate treatment soapsuds enema followed by hexylresorcinol enema (20-30 ml./kg. up to 1,200 ml.). Enema should be retained for 30 minutes before expulsion.

2-14. ASCARIASIS. The most common intestinal worm. Worldwide distribution. Infection is caused by ingestion of mature eggs in fecally contaminated food and drink. Eggs hatch and the larva penetrate the walls of the small intestines and migrate to the lungs. Adult worms are 20-40 cm. long.

S. and O. Fever, cough, hemoptysis (spitting or coughing up blood), rales, and other evidence of lung involvement. Rarely, the larva may go astray lodging in the brain, kidney, eye, spinal cord, or skin.

Heavy infections may also cause vague abdominal complaints and colic. With heavy infestations, especially if the worms are stimulated by certain oral medications or anesthetics, wandering may occur. Worms may be coughed up, vomited, or passed out through the nose. They may also cause mechanical blockage and inflammation by forcing themselves into the common bile duct, the pancreatic duct, the appendix, diverticula, and other sites.

Lab findings: Eggs in the stool; larva may occasionally be found in the sputum. CBC reveals eosinophilia.

A. Ascariasis lumbricoides. Differential diagnosis: Allergic disorders, other causes of pneumonitis, appendicitis, diverticulitis, etc.

P. Piperazine. Each ml. of syrup contains 100 mg. of piperazine hexahydrate, tablets contain 250-500 mg.

up to 14 kg. give 1 gm	once a day x 2 days
14-22 kg. give 2 gm	Heavy infections may
22-45 kg. give 3 gm	require 3 to 4 days
over 45 kg. give 3.5 gm	of treatment.

Alternate drugs are Pyrantel pamoate, mebendazole, levamisole, and bephenium hydroxynaphthoate.

2-15. STRONGYLOIDIASIS. Common in tropical and subtropical areas worldwide. Essentially an infection of humans but dogs may become infected. Larvae that are passed in the feces can remain alive for several weeks in certain soil conditions. They infect man by penetrating the skin and entering the bloodstream, and are carried to the lungs. They leave the bloodstream and ascend the bronchial tree. The larvae are then swallowed and are carried to the small intestines where they mature and lay eggs.

S. and O. Many cases are asymptomatic. Sensitized patients may develop linear, erythematous, or urticarial wheals that may be intensely pruritic or even hemorrhagic following entry of the larvae into the skin. During the migratory phase, vague symptoms develop including malaise, anorexia, fever, asthma, recurrent cough, and urticaria. Frequent gastrointestinal symptoms follow; diarrhea (may alternate with periods of normal bowel movement or constipation), nausea, vomiting, and diffuse colicky pain. In children there may be abdominal distention and persistent diarrhea accompanied by malabsorption syndrome plus weight loss and debilitation.

Lab findings: Eosinophilia normal to 50%, W.B.C. up to 20,000, and larvae or adult worms in the stools (allow the stool to stand 24-48 hours before examining).

A. Strongyloidiasis. Differential diagnosis: Epigastric pain may mimic peptic ulcer syndrome but with less relationship to meals. Can cause pneumonia. Skin invasion can resemble hookworm.

P. Drug of choice: Thiabendazole 25 mg./kg. (maximum 1.5 gm) b.i.d. x 2-3 days orally after meals.

Alternate drugs: Mebendazole, pyrantel pamoate, or levamisole.

2-16. ENTEROBIASIS (pinworms). Humans are the only host of this parasite. It occurs worldwide. Humans become infected by contaminated food, drink, or hands.

S. and O. Many patients are asymptomatic. Symptoms include pruritis of the perianal area, insomnia, restlessness, involuntary urination, and irritability, particularly in children. Mild gastrointestinal symptoms are also possible such as abdominal pain, nausea, vomiting, diarrhea, and anorexia.

Lab findings: W.B.C. normal except for modest eosinophilia (4-12%). To find eggs, apply scotch tape to the perianal skin and spread the tape over a slide for examination. This should be done on three consecutive days before the patient bathes or defecates. Adult worms should be looked for in the stool.

A. Pinworms.

P. Symptomatic patients should be treated and concurrent treatment of all household members should be considered. All bedding should be washed and personal hygiene should be stressed, e.g., careful washing of hands with soap and water after defecation and before meals, trim fingernails, avoid scratching rectal area, and keep hands away from the mouth. Eggs in a moist environment remain infective for 2-3 weeks, so it is best to repeat the medication every 2 weeks for 3 doses. Drug of choice is pyrantel pamoate 10 mg./kg. (maximum of 1 gm) in a single dose before or after meals. Repeat in 2 weeks. Alternates: Pyrvinium pamoate, mebendazole and piperazine citrate. Piperazine is last choice because the course of treatment requires 1 week.

2-17. HOOKWORM. Widespread in the tropics and subtropics. Infection of humans is through the skin in the same path as strongyloidiasis with the exception that hookworm eggs do not hatch in humans; they are passed in the stool.

S. and O. The first signs of hookworm infection is a pruritic erythematous dermatitis, either maculopapular or vesicular (ground itch) where the larvae invade the skin (allergic reactions to the invasion can occur and may be severe). Pulmonary signs are cough and bloody sputum. Two weeks or more after the skin invasion, abdominal symptoms including abdominal discomfort, flatulence, and diarrhea develop.

Lab findings: Eosinophilia present in the first few months of infection. Stool usually contains blood. (Guaiac test.) Anemia may be present depending on the number of worms. Eggs can be found in the stool; 4-5 ova per low power microscope field relates to about 5,000 eggs per gram of unconcentrated stool.

A. Hookworm.

P. Light infections in asymptomatic patients do not require treatment (up to 2,000 ova per gram of stool). Drug choice: Pyrantel pamoate 10 mg./kg./d. x 3 days orally in single dose, before or after meals.

Alternate drugs: Mebendazole 100 mg. b.i.d. x 3 days (do not use in pregnancy), bephenium hydrorynaphthoate 5 gm b.i.d. x 3 days on an empty stomach and withhold food for 2 hours; repeat in 1 week (for children less than 22 kg., cut dose in half)

2-18. FILARIASIS. Caused by one of two filarial nematodes that are transmitted by the bite of certain mosquitos. Widely distributed in the tropics and subtropics of both hemispheres and on Pacific islands. Over months the adult worms mature in or near the lymphatics or lymph nodes.

S. and O. Early manifestations are inflammatory with episodes of fever with or without inflammation of lymphatics and nodes, occurring at irregular intervals. Funiculitis (inflammation of the spermatic cord) and orchitis are common. Persistent lymph node enlargement may occur and abscesses may form at these sites. Later stages are obstructive and may not appear for months or years. Obstructive manifestations include hydrocele (accumulation of serous fluids in a saclike cavity), scrotal lymphedema, lymphatic varices, and elephantiasis. Elephantiasis may involve legs, genitalia, and less often arms and breasts.

Lab findings: Eosinophilia (10-30% or higher) in the early

stages. The count falls as the obstructive phase develops. Motile (mobile) larvae (microfilariae) are rare in the blood in the first 2-3 years, abundant after that and rare again in the advanced obstructive stage. Microfilariae should be microscopically looked for using wet thick smears of fresh anticoagulated blood.

A. Filariasis.

P. General measures: Bed rest during febrile and local inflammatory episodes. Antibiotic therapy to treat secondary infections. Suspension bandages for orchitis, epididymitis, and scrotal lymphedema. Treat mild limb edema with bed rest, elastic bandage wrap, and elevation of the affected part.

Surgical measures: Surgical removal of elephantoid scrotum, vulva, or breast should be considered. It is relatively easy and the results are usually satisfactory. Surgery for elephantiasis of a limb should be avoided. The surgery is difficult and results are poor.

Drug of choice: Diethylcarbamazine 2 mg./kg. orally after meals t.i.d. x 21-28 days. Headache, malaise, nausea, and vomiting may occur from the medication. Concurrent administration of an antihistamine and antiemetic may reduce the likelihood and intensity of allergic reactions.

Relapses may occur 3-12 months after treatment requiring several courses of treatment over 1-2 years.

Section II - Mycotic (Fungal)

2-19. COCCIDIOIDOMYCOSIS. Infection results from inhalation of arthrospores of Coccidioides immitis, a mold that grows in soil in arid regions of Southwest United States, Mexico, Central and South America. About 60 percent of infections are subclinical and unrecognized; incubation period 10-30 days.

S. Forty percent of patients develop mild to severe and prostrating symptoms that resemble those due to viral, bacterial, or other mycotic infections. Onset is usually that of a respiratory infection with fever and occasional chills, pleural pain (usually severe), muscular ache, backache, and headache (may be severe). Nasopharyngitis may be followed by bronchitis accompanied by a dry or slightly productive cough. Weakness and anorexia may become marked, leading to prostration. Symptoms of progressive coccidioidomycosis depend upon the site of dissemination. Any or all organs may be infected.

O. A morbilliform (measlelike) rash may appear 1-2 days after onset of symptoms. Arthralgia accompanied by periarticular swellings, often of the knees and ankles, is common. Erythema nodosum (painful red nodules on legs) may appear 2-20 days after onset of symptoms. Erythema multiforme (macular eruption with dark red papules or tubercules with no itching, burning, or rheumatic pain appearing in separate rings, concentric rings, disk-shaped patches, distributed elevations, and figured arrangements) may appear on the upper extremities, head, and thorax. Lab findings: May be moderate leukocytosis and eosinophilia. Sedimentation rate is elevated, returning to normal as infection subsides. There is a skin test available for coccidioidomycosis.

A. Coccidioidomycosis. Differential diagnosis: Viral,

bacterial, or other mycotic infections presenting flulike syndrome.

P. Bed rest and general symptomatic treatment until there is a complete regression of fever and a normal sedimentation rate. Amphotericin B has proven effective in some patients with disseminated disease, but because of its toxic properties, adult dose should not exceed 0.5-1 mg./kg. Therapy should begin with 1 mg./d. increasing by 5 mg. increments to 25-35 mg./d. or to 40-60 mg./d. in the acutely ill.

2-20. HISTOPLASMOSIS. Caused by Histoplasma capsulatum, a mold found in the soil in central and eastern United States, eastern Canada, Mexico, Central and South America, Africa, and Southeast Asia. Infection is presumably by inhalation of spores. May be carried by the blood to other parts of the body.

S. and O. Most cases are asymptomatic or mild and unrecognized. Symptomatic infections may present mild influenzalike characteristics lasting 1-4 days. In moderately severe cases, the patients have fever, cough, and mild chest pain lasting 5-15 days. Physical examination is usually negative.

Severe infections are divided into three groups: (1) Acute histoplasmosis frequently occurs in epidemics. Symptoms are marked prostration, fever, and occasional chest pain, but no particular symptoms relative to the lungs. X ray may show severe disseminated pneumonitis. Infection may last from 1 week to 6 months; it is rarely fatal. (2) Acute progressive histoplasmosis is usually fatal within 6 weeks or less. Fever, dyspnea, cough, weight loss, and prostration are usual sypmtoms. Diarrhea is usual in children. Mucous membrane ulcers of the oropharynx may be present. All the organs of the body are involved and liver and spleen nearly always enlarged. (3) Chronic progressive histoplasmosis is usually found in older patients with chronic obstructive lung disease. It closely resembles chronic tuberculosis; occasionally the patient will have both diseases. It appears to be primarily confined to the lungs, but all organs are involved in the terminal stage.

Lab findings: Sedimentation rate is elevated in moderate to severely ill patients. Leukopenia with normal differential count or neutropenia. Most patients with progressive disease show a progressive hypochromic anemia.

A. Histoplasmosis. Differential diagnosis: Mild cases--influenza; moderate--a typical pneumonia; severe cases--tuberculosis.

P. No specific therapy. Bed rest and symptomatic treatment for the primary form. Normal activity should not be resumed until fever has subsided. Amphotericin B has helped some patients (see coccidioidomycosis for treatment plan). Some milder forms of acute primary or early chronic disease respond to sulfadiazine therapy.

2-21. NORTH AMERICAN BLASTOMYCOSIS. A chronic systemic fungus infection caused by Blastomyces dermatitidis. Occurs more often in men. Found in central and eastern United States and Canada. A few cases have been found in Mexico and Africa.

S. and O. Mild or asymptomatic cases are rarely found. Little is known of the mildest pulmonary phase of this disease. Cough, moderate fever, dyspnea, and chest pain are evident in symptomatic cases. These may disappear or progress with bloody and purulent sputum production, pleurisy, fever, chills, loss of weight, and prostration. Raised verrucous (tumor of the epidermis) cutaneous lesions that have an abrupt downward sloping border are usually present in disseminated blastomycosis. The surface is covered with miliary (small lesions resembling millet seeds) pustules. The border extends slowly leaving a central atrophic scar. Only cutaneous lesions are found in some patients. Lesions are most frequently seen on the skin, in bones, and in the genitourinary system, but any or all organs or tissues in the body can be attacked.

Lab findings: Usually leukocytosis, hypochromic anemia, and elevated sedimentation rate. Organism can be found in lesions. It is a thick-walled cell that may have a single bud.

A. North American blastomycosis. Differential diagnosis: Epididymitis, prostatitis, other diseases attacking bone or skin.

P. No specific treatment but amphotericin B (see coccidioidomycosis for treatment schedule). Surgical excision of cutaneous lesions may be successful. Careful follow-up for early evidence of relapse should be made for several years so therapy may be resumed if needed.

2-22. PARACOCCIDIOIDOMYCOSIS (South American Blastomycosis). Found only in South or Central America or Mexico. Caused by Paracoccidioides brasiliensis.

S. and O. Ulceration of nasopharynx usually the first symptom. Papules ulcerate and enlarge both peripherally and deeper into the subcutaneous tissue. Eventually may result in destruction of the epiglottis, vocal cords, and uvula with extension to the lips and face. Eating and drinking are extremely painful. Skin lesions of variable appearance may occur on the face. They may have a necrotic central crater with a hard hyperkeratotic border. Lymph node enlargement may be the presenting symptom or may follow mucocutaneous lesions. Lymph nodes eventually ulcerate and rupture through the skin. Some patients may present with gastrointestinal disturbances, including enlargement of liver and spleen, but symptoms are vague. Extensive ulceration of the upper gastrointestinal tract prevents sufficient intake and absorption of food causing malnutrition. Death may result from respiratory failure or malnutrition.

Lab findings: Elevated sedimentation rate, leukocytosis with neutrophilia showing a shift to the left, and sometimes eosinophilia and monocytosis. The fungus is a spherical cell that may have many buds arising from it.

A. Paracoccidioidomycosis.

P. Amphotericin B (see coccidioidomycosis for treatment plan) has had considerable success in hospitalized patients. Sulfadiazine (2-4 gm) daily or "Triple Sulfa" (1 gm) daily has been used for control and occasional cures have been reported following months or years of treatment. Relapses may occur when the drug is stopped. Drug toxicity with prolonged high dosage is common. Rest and supportive care help in promoting a favorable response.

2-23. See Chapter 1, Section I, Integumentary System for sporotrichosis, dermatophyte infections (ringworm, athlete's foot, dandruff, etc.), and chromomycosis.

2-24. CANDIDIASIS (moniliasis, thrush). A yeast found normally in the mouth, vagina, and feces of most people. Overgrowth does not occur unless the "balance" of the oral flora is disturbed by debilitating or acute illness or in those being treated with antibiotics. Overgrowth is also favored by diabetes, iron deficiency anemia, and immunosuppressed status.

S. and O. Creamy-white curdlike patches anywhere in the mouth. Adjacent mucosa is usually erythematous, and scraping the lesion often uncovers a raw, bleeding surface. Commonly, a candidal lesion may appear as a slightly granular or irregularly eroded erythematous patch. Pain is usually present but fever and lymphadenopathy are uncommon. Concomitant candidiasis of the gastrointestinal tract (including the pharynx and esophagus) may occur. Vaginal overgrowth (see Chapter 7, Gynecology).

Systemic candidal infections are of two types: Endocarditis that almost always affects previously damaged heart valves, usually follows heart surgery or inoculation by contaminated needles or catheters. Splenomegaly and petechiae are usual, and emboli are common. Upper gastrointestinal tract candidiasis is the usual source in the other type of systemic infection. Dissemination follows antibiotic or cytotoxic chemotherapy for serious debilitating disease. The kidneys, spleen, lungs, liver, and heart are most commonly involved. Fungiuria is usual in renal disease.

Lab findings: Candida albicans is seen as a gram-positive budding cell and a pseudomycelium and is the most common cause of systemic disease.

A. Candidiasis. Differential diagnosis: Other systemic diseases depending on which area of the body is affected and other fungal skin infections.

P. Amphotericin B IV (as for coccidioidomycosis) is necessary for serious systemic infection. When combined with rifampin or flucytosine (Ancobon) 150 mg./kg./d. orally, lower doses of amphotericin B can be used and still prevent emergence of resistant organism.

Oral, gastrointestinal, and cutaneous lesions should be treated with amphotericin B, nystatin, or miconazole mouthwash, tablets, or lotions. Gentian violet, 1% in 10-20% alcohol, is also effective for oral, cutaneous, and vaginal lesions. Antibiotic therapy should be discontinued if possible. All patients with candidiasis should be checked for diabetes.

2-25. CRYPTOCOCCOSIS. An encapsulated budding yeast that is found worldwide in soil and on dried pigeon dung. Infection is acquired by inhalation.

S. and O. In the lungs, the infection may remain localized, heal, or disseminate. Upon dissemination, lesions may form in any part of the body; the most common part involved is the C.N.S. and is the usual cause of death. Generalized meningoencephalitis occurs more frequently than localized granuloma in the brain or spinal cord. Solitary localized lesions may develop in the skin and, rarely, in bones or other organs. Pulmonary cryptococcosis presents no specific signs or symptoms. Many patients are asymptomatic, others may present with low-grade fever, pleural pain, and cough possibly with sputum production. C.N.S. involvement usually presents a history of recent URI or pulmonary infection. Usually the first and most prominent symptom is increasingly painful headaches. Vertigo, nausea, anorexia, ocular disorders, and mental deterioration develop. Neck rigidity is present, and Kernig's and Brudzinski's signs are positive. Patellar and achilles reflexes are often diminished or absent. Acneiform lesions enlarge slowly and ulcerate, often coalescing with other lesions to cover a large area.

Lab findings: Mild anemia, leukocytosis, and increased sedimentation rate.

A. Cryptococcosis. Differential diagnosis: Other systemic fungal infections with C.N.S. involvement.

P. Combination of amphotericin B (see coccidioidomycosis for dosage) and flucytosine (Ancobon), 150 mg./kg./d. in 6 hourly doses, may be curative in a 6-week regimen.

Section III - Bacterial

2-26. General. Bacteria are the most common disease causing organisms. They cause a wide variety of infections that can be located anywhere on or in the body.

2-27. STREPTOCOCCAL INFECTIONS.

a. Beta-hemolytic group A streptococci are the most common cause of exudative pharyngitis, and they also cause skin infections (impetigo). Respiratory infections are transmitted by droplets; skin infections by contact. Either may be followed by suppurative and nonsuppurative (rheumatic fever, glomerulonephritis) complications. Beta-hemolytic group B streptococci are often carried in the female genital tract and thus may infect the newborn. They are a common cause of neonatal sepsis and meningitis and may be associated with respiratory distress syndrome.

b. Streptococcal sore throat (strep throat).

S. Sudden onset of fever, sore throat, severe pain on swallowing, malaise, and nausea. Children may vomit or convulse. If scarlet fever rash occurs, the skin is diffusely erythematous, with superimposed fine red papules. The rash is most intense in the groin and axillas, blanches on pressure, and may become petechial. It fades in 2-5 days, leaving a fine desquamation.

O. Tender, enlarged cervical lymph nodes; the pharynx, soft palate, and tongue are red and edematous; and there may be a purulent exudate. In scarlet fever, the face is flushed with circumoral pallor, and the tongue is coated with protrusions of enlarged red papillae (strawberry tongue). CBC showing leukocytosis with an increase in polymorphonuclear neutrophils. Smears of the exudate from the throat show streptococci. Complications of streptococcal sore throat include sinusitis, otitis media, mastoiditis, peritonsillar abscess, suppuration of cervical lymph nodes, reheumatic fever, and glomerulonephritis.

A. Streptococcal sore throat. Differential diagnosis: Streptococcal sore throat resembles (and cannot be reliably distinguished clinically from) the pharyngitis caused by adeno-viruses, herpes viruses, and occasionally other viruses. It also is commonly confused with infectious mononucleosis, diphtheria, candidiasis, and necrotizing ulcerative gingivostomatitis.

P. Antibiotic therapy is often given without proof of streptococcal origin if fever and leukocytosis accompany a sore throat with tender cervical lymph nodes.

(1) Benzathine penicillin G 1.2 million units IM as a single dose or procaine penicillin G 300,000 units IM daily x 10 days.

(2) Penicillin V 400,000 units q.8h. x 10 days.

(3) Patients hypersensitive to penicillin may be treated with erythromycin 500 mg. q.i.d. x 10 days.

(4) General measures include aspirin and gargling with warm saline solution to relieve sore throat. Bed rest and forced fluids until the patient is afebrile.

c. Rheumatic fever. Triggered by group A beta-hemolytic streptococcus producing a first attack of rheumatic fever in 0.3 percent of untreated or inadequately treated children. If a child has rheumatic fever once, his chances of reinfection within the next 5 years are 50 percent. Usually, the clinical manifestations of an attack of rheumatic fever tend to repeat themselves in subsequent attacks. The peak period of risk for children is 5-15 years of age.

S. and O. It takes two major or one major and two minor manifestations to justify a presumptive diagnosis of rheumatic fever. Major manifestations are:

(1) Active carditis (any one of the following).

(a) Significant new murmurs that are clearly mitral or aortic insufficiency.

(b) Pericarditis (pericardial friction rub or evidence of pericardial effusion).

(c) Evidence of congestive heart failure.

(2) Polyarthritis. Two or more joints <u>must</u> be involved either simultaneously or in a migratory fashion.

(3) Subcutaneous nodules. Nontender and freely movable under the skin, a few millimeters to 2 cm. in diameter, most commonly found over joints, scalp, and spinal column, and usually seen only in severe cases.

(4) Erythema marginatum. Usually occurs only in severe cases and is often mistaken for other types of skin lesions. It is a macular erythematous rash with a circinate border appearing primarily on

the trunk and extremities; the face is usually not involved.

(5) Sydenham's chorea. Progressively more severe emotional instability, involuntary movements, and muscular weakness often followed by muscular incoordination and slurring of speech. Involvement is not uncommonly limited to one side. Individual attacks are self-limiting, but may last up to 3 months.

Minor manifestations of rheumatic fever are:

(1) Fever: Usually low grade but occasionally 103-104 degrees F.

(2) Polyarthralgia: Pain in two or more joints without heat, swelling, and tenderness.

(3) History: Prior history of acute rheumatic fever or recent scarlet fever.

(4) Accelerated sedimentation rate.

(5) Positive throat culture or smear for group A streptococcus. Associated findings may include abdominal, back, and precordial pain; erythema multiforme, malaise, vomiting, nontraumatic epistaxis (nose bleed), weight loss, and anemia.

In the absence of carditis, rheumatic fever lasts on the average 89 - 27 days. With carditis, rheumatic fever lasts on the average 124 - 68 days.

A. Rheumatic fever. Differential diagnosis: Other causes of carditis, arthritis, and skin lesions. Other debilitating diseases, e.g., mononucleosis.

P. Therapy is divided into short-term and long-term treatment.

(1) Short-term therapy ranges from saving the life of a patient with severe carditis to relieving joint discomfort.

(a) Streptococcal infection must be eradicated. Benzathine penicillin G, in a single IM injection 0.6-1.2 million units, depending on patient weight, or 125-250 mg of pencillin orally q.i.d. x 10 days. Alternate is erythromycin 250 mg. orally q.i.d. x 10 days.

(b) Aspirin (in the absence of severe carditis with congestive heart failure) 100 mg./kg./d. orally divided into 4 doses. Maximum dose regardless of weight is 5,000 mg./d. (four 5 gr. aspirin tablets q.i.d.). After 1 week reduce dosage to 50 mg./kg./d. in 4 doses and continue for at least 1 month.

(c) Congestive heart failure therapy (see Chapter 1, Section IV, The Circulatory System).

(d) Corticosteroids should be used for all patients with congestive heart failure and/or carditis. Dosage: prednisone 2 mg./kg./d. x 2 weeks orally, then 1 mg./kg./d. x 1 week, begin aspirin 50 mg./kg./d. on the third week and continue for 8 weeks.

(e) Strict bed rest is not required for patients with arthritis and mild carditis. Bed-to-chair with bathroom privileges and meals at the table for patients without severe carditis is all that is required. Strict bed rest should be maintained for patients with severe carditis at least until corticosteroid therapy is completed. Both should have gradual indoor ambulation followed by modified outdoor activity after symptoms have disappeared. This should last at least 2 months and the child should not return to school while there is clear evidence of rheumatic activity.

(f) Symptomatic treatment as necessary.

(2) Long-term therapy is aimed toward those patients who had carditis and/or congestive heart failure during the clinical course of rheumatic fever. At the present, antibacterial therapy is a lifetime undertaking to prevent recurrence. Benzathine penicillin G 1.2 million units IM once a month for life, or sulfadiazine 500 mg. in a single dose daily for patients under 60 lbs and 1 gm orally daily in a single dose for patients over 60 lbs, or erythromycin 250 mg. b.i.d. orally for patients allergic to penicillin and sulfonamides.

2-28. DIPHTHERIA. See Chapter 6, Pediatrics.

2-29. MENINGITIS.

a. General considerations. Meningitis is caused by numerous organisms. Even fungal and viral infections can cause meningitis. The most common causes of bacterial meningitis are meningococcal, pneumococcal, streptococcal, staphylococcal, Haemophilus influenzae, and tubercular infections. All but tuberculous meningitis are similar in sign and symptoms and treatment.

b. Meningococcal meningitis. About 15-40 percent of the population are nasopharyngeal carriers of meningococci, but few develop the disease. Infection is transmitted by droplets.

S. High fever, chills, and headache; back, abdominal, and extremity pain; and nausea and vomiting are present. In severe cases, rapidly developing confusion, delirium, and coma occur. Twitch or frank convulsions may also be present.

O. Petechial rash of skin and mucous membranes is found in most cases. Petechiae may vary from pinhead size to large ecchymoses or even areas of skin gangrene that may later slough if the patient survives. These petechiae usually fade in 3-4 days. Neck and back stiffness with positive Kernig (sitting or lying with the thigh flexed upon the abdomen, the leg cannot be completely extended) and Brudzinski sign. (In meningitis, flexion of the neck usually results in flexion of the hip and knee. Also when passive flexion of the lower limb on one side is made, a similar movement will be seen in the opposite limb.) Shock due to the effects of endotoxin may be present and is a bad prognostic sign.

CBC shows usually marked leukocytosis early in the course of the disease. Urine may contain protein, casts, and red cells. Lumbar puncture reveals a cloudy to frankly purulent cerebrospinal fluid, with elevated pressure, increased protein, and decreased glucose content. The fluid usually contains numerous white cells and gram-negative intracellular diplococci. The absence of organisms in a gram-stained smear does not rule out the diagnosis.

A. Meningococcal meningitis. Differential diagnosis: Other meningitides.

P. Antibacterial therapy by IV route.must be started immediately. Aqueous penicillin G 24 million units/24 hours for adults and 400,000 units per kg./24 hours for children is the drug of choice. One-fourth of the dose is given rapidly IV and the rest by continuous drip. If the patient is allergic to penicillin, chloramphenicol 100 mg./kg. daily is the preferred alternate. Treatment should continue for 7-10 days by IV route. If the possibility of Haemophilus influenzae meningitis has not been ruled out, give both sodium ampicillin 300 mg./kg. daily IV (1/4 of the dose initially and the remainder in divided doses every 4 hours) and chloramphenicol (same as before) (separately, not in mixed doses). General measures include Ringer's lactate IV drip for maintenance and to prevent hypovolemic shock. Monitor vital signs closely. If patient survives the first day, the prognosis is excellent.

2-30. TYPHOID FEVER. Caused by the gram-negative rod Salmonella typhi. Infection is transmitted by consumption of contaminated food or drink. The sources of most infections are chronic carriers with persistent gallbladder or urinary tract infections. The incubation period is 5-14 days.

S. Onset is usually insidious but may be abrupt, especially in children, with chills and a sharp rise in temperature. Usually the patient develops increasing malaise, headache, cough, general body aching, sore throat, and nosebleeds. Frequently there is abdominal pain, constipation or diarrhea, and vomiting. During this period, the fever ascends in a stepladder fashion; the maximum temperature each day is slightly higher than the previous day. Temperature is generally higher in the evening than the morning. After 7-10 days the fever stabilizes and the patient becomes very sick. "Pea soup" diarrhea or severe constipation or marked abdominal distention is common. In severe cases, the patient lies motionless and unresponsive, with eyes half shut and appearing wasted and exhausted (the "typhoid state"), but can usually be aroused to carry out simple commands. If the patient survives this portion and no complications occur, he gradually improves. Fever declines in a stepladder fashion to normal in 7-10 days and with it the other symptoms gradually disappear. Relapses may occur as late as 1-2 weeks after temperature returns to normal, but they are usually milder than the original infection.

O. Early physical findings are slight. Later, splenomegaly, abdominal distension and tenderness, relative bradycardia, dicrotic (double wave) pulse, and occasionally systolic murmur and gallop rhythm appear. During the second week of the disease, a rash (rose spots) appears principally on the trunk (pink papules 2-3 mm. in diameter that fade on pressure) and disappears over a period of 3-4 days. Leukopenia and moderate anemia are the rule. The organism may be found in the stool after the first week or possibly may be found in the urine. Blood, stool, or urine cultures are usually positive after the first week.

A. Typhoid fever. Differential diagnosis: Tuberculosis, viral pneumonia, psittacosis, infective endocarditis, brucellosis, or Q fever.

P. Active immunization should be provided for household contacts of typhoid carrier, travelers to endemic areas, and during epidemic outbreaks. Food and water should be protected and waste should be adequately disposed of. Specific measures include ampicillin 100 mg./kg. daily IV or 4-250 mg. capsules every 4 hours orally, or chloramphenicol 1 gm q.6h. orally or IV until fever disappears, then 500 mg. q.6h. for 2 weeks. IV fluids may be necessary to supplement oral intake and maintain urine output; 100 mg. hydrocortisone q.8h. may help severely toxic patients. Strict stool and urine isolation techniques must be observed. Treatment of carriers is usually ineffective, but a trial of ampicillin first then chloramphenicol should be tried. Cholecystectomy may be effective.

2-31. CHOLERA. An acute diarrheal disease caused by vibrio cholerae or related vibrios. The infection is caused by ingestion of food or drink contaminated by feces from cases or carriers. Cholera is fatal in 50 percent of all untreated patients. The incubation period is 1-5 days, but only a small minority of those exposed become ill.

S. Typical cases have an explosive onset of frequent, watery stools that soon lose all fecal appearance and odor. The stool is grayish, turbid, and liquid, containing degenerated epithelium cells and mucus, but rarely gross pus or blood. The patient can lose up to 1 liter per hour. Vomiting may also occur early.

O. The patient rapidly becomes dehydrated and acidotic, with sunken eyes, hypotension, subnormal temperature, rapid and shallow breathing, muscle cramps, oliguria, shock, and coma. Hematocrit will rise sharply due to loss of plasma resulting in a concentration of red cells. The vibrios can easily be cultured from the stool and might possibly be found using Gram's stain of stool specimens.

A. Cholera. Differential diagnosis: Other causes of severe diarrhea, particularly those due to shigellae, viruses, E. coli enterotoxins and protozoa in endemic areas.

P. Water and electrolyte loss must be restored promptly and continuously, and acidosis must be corrected. Diarrheal loss and hemoconcentration must be measured continuously. In moderately ill patients, it may be possible to provide replacement by oral fluids given in the same volume as that lost. (See Chapter 18, IV Therapy.) Those unable to take fluid by mouth require IV fluid replacement. Tetracycline 500 mg. q.6h. x 3-5 days should also be given. Effective decontamination of excreta is essential, but strict isolation of patients is unnecessary and quarantine is undesirable.

Prevention: Cholera vaccine gives only limited protection and is of no value in controling outbreaks. In endemic areas, all water, other drinks, food, and utensils must be boiled or avoided.

2-32. BACILLARY DYSENTERY. See Chapter 1, Section V, Digestive System.

2-33. GAS GANGRENE. Produced by entry of one of several clostridia into devitalized tissues. These gram-positive rods grow and produce toxins under anaerobic conditions.

S. Onset usually sudden with rapidly increasing pain in the affected area. The wound becomes swollen and the surrounding skin is pale. This is followed by a discharge of a brown to blood-tinged, serous, foul-smelling fluid from the wound. As the disease advances, the surrounding tissue changes from pale to dusky and finally becomes deeply discolored, with coalescent, red, fluid-filled vesicles. In the last stages of the disease, severe prostration, stupor, delirium, and coma occur.

O. The increasing pain is accompanied by a fall in blood pressure. Temperature may be elevated, but not proportionate to the severity of infection. Gas may be palpable in the tissues. In clostridial sepsis, hemolysis and jaundice are common, often complicated by renal failure. Gram's stain of the exudate should show the organism and is a valuable clue, but the clinical picture must be present to make the diagnosis.

A. Gas gangrene. Differential diagnosis: Other infections that cause gas formation, e.g., enterobacter, Escherichia, and mixed anaerobic infections including Bacteroides and Peptostreptococcus.

P. Antibiotic therapy in the form of penicillin, chloramphenicol, or chlortetracycline should be started promptly in heroic doses. Massive debridement of all involved tissue. Frequently gas in the subcutaneous tissue or fascial planes extends beyond the area of muscle involvement. In such cases the overlying skin should be incised widely and the necrotic fascia excised. Careful and complete debridement of all wounds and good wound care will eliminate almost all chance for gangrene to develop.

2-34. TETANUS. An acute central nervous system intoxication caused by toxins produced by the slender, spore-forming, gram-positive anaerobic bacillus Clostridium tetani that are found mainly in the soil and in the feces of animals and humans and that enter the body by wound contamination. In the newborn, infection often enters through the umbilical stump. Incubation period is 5-15 days.

S. Occasionally, the first symptom is pain and tingling at the wound site followed by spasticity of the nearby muscle groups; this may be all that happens. Usually the presenting symptoms are stiffness of the jaw, neck stiffness, difficulty in swallowing, and irritability. Hyperreflexia develops later, with spasms of the jaw muscles (trismus) or facial muscles and rigidity and spasm of muscles of the abdomen, back, and neck.

O. Painful tonic convulsions caused by minor stimuli (any loud noise, etc.) are common. The patient is awake and alert during the entire course of the illness. During convulsions, the glottis and the respiratory muscles go into spasm so that the patient is unable to breath, and cyanosis and asphyxia may ensue. Temperature is only slightly elevated. Although there is usually a leukocytosis, the diagnosis of tetanus is made clinically.

A. Tetanus. Differential diagnosis: Other types of acute C.N.S. infections and strychnine poisoning should also be considered.

P. Active immunization with tetanus toxoid should be universal. Adequate debridement of wounds and a booster tetanus immunization is the most important preventive measure. Specific treatment: Give tetanus immune globulin (human) 5,000 units IM. If not available, test for sensitivity to horse serum and give 100,000 units tetanus antitoxin IV. Place patient at bed rest and minimize stimulation. Sedation and anticonvulsant therapy is essential. Penicillin is of value but should not be substituted for antitoxin. IV fluids as necessary. Tracheostomy and/or assisted respiration may be required. Mortality rate is about 40 percent higher in children and very old people.

2-35. BOTULISM. See Chapter 1, Section V, Digestive System.

2-36. ANTHRAX. A disease of sheep, cattle, horses, goats, and swine caused by Bacillus anthracis, a gram-positive spore-forming aerobe transmitted to humans by entry through broken skin mucous membranes or by inhalation. Uncommon, but most apt to occur in farmers, veterinarians, and tannery and wool workers.

S. Cutaneous anthrax. An erythematous papule appears on the exposed area of skin and becomes vesicular with a purple to black center. The area around the lesion is swollen or edematous and surrounded by vesicles. The center finally forms a necrotic eschar and sloughs. Malaise, headache, nausea, and vomiting may be present.

Pulmonary anthrax (woolsorter's disease): Fever, malaise, headache, labored or difficult breathing (dyspnea), and cough.

O. Cutaneous anthrax. Regional adenopathy and variable fever may be present. After eschar sloughs, sepsis may occur at times manifested by shock, cyanosis, sweating, and collapse. Hemorrhagic meningitis may occur. Anthrax sepsis may occur without a skin lesion.

Pulmonary anthrax: Congestion of the nose, throat, and larynx; and auscultatory or X ray signs of pneumonia.

Lab findings: White count may be elevated or low. Smears of skin lesions show gram-positive encapsulated rods.

A. Anthrax. Differential diagnosis: Rarely gram-positive spore-forming aerobic bacilli other than B. anthracis can produce similar disease.

P. Penicillin G 10 million units IV daily; or in mild localized cases tetracycline 500 mg. q.6h. x 10 days.

2-37. TULAREMIA. An infection of wild rodents, particularly rabbits and muskrats, transmitted to humans by contact with animal tissue (e.g., trapping and skinning rabbits, etc.), by the bite of certain ticks and biting flies, by eating infected undercooked meat, or by drinking contaminated water. Incubation period is 2-10 days.

S. Fever, headache, and nausea begin suddenly, and a papule develops at the site of inoculation and soon ulcerates. Lesion may be on the skin of an extremity or in the eye. If ingested, it may manifest as gastroenteritis, stupor, and delirium. There may be rashes, generalized aches, and prostration.

O. Regional lymph nodes become enlarged and tender and may suppurate (to form pus). In any type of involvement, the spleen may be enlarged. Asymptomatic infection is not rare. W.B.C. may be slightly elevated or normal. Cultures of blood, lesion, or lymph node aspirate require special culture media. There is a delayed type skin test (read in 48 hrs) that can be used.

A. Tularemia. Differential diagnosis: Rickettsial and meningococcal infections, cat scratch fever, infectious mono, and various pneumonias and fungal diseases.

P. Streptomycin 500 mg. q.6-8h. IM, together with tetracycline 500 mg. q.6h. until 5 days after patient is afebrile. Adequate fluid intake is essential and O_2 therapy may be necessary. Drainage of fluctuant lymph nodes may be needed and is safe after proper antibiotic therapy for several days.

2-38. PLAGUE. An infection of wild rodents with Pasteurella pestis, a small gram-negative rod. Transmitted from rodent to rodent and to humans by the bites of fleas. If a plague victim develops pneumonia, the infection can be transmitted by droplets and an epidemic may start. The incubation period is 2-10 days.

S. Usually sudden onset with high fever, malaise, intense headache, and generalized muscular ache. The patient appears profoundly ill and very anxious. Delirium may ensue. With systemic spread, the patient may rapidly become severely septic and comatose with purpuric spots (black plague) appearing on the skin.

O. Tachycardia is usually noted with onset of symptoms. If pneumonia develops, tachypnea, productive cough, blood-tinged sputum, and cyanosis also occur. Meningeal signs may develop; a pustule or ulcer at the site of inoculation and signs of lymphangitis may occur. Axillary, inguinal, or cervical lymph nodes become enlarged and tender and may eventually suppurate and drain. Primary plague pneumonia from droplets coughed by another patient with plague pneumonia is a fulminant pneumonitis with bloody, frothy sputum and sepsis. It is usually fatal unless treatment is started within a few hours of onset.

Lab findings: W.B.C. 12-20,000; the plague bacillus may be found in smears from aspirates of buboes using Gram's stain.

A. Plague. Differential diagnosis: Lymphadenitis accompanying staph or strep infections of an extremity, lymphogranuloma venereum, syphilis, or tularemia. Systemic manifestations resemble those of enteric or rickettsial fevers, malaria, or flu.

P. Therapy must be started promptly when plague is suspected. Streptomycin 1 gm. IM q.6h. x 2 days then 500 mg. q.6-8h. tetracycline 500 mg. q.6h. is given at the same time. IV fluids, pressor drugs, oxygen, and tracheostomy are used as required.

2-39. LEPROSY (Hansen's disease). A chronic infectious disease caused by the acid-fast rod Mycobacterium leprae. Mode of transmission is unknown; probably involves prolonged exposure in childhood; adults rarely become infected (e.g., by tattooing). Endemic in tropical and subtropical Asia, Africa, Central and South America, the Pacific regions and southern USA.

S. & O. Onset is insidious, lesions involve skin, superficial nerves, nose, pharynx, larynx, eyes, and testicles. May occur as pale anesthetic macular lesions 1-10 cm. in diameter, discrete erythematous infiltrated nodules 1-5 cm. in diameter, or diffuse skin infiltration. Neurologic disturbances are manifested by nerve infiltration and thickening, with resultant anesthesia, neuritis, paresthesia, trophic ulcers, bone reabsorption, and shortening of the digits. In untreated cases, the disfigurement may be extreme. Leprosy is clinically and by laboratory tests divided into two types: lepromatous and tuberculoid. In the lepromatous type, the course is progressive and malignant with abundant acid-fast bacilli in the skin lesion and a negative lepromin skin test. The tuberculoid type is benign and nonprogressive with severe asymmetrical nerve involvement of sudden onset with few bacilli in the lesions and a positive lepromin skin test. Eye involvement (keratitis and iridocyclitis), nasal ulcers, nose bleeds, anemia, and lymphadenopathy may occur.

A. Leprosy. Differential diagnosis: Skin lesions resemble those of lupus erythematosus, sarcoidosis, syphilis, erythema nodosum, erythema multiforme, and vitiligo.

P. Untreated lepromatous leprosy is progressive and fatal in 10-20 years. In tuberculoid leprosy, spontaneous recovery usually occurs in 1-3 years; however, it may produce crippling deformities. With treatment, lepromatous leprosy regresses slowly (over a period of 3-8 years). Recovery from tuberculoid leprosy is more rapid. Return of symptoms is always possible and it is safe to assume that the bacilli are never totally eradicated. The treatment of leprosy is very complicated, requiring numerous drugs (dapsone, amithiozone, thalidomide, rifampin, clofazimine and corticosteroids) in increasing doses over a period of years or indefinitely. All of this necessitates evacuation to a hospital or area better equipped to handle these cases.

2-40. TUBERCULOSIS. Caused by acid-fast Mycobacterium tuberculosis and characterized by the formation of tubercles in the lung. Occurs almost exclusively by inhalation of airborne droplets from the cough of a person with tubercle bacilli in the sputum. Ingestion of milk containing tubercle bacilli (unpasteurized) is another mode of transmission. The danger of infection from contaminated surfaces is negligible. The first or primary infection is usually a self-limiting disease in children that escapes detection. A few patients develop progressive primary tuberculosis. Another small percentage develop progressive pulmonary disease. Primary infections occurring in adults may evolve into progressive pulmonary disease without the characteristic changes of primary disease seen in children. Most people who are infected at any age do not develop the disease. Malnutrition, diabetes, measles, chronic corticosteroid treatment, silicosis, and general debility favor progression of infection into progressive pulmonary disease.

S. Symptoms may be absent or mild and nonspecific in the presence of active disease. The most frequent symptoms, when present, are cough, malaise, easy fatigability, weight loss, low-grade afternoon fever, night sweat, and pleuritic pain. Cough, when present, has no specific characteristics. Patients with pulmonary tuberculosis occasionally present with symptoms due to extra pulmonary complications such as laryngeal, renal, intestinal, or C.N.S. involvement.

O. Pulmonary signs may be difficult to elicit even in the presence of active disease. Fine persistent rales over the upper lobes may be found. These are best heard after a slight cough. Advanced disease may lead to retraction of the chest wall, deviation of the trachea, wheezes, rales, and signs of pulmonary consolidation. Pulmonary TB cannot be ruled out by physical examination only. A chest X ray is the minimum diagnostic requirement. Lab findings: Sputum smears are positive when bacteria count is high but should be confirmed with culture. Tine test may be used for screening, but PPD 0.1 cc. 1.0 is more accurate. These tests are only for screening of patients, not for diagnostic purposes. Patients with positive skin tests should have chest X rays.

A. Pulmonary tuberculosis. Differential diagnosis: TB can mimic almost any pulmonary disease such as bacterial or viral pneumonias, lung abscess, pulmonary mycoses, bronchogenic carcinoma, sarcoidosis, and "atypical" (nontuberculosis) mycobacterial infections. Negative tine or PPD test make diagnosis of TB very unlikely.

P. Prevention: Patients with active TB should be isolated during the first 2 weeks of treatment and taught to cover their mouth and nose with disposable tissue during coughing. Close contacts must have skin test and if positive, chest X rays. If negative they should be retested in 2 months. If contact is positive and chest X ray is negative, they should receive isoniazid treatment for 1 year. Infants and children who are in close contact should be given isoniazid even if skin tests are negative, but their treatment can be discontinued if the skin test is still negative 3 months after exposure is discontinued. Persons who convert from negative to positive within 2 years who have negative X rays should receive isoniazid for 1 year. Positive reactors with negative X rays with high risk factors (e.g., prolonged corticosteroid therapy for other diseases, Hodgkin's disease, leukemia, diabetes, and silicosis) should receive isoniazid for 1 year. Preventive treatment with isoniazid consists of 300 mg. daily (10 mg./kg. daily for children) for 1 year.

Treatment for active TB

Drug	Adult Dose	Comments
Isoniazid (NH)	5-10 mg./kg. daily orally	With the sole exception of preventive treatment, this should be used only in combination with other drugs.
and		
Streptomycin	1 gm IM daily or twice weekly	
and		
ethambutol	15 mg./kg. daily orally	
or		
Aminosalicylic acid(PAS)	4-5 gm orally t.i.d. after meals	Use only when ethambutol is not available
or Isoniazid	same as above	
and		
Rifampin	600 mg. daily orally	

Most authorities advise a minimum of 12 months of treatment after it has been shown X ray lesions are stable, no cavitation is present, and cultures are negative (control is usually achieved in 2-3 months).

Severe cases may require surgery. Because of the complications, special tests, and prolonged treatment, it is best to evacuate these patients if possible.

Section IV - Viral

2-41. GENERAL. Viruses are extremely small organisms that cannot be seen under a normal microscope. Viruses cause a variety of important infectious diseases; among these are the common cold, yellow fever, hepatitis, and the majority of the infections of the upper respiratory tract.

2-42. MEASLES (Rubeola). An acute systemic viral infection transmitted by inhalation of infective droplets. One attack confers permanent immunity. Communicability is greatest during the preemptive stage, but continues as long as the rash remains. Incubation period is 10-14 days.

S. Fever often as high as 104-105 degrees F., coryza (nasal obstruction, sneezing, sore throat), persistent and nonproductive cough, malaise (may be marked), and conjunctivitis with redness, swelling, photophobia, and discharge. Koplik's spots (small red spots with bluish-white centers on the oral mucosa and often on the inner conjunctival folds and vaginal mucous membrane) appear about 2 days before the rash and last 1-4 days. Rash usually appears first on the face and behind the ears 4 days after the onset of symptoms.

O. The pharynx is red and a yellowish exudate may appear on the tonsils. The tongue is coated in the center and the tip and margins are red. Moderate generalized lymphadenopathy is common; splenomegaly occurs occasionally. The initial lesions of the rash are pinhead-sized papules that coalesce to form the brick-red irregular blotchy maculopapular rash and that may further coalesce, in severe cases, to form an almost uniform erythema on some areas of the body. By the second day, the rash begins to coalesce on the face as it appears on the trunk. On the third day, the rash begins to coalesce on the trunk as it appears on the extremities and begins to fade on the face. Thereafter, it fades in the order of its appearance. Hyperpigmentation remains in fair-skinned individuals and severe cases.

A typical measles is a rarely occurring syndrome in children or adults who have received inactive or live measles vaccine and as a result have developed hypersensitivity rather than protective immunity. When infected with mild measles virus, they develop high fever, unusual rashes (papular, hemorrhagic), arthralgias, and pneumonitis, often with severe illness and a substantial mortality rate. Leukopenia is usually present unless there is a secondary bacterial infection. Complications include encephalitis, bronchopneumonia or bronchiolitis, and secondary bacteria infections.

A. Measles. Differential diagnosis: Rubella, chickenpox, smallpox, infectious mononucleosis, enterovirus infections, and drug eruptions.

P. Isolate the patient for the week following onset of rash and keep at bed rest until afebrile. Give aspirin, saline eye sponges, vasoconstrictor nose drops, and sedative cough mixture as necessary; treat complications as needed.

Prevention: Multiple virus vaccines are available (measles,

mumps, rubella) and can be used for prevention in the first 24 hours after exposure.

2-43. RUBELLA (German measles). A systemic viral infection transmitted by inhalation of infective droplets. Only moderately communicable. One attack usually confers permanent immunity. Disease can be transmitted for 1 week before rash appears. Incubation period is 14-21 days.

S. Fever and malaise, usually mild, with tender suboccipital adenitis may precede eruption by 1 week. Symptoms of mild head cold may be present. Joint pains occur in 25 percent of adult cases. Symptoms usually subside in about 7 days. A fine, pink maculopapular rash appears on face, trunk, and extremities in rapid progression, usually lasting one day in each area. Rubella without the rash is as common as with the rash.

O. Posterior cervical and postauricular lymphadenopathy is very common. Redness of the palate and throat, sometimes blotchy, may be noted. Diagnosis can be suspected when there is epidemiologic evidence of rubella in the area. CBC may show leukopenia early and may be followed by an increase in plasma cells.

Complications: In pregnancy, risk to the fetus is high in the first trimester and continues into the second trimester. An infant acquiring rubella in uterus may be normal at birth, but more likely will have a wide variety of manifestations including growth retardation, maculopapular rash, thrombocytopenia (abnormal decrease in number of blood platelets), cataracts, deafness, congenital heart defects, organomegaly (enlargement of organs), and many other manifestations.

A. Rubella. Differential diagnosis: Infectious mononucleosis, echovirus infections, and coxsackievirus infections.

P. Symptomatic treatment: Aspirin, fluids, rest. Rubella is mild and rarely lasts more than 3-4 days. Congenital rubella has high mortality rate and congenital defects require years of medical and surgical management.

Prevention: Live attenuated rubella virus vaccine offers complete protection. Birth control must be practiced by women for at least 3 months after the use of the vaccine.

2-43. HERPES ZOSTER (Shingles). See Chapter 1, Section I, Integumentary System.

2-44. VARICELLA (Chickenpox). See Chapter 6, Pediatrics.

2-45. VARIOLA (Smallpox). An acute, contagious, systemic viral disease. Transmitted by direct contact with infected patient or handling of contaminated articles. Thought to be eradicated worldwide as of 1979 through the efforts of the W.H.O. using smallpox vaccination. Incubation period is 7-17 days, usually 10-12 days to onset of illness, and 2-4 more days to onset of rash.

S. Abrupt onset with chills, headaches (usually frontal), intense lumbar pain, fever (up to 104 degrees F. or higher), nausea, or more frequently vomiting. Fever falls sharply on evening of third or morning of fourth day, often to normal, and eruption appears as temperature falls. Normally, rash starts first on face and soon after, on extremities and to lesser extent on trunk.

O. Rash is of the same character in any general location, in this respect, differing markedly from rash of chickenpox. Rash is initially macules; about the second day they become papules that become vesicles from the third to fifth day. The vesicles increase in size and by the seventh to eighth day become well developed pustules. Finally scabs form. These scabs fall off in about 3 or 4 weeks. The lesions of smallpox are deep-seated with a thick protective covering and do not rupture easily. The lesion does not collapse when pricked by a needle. Recovery in untreated cases is doubtful.

A. Smallpox. Differential diagnosis: Chickenpox, herpes zoster.

P. Absolute isolation of patient in a screened but well ventilated room until all scabs and crusts have disappeared. Symptomatic treatment is forced fluids, aspirin. Do not use ointments on the skin before the drying up is complete as it increases the likelihood of abscess formation. Close attention must be given to the eyes; if necessary, they may be irrigated several times a day with 2% sodium bicarbonate solution. Weak iodine or weak permanganate baths can be used on the skin for cleansing and as a deodorant.

Successful vaccination against smallpox is an absolute preventive, but this should be repeated during an epidemic or when an individual has been exposed.

2-46. MUMPS (Endemic parotitis). See Chapter 6, Pediatrics.

2-47. POLIOMYELITIS. Three antigenically distinct types are recognized, with no cross immunity between them. Probably acquired by respiratory droplet route or by ingestion. Incubation period is 5-35 days (usually 7-14 days). Infectivity is maximal during the first week. Since the introduction of effective vaccine, poliomyelitis has become rare in the developed areas of the world.

S. and O.

(1) Abortive poliomyelitis: Headache, fever, vomiting, diarrhea, constipation, and sore throat.

(2) Nonparalytic poliomyelitis: Headache; neck, back, and extremity pain; lethargy; and irritability are present. Muscle spasm in extensors of neck and back is always present and usually present in the hamstring muscles. Muscle spasm is variably present in other muscles. Spasm may be seen when patient is at rest or elicited by putting each muscle through the maximum range of motion. Resistance to neck flexion is noted after a varying range of free flexion. Straight leg raising is less than 90 degrees. The muscles may be tender to palpation.

(3) Paralytic poliomyelitis: May occur at any time during the febrile (feverish) period. Symptoms of nonparalytic poliomyelitis plus tremor and muscle weakness. Paresthesia and urinary retention are noted occasionally. Constipation and abdominal distention are common. Paralytic poliomyelitis may be divided into two forms that may coexist. Spinal poliomyelitis (weakness of muscles supplied by spinal nerves) and bulbar poliomyelitis (weakness of muscles supplied by cranial nerves and variable

"encephalitis" symptoms). Other symptoms include diplopia (double vision) (uncommon), facial weakness, dysphasia (speech impairment), nasal voice, weakness of the sternocleidomastoid and trapezius muscles (difficulty in chewing, inability to swallow or expel saliva), and regurgitation of fluids through the nose. The most life threatening aspect is respiratory paralysis. Paralysis may quickly become maximal or progress over several days until temperature becomes normal. Deep tendon reflexes are diminished or lost, often asymmetrically. Lethargy or coma may be due to encephalitis or hypoxia, most often caused by hypoventilation.

Lab findings: W.B.C. may be normal or slightly elevated.

A. Poliomyelitis. Differential diagnosis: Other forms of aseptic meningitis due to other enterovirus (muscle tenderness and spasm, if present, point to polio) is very difficult to distinguish from polio. Acute infectious polyneuritis (Guillain-Barre) and tick bite paralysis may initially resemble poliomyelitis.

P. Symptomatic: Maintain comfortable but changing positions on a firm mattress with footboard, sponge rubber pads or rolls, sandbags, and light splints. Hotpacks for the extremities and analgesic drugs usually control muscle spasm and pain. IV therapy may be needed to prevent dehydration. Indwelling catheter may be required. Intestinal hypoactivity may lead to fecal impaction. Cases of bulbar poliomyelitis involving respiratory muscles require intensive care. Attention must be focused on maintaining a clear airway, handling secretions, preventing respiratory infections, and maintaining adequate ventilation. Assisted ventilation and tracheostomy are often required.

Prevention of deformities is best accomplished by avoiding active exercise during febrile period and substituting passive range of motion exercises and frequent changes of position. As soon as fever subsides, early mobilization and active exercise should be started. Early bracing and splinting for therapeutic purposes are recommended.

Prevention: Oral live virus vaccine (Sabin), the trivalent form is preferable for immunizing children and infants. Adults who are exposed to poliomyelitis or plan to travel in endemic areas should receive the oral vaccine also.

2-48. DENGUE (Breakbone fever, dandy fever). Viral disease transmitted by Aedes mosquito. Occurs only in active mosquito season (warm weather). Incubation period 3-15 days (usually 5-8 days).

S. Sudden onset of high fever, chilliness, severe aching (breakbone) of the head, back, and extremities, accompanied by sore throat, prostration, and depression. Initial febrile phase lasts 3-4 days, usually followed by remission of a few hours to 2 days. A rash appears in 80 percent of cases during remission or during second febrile phase that lasts 1-2 days and is accompanied by similar but milder symptoms.

O. May be conjunctival redness and flushing or blotching of the skin. Rash may be scarlatiniform, morbilliform, macropapular, or petechial, appearing first on dorsum of hands and feet and spreads to the arms, legs, trunk, and neck, but rarely to the face. Rash lasts 2 hours to several days and may be followed by peeling: Petechial rashes and gastrointestinal hemorrhages occur in a high portion of cases in Southeast Asia.

Lab findings: Leukopenia is characteristic.

A. Dengue. Differential diagnosis: Before the rash appears, it is difficult to distinguish from malaria, yellow fever, or influenza.

P. Symptomatic treatment: Treat shock, give salicylates as required, forced fluids, gradual restoration of activity during prolonged convalescence.

Prevention: Mosquito control. An effective vaccine has been developed but has not been produced commercially.

2-49. COLORADO TICK FEVER. An acute viral infection transmitted by tick bites, limited to western USA and most prevalent during tick season (March to August). Incubation period 3-6 days.

S. Abrupt onset of 102-105 degree F. fever, sometimes with chills. Severe myalgia, headache, photophobia, anorexia, nausea, vomiting, and generalized weakness.

O. Abnormal findings are limited to an occasional faint rash. Fever lasts 3 days followed by remission of 2-3 days, and then by full recurrence of symptoms for 3-4 days. Occasionally, there may be 2-3 bouts of fever. Lab findings: Leukopenia (2,000-3,000 W.B.C. with a shift to the left.

A. Colorado tick fever. Differential diagnosis: Influenza, Rocky Mountain spotted fever, and other acute leukopenic fevers.

P. Symptomatic treatment: Aspirin or codeine may be given for pain.

2-50. RABIES. See Chapter 12, Bites.

2-51. YELLOW FEVER. Transmitted by Aedes and jungle mosquitoes. Endemic to Africa and South America. Incubation period is 3-6 days.

S. Mild form: Malaise, headache, fever, retro-orbital pain, nausea, vomiting, and photophobia. Severe form: Same symptoms with sudden onset and then severe pains throughout the body, extreme prostration, bleeding into the skin and from mucous membranes, "coffee ground" vomitus, and jaundice, followed by a period of calm on about the third day when the temperature returns to normal. Then fever returns, bleeding, and later delirium.

O. Mild form: Bradycardia may be present. Severe form: Tachycardia, oliguria, erythematous face, and conjunctival redness during congestive phase. After the period of calm; bradycardia, hypotention, jaundice, and hemorrhages (gastrointestinal tract, bladder, nose, mouth, subcutaneous).

Lab findings: Proteinuria sometimes as high as 5-6 gm/L. and disappears with recovery; hematuria and leukopenia occurs, although it may not be present at the onset.

A. Yellow fever. Differential diagnosis: Mild form is difficult to distinguish from hepatitis, leptospirosis, and other forms of jaundice on clinical evidence alone.

P. Symptomatic treatment: Liquid diet, limiting food to high-carbohydrate, high-protein liquids as tolerated; IV glucose and normal saline as required; analgesics and sedatives as required; and saline enemas for constipation.

Prevention: Mosquito control and live virus vaccine for persons living in or traveling to endemic areas.

Prognosis: Mortality is high in severe form, with death occurring most commonly between the sixth and ninth days. In survivors, temperature returns to normal by seventh or eighth day.

2-52. INFLUENZA. See Chapter 1, Section IX, Eye, Ear, Nose, and Throat.

2-53. VIRAL HEPATITIS.

a. Hepatitis A ("infectious" or short incubation period hepatitis) is a generalized viral infection in which liver involvement dominates the clinical picture. It may occur sporadically or in epidemics. Transmission is usually by fecal-oral route; however, it may be transmitted (rarely) by contaminated needle stick or transfusion. There is no known carrier state with hepatitis A.

b. Hepatitis B ("serum" or long incubation period hepatitis) usually transmitted by inoculation of infected blood or blood products but can be spread by oral or sexual contact. Fecal-oral transmission has also been documented. Approximately 5-10 percent of infected individuals become carriers. The incubation period is 6 weeks to 6 months. The clinical picture is similar in Type A and B hepatitis but in Type B, the onset tends to be more insidious.

S. Clinical picture is extremely variable from asymptomatic infection without jaundice to a fulminating disease and death in a few days.

Prodromal phase: Onset varies from abrupt to insidious with general malaise, myalgia, arthralgia, easy fatigability, upper respiratory symptoms (nasal discharge, pharyngitis), and severe anorexia. Nausea and vomiting are common and diarrhea or constipation may occur. Fever usually present but rarely more than 103.1 degrees F. Return of temperature to normal often coincides with onset of jaundice. Chills or chilliness may mark an acute onset. Abdominal pain usually mild and constant in upper right quadrant or right epigastrium often aggravated by jarring or exertion. A distaste for smoking paralleling anorexia may occur early.

Icteric (jaundice) phase: Usually occurs after 5-10 days but may appear at same time as initial symptoms. There is often an intensification of prodromal symptoms with onset of jaundice. <u>Some</u> patients <u>never</u> develop jaundice.

Convalescent phase: Gradual improvement over a 3-16 week period. Most patients recover fully.

O. Hepatomegaly: Rarely marked - present in over half of cases. Liver tenderness is usually present. Splenomegaly is present in 15 percent of cases, and soft enlarged lymph nodes, especially in cervical or epitrochlear area, may occur. Signs of general toxemia vary from minimal to severe.

Lab findings: W.B.C. is normal to low (abnormal or "atypical" lymphocytes may suggest mononucleosis; mono spot test may be positive). Mild proteinuria is common and bilirubinuria often precedes jaundice.

A. Hepatitis. Differential diagnosis: Infectious mononucleosis, cytomegalic inclusion, leptospirosis, secondary syphilis, Q fever, and drug-induced liver disease. Distinguish prodromal phase from influenza, URI, and prodromal stages of the exanthematous diseases. In obstructive phase, rule out other obstructive lesions such as choledocholithiasis.

P. Symptomatic treatment: Bed rest at patient's option, forced fluids (or IV 10% dextrose if nausea and vomiting are significant problems), avoid morphine sulfate, drugs that have to be broken down by the liver, and hepatotoxic agents. Steroids have no value in hepatitis treatment. Patients should avoid strenuous exercise and alcohol. Strict isolation is not necessary, but handwashing after bowel movements is required. Thorough handwashing after handling contaminated utensils, bedding, or clothing is essential. Disinfection of feces is necessary when waterborne sewage disposal is not available. Give 5 cc. of gamma globulin (GG) to all close contacts of infected patients.

2-54. INFECTIOUS MONONUCLEOSIS. An acute infectious disease due to EB herpes virus. Universal in distribution and may occur at any age but usually occurs between ages of 10-35, either in epidemic form or sporadic cases. Probably transmitted by respiratory droplets. Incubation period is probably 5-15 days.

S. Symptoms are varied in type and severity. Fever, sore throat, and toxic symptoms (malaise, anorexia, and myalgia) occur frequently in early phase of the illness. A macular to maculopapular or occasionally petechial rash occurs in less than 50 percent of cases. Exudative pharyngitis, tonsillitis, or gingivitis may occur. Common manifestations are easy fatigability, nausea, jaundice (from hepatic involvement), headache, neck stiffness, photophobia, neuritis, and occasionally even Guillain-Barre syndrome (see Chapter 1, Section VII, Nervous System) (from C.N.S. involvement), chest pains, dyspnea, and cough (from pulmonary involvement).

O. Discrete, nonsuppurative, slightly painful, moderately enlarged lymph nodes especially those of the posterior cervical chain Splenomegaly in 50 percent of cases. Hepatomegaly is common; and myocardial involvement with arrhythmias and tachycardia.

Lab Findings: Initially there is a granulocytopenia (decrease in number of neutrophils, basophils, and eosinophils) followed within 1 week by a lymphocytic leukocytosis (increase in lymphocytes and total number of white cells). Many lymphocytes are atypical, i.e., larger than normal adult lymphocytes, stain more darkly, and frequently show vacuolization (look like small air bubbles) of the cytoplasm and nucleus. Mononucleosis spot test will be positive.

A. Mononucleosis. Differential diagnosis: Hepatitis, streptococcal tonsillitis, diphtheria, rubella, toxoplasmosis, and, with C.N.S. involvement, meningitis.

P. Symptomatic treatment: Patient requires support and reassurance because of frequent feeling of lassitude and duration of symptoms. If diagnosis is well established, a short course of corticosteroids can give symptomatic relief to severely ill patients. In uncomplicated cases, the fever disappears in 10 days and the lymphadenopathy and splenomegaly in 4 weeks. In some cases the illness may linger for 2-3 months, especially the lassitude and easy fatigability.

Section V - Rickettsial and Spirochetal

2-55. RICKETTSIA. Are between viruses and bacteria in size and are usually transmitted by arthropods (lice, fleas, ticks, mites), which serve as vectors.

a. Epidemic louse-borne typhus. Due to infection with Rickettsia prowazekii, a parasite of the body louse that ultimately kills the louse. Transmission occurs when a louse sucks blood from an infected individual; the louse then sucks blood from another individual and defecates at the same time; then the individual in scratching the bite rubs the infected feces into the bite wound. Dry, infectious louse feces may also be inhaled and result in human infection.

An individual who recovers from clinical or subclinical typhus may carry R. prowazekii in his lymphoid tissue for many years and even have a recurrence of typhus without exposure to lice or the infectious agent. During such a recurrence, he can serve as a source of infection for lice.

S. Prodromal malaise, cough, headache, and chest pains after 10-14 day incubation period, followed by an abrupt onset of chills, high fever, and prostration, with influenza-like symptoms, progressing to delirium and stupor. The fever is unremitting for many days, and the headache is intractably severe.

O. Conjunctivitis, flushed face, rales at lung bases, and often splenomegaly, a macular rash (that soon becomes papular) appears first in the axillas and spreads over the trunk and then the extremities. Rarely involves the face, palms, or soles. The rash becomes hemorrhagic and hypotension becomes marked in severely ill patients. There may be renal insufficiency, stupor, and delirium. Improvement begins in 13-16 days after onset with rapid drop of fever in spontaneous recovery.

Lab findings: W.B.C. is variable. Proteinuria and hematuria occur commonly.

A. Epidemic louse-borne typhus. Differential diagnosis: Murine typhus.

P. Tetracycline 250-500 mg. q.i.d. x 10 days or Vibramycin 200 mg. the first day followed by 100 mg. a day x 10 days. Alternate is chloramphenicol. Prevention consists of louse control with insecticides, particularly clothing and bedding, and frequent bathing. Immunization provides good protection against the severe disease but does not prevent infection or mild disease.

b. Endemic flea-borne typhus (murine typhus). Caused by Rickettsia typhi (R. mooseri), a parasite of rats. Transmitted to humans by bite from an infected flea that releases infected feces while sucking blood.

S. and O. Flea typhus resembles recurrent epidemic (Brill's disease) in that it has a gradual onset, fever and rash are of shorter duration (6-13 days), and the symptoms are less severe. The rash is maculopapular mainly on the chest and fades fairly rapidly. Even without antibiotics it is a mild disease.

A. Murine typhus. Differential diagnosis: Recurrent epidemic typhus.

P. Antibiotic therapy (same as for epidemic louse-borne typhus).

Prevention: Control fleas and rats. Apply insecticides to rat runs, nests, and colonies and then poison or trap the rats.

c. Rocky Mountain spotted fever (Queenland tick typhus in Australia, Boutonneuse fever in Africa). All are caused by related Rickettsia. Rickettsii organisms through the bite of infected hard ticks. Rickettsia are often transmitted from one generation of ticks to the next without passage through an intermediate host.

S. The patient develops anorexia, malaise, nausea, headache, and sore throat 3-10 days after an infectious tick bite, progressing with chills; fever; aches in bones, joints, and muscles; nausea and vomiting; restlessness; insomnia and irritability. Delirium, lethargy, stupor, and coma may appear.

O. Face is flushed and conjunctivas injected. After 2-6 days of fever, a rash appears starting on the wrists and ankles spreading to the arms, legs, and trunk. The rash is initially small, red, and macular; over 2-3 days it becomes larger and petechial. Hepatomegaly, splenomegaly, jaundice, gangrene, myocarditis, or uremia may occur.

Lab findings: Leukocytosis, proteinuria, and hematuria are common.

A. Rocky Mountain spotted fever. Differential diagnosis: Measles, typhoid, or meningococcemia. Many other infections have similar early signs and symptoms.

P. Response to tetracycline or chloramphenicol is prompt if started early.

Prevention: Protective clothing, insect repellent, and buddy system checking for ticks at frequent intervals help.

d. Scrub typhus (Tsutsugamushi disease). Caused by Rickettsia Tsutsugamushi, a parasite of rodents that is transmitted by the bite of mite larva. The mite larva spends most of its life cycle on vegetation, and when an animal or human brushes against the vegetation, the larva drops onto them.

S. Incubation period of 1-3 weeks after bite by mite larva. Malaise, chills, severe headache, and backache. A papule develops at the site of the mite bite that vesicates and forms a flat black eschar.

O. Regional draining lymph nodes are enlarged and tender. There may be generalized adenopathy. Gradually rising fever with a generalized macular rash developing at the end of first week and is most marked on the trunk. During the second week of fever, pneumonitis, encephalitis, myocarditis, and cardiac failure may occur. The patient appears confused, out of contact with the environment, and dulled in sensitivity.

A. Scrub typhus. Differential diagnosis: Leptospirosis, typhoid, dengue, malaria, and other rickettsial infections.

P. A tetracycline or chloramphenicol.

Prevention: Repeated area application of long-acting miticide and/or insect repellents on clothing or skin.

e. Rickettsialpox. Caused by Rickettsia akari, a parasite of mice, and transmitted by mites. The disease is fairly mild and self-limited.

S. and O. Incubation of 7-12 days with sudden onset of chills, fever, headache, photophobia, and disseminated aches and pains. Primary lesion at bite site is a red papule that vesicates and forms a black eschar. A widespread papular eruption appears 2-4 days after the onset of symptoms, becomes vesicular, and forms crusts that are shed in about 10 days.

A. Rickettsialpox. Differential diagnosis: Chickenpox or smallpox.

P. A tetracycline or chloramphenicol.

Prevention: Apply insecticide to mice runs and nests, then eliminate the mice.

f. Trench fever. A self-limited louse-borne relapsing febrile disease caused by Rickettsia quintana. Humans appear to be only animal reservoir. Occurs in epidemic form in louse-infested troops and civilians during wars and in endemic form in Central America.

S. Abrupt onset of fever lasting 3-5 days, often followed by relapses. Weakness; severe pain behind the eyes and in the back and legs.

O. Lymphadenopathy, splenomegaly, and a transient maculopapular rash may appear.

A. Trench fever. Differential diagnosis: Dengue, leptospirosis, malaria, relapsing fever, and typhus.

P. A tetracycline or chloramphenicol. The illness is self-limiting and recovery regularly occurs without treatment.

g. Q fever. Caused by Coxiella burneti, a parasite of cattle, sheep, and goats. Transmitted to humans by inhalation of contaminated dust or droplets or by ingestion of infected milk. It is excreted by cattle, goats, and sheep through feces, milk, and placenta. Coxiella is relatively resistant to pasteurization in milk. Spread from human to human is rare, but fetal infection can occur.

S. Incubation of 1-3 weeks with developing headache, prostration, muscle pains, and occasionally with a nonproductive cough, abdominal pains, or jaundice.

O. Physical signs of pneumonitis are slight. Hepatitis may be severe and endocarditis occurs rarely. Occasionally signs of encephalopathy are present. The clinical course may be acute, chronic, or relapsing.

Lab findings: Leukopenia is often present.

A. Q fever. Differential diagnosis: Atypical pneumonia, hepatitis, brucellosis, tuberculosis, psittacosis, and other animal-borne diseases must be considered.

P. Tetracyclines can suppress symptoms and shorten the clinical course, but do not always eradicate the infection. Even in untreated cases, the mortality rate is negligible.

Prevention: Based on detection of infection in livestock, treatment and reduction in contact with the animal and dust contaminated by them, and effective pasteurization of milk.

2-56. SPIROCHETAL.

a. Syphilis. See Chapter 2, Section VI, Venereal.

b. Yaws (Frambesia, pian, bouba, parangi, domaria). An acute and chronic relapsing, contagious, nonvenereal, spirochetal disease caused by Treponema pertenue, which is morphologically indistinguishable from Treponena pallidum. Restricted to the tropical zones; the highest incidence is among native populations whose level of personal hygiene is low. It is predominately a disease of childhood, but transmission from child to mother by contact is frequent.

S. and O. Incubation period of 2-8 weeks. Initial lesion (mother yaw) appears at the site of implantation. It resembles the typical granulomatous secondary lesion, except it is often larger and healing takes longer. It is frequently still present when the secondary eruption appears. There is aching of the limbs, joint pains, and often an irregular fever is present. There may be enlargement of the regional lymph nodes. A few weeks to 4 months later the secondary or generalized stage begins with the appearance of secondary lesions scattered over the surface of the body. These lesions may involve the palms of the hands and/or the soles of the feet. The lesions are usually elevated, apparently granulomatous papules varying from a few to 50 mm. or more in diameter and tend to be round or oval. Initially the surface is composed of greatly proliferated epithelium exuding clear serum that contains concentrations of spirochettes. Later, a yellow crust forms (may be discolored by debris). In young children suffering from anemia or malnutrition, the lesions may appear as erosions with bright pink borders and whitish centers. Successive eruptions often appear before the preceding ones heal. These later lesions tend to be most numerous around the lips, axillae, genitalia, and anus. These recurring eruptions may continue for 2-3 years and lesions about the lips or on the soles of the feet may recur after many years. Healing of the secondary lesions leave only slight scarring that is never permanently atrophic and pigmented.

Nondestructive lesions of the bones are frequent in the secondary stage. They develop rapidly and resolve spontaneously in a few weeks or months, but the periosteal reaction may cause thickening of the bone resulting in deformities.

The tertiary stage of yaws usually does not appear until after a relatively or completely symptom-free period of several years. Most commonly it begins during the third or fourth decades of life. In this stage, resolution and spontaneous cure may occur, or the disease become latent, with the subsequent appearance of relapsing tertiary lesions. The tertiary lesions are of three types: (1) extensive, spreading, superficial, and relatively clean ulcerations that gradually heal from the center; (2) cutaneous and subcutaneous nodules that break down forming deep, indolent ulcers with irregular bases (these heal from the margin and isolated islands in the base, causing atrophic scars that may be unpigmented in the early stages but later are often deeply pigmented and may cause severe contractures); (3) hyperkeratotic lesions of the soles of the feet and less commonly of the palms of the hands ("Crab Yaws") causing extensive thickening of the skin with fissures and ulcerations (painful and a source of severe disability).

Destructive bone and periosteal lesions most commonly involving the tibia, other long bones, and the hands are frequent. These are usually single or few in number and develop slowly. They may extend through the subcutaneous tissue and skin, producing chronic ulceration that responds slowly to treatment. The lesions are accompanied by local swelling, tenderness, and pain. These lesions can also occur on the skull, clavicles, scapulae, sternum, hard palate (can cause extensive destruction of the structure of the nose), and joints.

Lab findings: Spirochetes can usually be found by Giemsa's stain of exudates from lesions under darkfield examination. (India ink stain of slide also works.) Serum test for syphilis is positive.

A. Yaws. Differential diagnosis: The mucocutaneous lesions of leishmaniasis, the ulcerating lesions of leprosy, tuberculosis, and the late lesions of syphilis.

P. Treatment for the various stages of yaws is the same as for the various stages of syphilis (see Chapter 2, Section VI, Venereal).

c. Endemic syphilis. An infectious, chronic, nonvenereal infection of the intermediate tropical and temperate climates caused by Treponema pallidum (?), morphologically indistinguishable from the spirochetes of syphilis or yaws. Some authorities think that syphilis and endemic syphilis are the same disease. It occurs in localized areas in backward regions where socioeconomic levels are low and advanced education is lacking. When modern civilization reaches endemic areas through the construction of highways or development of an oil field, endemic syphilis disappears and venereal syphilis appears. It is primarily an early childhood disease and is spread by direct contact.

S. and O. Primary lesions consist of eruptions of the skin or mucous membranes, but are seldom recognized. Eruptions in the mouth are usually first, followed by moist papules in the folds of the skin. These lesions often resemble those of secondary syphilis. The late stage may appear within a few years after onset or be delayed for many years. It is characterized by plantar and palmar lesions, patchy pigmentation of the skin, and destructive lesions of the long bones, nose, and throat. Cardiovascular lesions are fairly common but involvement of the eyes, central nervous system, tabes, and paresis is rare.

Lab finding: Spirochetes may be found in wound aspirates using dark-field examination and serum test for syphilis is positive.

A. Endemic syphilis.

P. Same as yaws and syphilis (see Chapter 2, Section VI, Venereal).

d. Pinta (Mal del pinto, carate, azul, tina, lota, empeines). An acute and chronic nonvenereal disease caused by a spirochete (Treponema carateum) that is also morphologically indistinguishable from T. pallidum. Found in Central and South America, Mexico, and Cuba. Most frequent in the young and occurs most frequently in low lying and wooded areas, usually near rivers, where relative humidity is 80 percent or more and temperature is between 79 to 86° F. These people's primitive way of life and wearing of few clothes appear to promote their contacting pinta.

S. and O. Characterized by a superficial nonulcerative primary lesion, a secondary eruption, and late depigmentation and hyperkeratosis of the skin. The hands and wrists are most frequently involved, but feet and ankle involvement is common. Neurologic and cardiovascular involvement is fully as significant in late pinta as in syphilis.

Lab findings: Positive darkfield examination and STS.

A. Pinta. Differential diagnosis: Yaws, syphilis.

P. Same as for syphilis (see Chapter 2, Section VI, Venereal).

e. Relapsing fever (tick fever, famine fever, spirillum fever, febris recurrens, kimputu, garapata disease, and many others). Caused by the Borrelia species of spirochete and transmitted by tick bite or by crushed lice through abraded skin. Louse-borne relapsing fever has disappeared from the US but occurs in parts of South America, Europe, Asia, Africa, and Australia. Tick-borne relapsing fever is found in western US and Canada, Mexico, Central and South America, Europe, Africa, and Asia. Louse-borne relapsing fever is frequently found concomitantly with epidemic louse-borne typhus. Incubation period is from 2-10 days, but may be as long as 3 weeks.

S. Abrupt onset of fever (up to 104-105° F. or higher), chills, vertigo, severe headache, nausea, and vomiting. Transitory erythematous or petechial eruptions are common during the initial fever. Usually most pronounced about the neck and shoulder girdle and later extending to the chest and abdomen. Initial fever usually lasts 3-10 days. After an interval of 1-2 weeks, a relapse occurs, often somewhat milder. There may be 3-10 relapses before recovery.

O. Tachycardia occurs with the onset. Delirium occurs with high fever, and there may be various neurologic and psychic abnormalities. A slight icteric tint of the sclerae is common and marked jaundice may occur in severe cases. Hepatomegaly and splenomegaly may develop.

Lab findings: During episodes of fever, large spirochetes are seen in blood smears stained using Wright's or Giemsa's stain. Mild anemia and thrombocytopenia are common, but W.B.C. is usually normal.

A. Relapsing fever. Differential diagnosis: Malaria, leptospirosis, meningococcemia, yellow fever, typhus, or rat-bite fever.

P. Give 0.5 gm tetracycline or erythromycin in a single dose orally; 600,000 units of procaine penicillin G IM can also be used.

f. Rat-bite fever (sodoku). Uncommon acute infectious disease caused by a spirochete (Spirillum minus) that is transmitted by the bite of a rat.

S. The original rat bite heals rapidly unless secondarily infected. After an incubation period of one to several weeks, the bite site becomes swollen, indurated, painful, assumes a dusky purplish hue, and may ulcerate. Fever, chills, malaise, myalgia, arthralgia, and headache are present. After a few days, the local and systemic symptoms subside only to reappear in 24-48 hours. After the first few relapses, only the fever returns on this 24-48-hour cycle and may persist for weeks.

O. Regional lymphangitis and lymphadenitis are present. Splenomegaly may occur. A sparse, dusky-red maculopapular rash may appear on the trunk and extremities.

Lab findings: Spirochete may be found in aspirated lymph node material or in the ulcer exudate under darkfield examination. Leukocytosis is often present and STS is often falsely positive.

A. Rat-bite fever. Differential diagnosis: Streptococcal rash, tularemia, relapsing fever.

P. Give 300,000 units procaine penicillin IM q.12h. x 7 days.

g. Leptospirosis (Fort Bragg fever, Weil's disease, swineherd's disease). An acute and often severe infection caused by several Leptospira species. Leptospirosis is found worldwide. It is transmitted by ingestion of food or drink contaminated by rodents, cattle, or pigs. The disease can also be acquired by direct contact through minor skin lesions, and probably via the conjunctiva, and also through bathing in contaminated water. Incubation period is 2-20 days.

S. Sudden onset of fever (102-104o F.), chills, abdominal pains, vomiting, nausea, myalgia (especially of the calf muscles), and unrelenting frontal headache. Photophobia, sore throat, cough, and diarrhea are common. Petechial and maculopapular rashes may occur. Usually all signs and symptoms disappear within 3-4 days, but some patients may be ill for weeks. In some cases symptoms disappear for 1-3 days, then the fever and any of the initial symptoms may return.

O. Conjunctiva is markedly reddened. The liver can be palpated in 50 percent of the cases and jaundice is present about the fifth day. Capillary hemorrhages and purpuric skin lesions may appear. Meningeal irritation and associated findings of aseptic meningitis may occur.

Lab findings: W.B.C. may be normal or as high as 50,000 with neutrophilia. Urine may contain bile, protein, casts, and red cells. Spirochete may be found in urine from the tenth day to the sixth week. It can also be found in blood smears using dark-field examination during the first 10 days.

A. Leptospirosis. Differential diagnosis: Hepatitis, yellow fever, relapsing fever.

P. Give 600,000 units procaine penicillin IM q.3h. x 24h. then q.6h. x 6 days, or 500 mg. tetracycline q.6h. x 7 days.

Section VI - Veneral

2-57. Venereal diseases are contagious diseases most commonly acquired through sexual intercourse or other genital contact.

2-58. GONOCOCCAL INFECTIONS (clap, dose). A specific infection of the genitourinary tract caused by Neisseria gonorrhoeae. Extragenital infections (rectal, oral, skin, and eye infection of the newborn) do occur, but not as frequently.

S. In the male, incubation 2-7 days after contact; average is 3 days. A transient mucoid urethral discharge develops that becomes a profuse, thick, greenish, purulent urethral excretion. Painful urination is the outstanding symptom. Both the discharge and the painful urination may be severe, moderate, or even absent. About 10 percent of all cases have no S or S. Rectal infections are most often asymptomatic and the result of direct implantation of infection almost always by homosexual activity. The most common complication of untreated gonorrhea is urethral strictures; others include inguinal lymphadenitis, seminal vesiculitis, epididymitis, or prostatitis.

In the female, 80-90 percent are asymptomatic, but can continue to spread the infection. In the female, dysuria or vaginal discharge is the most frequent S or S, but may be so mild as to be unnoticed. Rectal infection can be caused by contamination from cervical discharge or rectal intercourse. Complications in the female are local spread of gonorrhea causing an inflammation of the vulvovaginal gland and/or fallopian tube. This spread may continue from the fallopian tubes into the peritoneal cavity.

In both male and female, but usually female, the infection may spread through the blood and may present in varied ways depending on the area or organs the infection attacks. The most common are arthritis, skin eruptions, meningitis, endocarditis, or conjunctivitis (via blood or by contamination from genital secretion).

O. Typical intracellular gram-negative diplococci are found in the smear of the urethral discharge or cultured from any site, particularly the urethra, cervix, or rectum. It is possible to gram stain smears from urethra, cervix, or rectum and find the organism, but a negative finding does not rule out gonorrhea. History and S and S can make the diagnosis.

A. Gonorrhea. Differential diagnosis: Nonspecific urethritis (50 percent caused by chlamydiae), trichomonal and candidal vaginitis, and cervicitis. The many agents causing salpingitis, pelvic peritonitis, arthritis, proctitis, and skin lesions must be considered also.

P. Uncomplicated gonorrhea: 1 gm probenecid orally; 4.8 million units aqueous procaine penicillin G IM in 2 or more sites.

Alternative: Give 3.5 gm ampicillin together with 1 gm probenecid orally at one time. NEVER TREAT GONORRHEA WITH BENZATHINE PENICILLIN G. If allergic to penicillin, give 1.5 gm tetracycline orally stat., then 0.5 gm orally q.i.d. x 4 days or spectinomycin 2 gm IM at one time. Watch for penicillin-resistant gonorrhea. Do a followup 7 days after completion of treatment. Treat complications with spectinomycin 2 gm IM. If after followup gonorrhea is still present, think of reinfection and give spectinomycin 2 gm IM again. If spectinomycin resistant, give cefoxitin 2 gm IM with 1 gm probenecid P.O. Alternates are tetracycline or erythromycin 0.5 gm orally q.i.d. x 10 days.

2-59. SYPHILIS. Causative agent is Treponema pallidum, a spirochete capable of infecting any organ or tissue in the body. Transmission occurs most frequently during sexual contact, but may be extragenital. The clinical course of untreated syphilis is divided into 4 stages: primary (early), secondary, latent (hidden), and tertiary (late) syphilis. The lesions associated with primary and secondary syphilis are self-limiting and resolve with few or no residual. Tertiary syphilis may be very destructive and permanently disabling and may lead to death. In general, if untreated, one-third of the people infected will undergo spontaneous cure, one-third will remain in latent stage for life, and one-third will develop serious late (tertiary) lesions.

Syphilis can be clinically cured in all of the stages, but the killing of the treponemes can cause Jarisch-Herxheimer reaction. This reaction is thought to be caused by the rapid release of antigenic materials from lysed treponemes. There may be a local and general reaction. The local reaction consists of intensification of the lesions (rashes become more pronounced, chancre becomes edematous). Systemically, frequently the temp rises to 101-102° F., occasionally as high as 104° F. Some patients have convulsions or increasing agitation requiring restraints or sedatives. Reaction usually occurs within 12 hours of treatment and usually lasts only a few hours, rarely more than 24 hours. This reaction is usually benign and of itself is not reason to discontinue treatment.

a. Primary syphilis.

S. A 10-90-day incubation period, then a primary chancre develops. This is a painless superficial ulcer with a clean base and firm indurated margins. Chancres are usually singular, but multiple lesions are not rare. Bacterial secondary infection may occur causing pain. Most frequently located on the penis, labia, cervix, or anorectal region. Occasionally found on lip, tongue, or tonsil and rarely on breast or finger. Press the edges of the primary lesion an you will feel a round pealike ball. The lesion will heal by itself, but may cause a scar. The primary chancre may pass unrecognized.

O. Enlarged regional lymph nodes that are rubbery, discrete, and nontender. Smear from lesion stains the spirochete pink using Giemsa's stain and black using silver impregnation method under dark-field illumination. The spirochete is somewhat hard to find and may require numerous smears before it is found. A serologic test for syphilis (STS) is the best test. These tests usually turn positive 1-3 weeks after the appearance of the primary lesion. If the initial STS and dark-field examination are negative, the STS should be repeated once weekly for 4 weeks.

A. Primary syphilis. Differential diagnosis: chancroid, genital herpes, lymphogranuloma venereum, or neoplasm.

P. Benzathine penicillin G 1.2 million units in each buttock for a total of 2.4 million units once. Only if patient is allergic to penicillin should tetracycline or erythromycin be used. Tetracycline 500 mg. orally q.i.d. x 15 days. Erythromycin 500 mg. orally q.i.d. x 20 days.

b. Secondary syphilis.

S. Generally appears a few weeks to 6 months after primary chancre. The most common manifestations are skin and mucosal lesions. The skin lesions are usually bilaterally symmetrical and are nonpruritic, macular, papular, pustular, or follicular (or any combination of these). Lesions are usually generalized but often involve the palms of the hands and the soles of the feet. The mucosal lesions range from ulcers and papules of the lips, mouth, throat, genitalia, and anus (mucous patches) to a diffuse redness of the pharynx. Mucous membrane and skin lesions are highly infectious during this stage. Meningeal, hepatic, renal, bone and joint invasion with resulting cranial nerve palsies, jaundice, nephrotic syndrome, and periostitis may occur. The lesions of secondary syphilis will heal spontaneously, but may relapse if undiagnosed or inadequately treated. These relapses may include any of the findings of secondary syphilis, but unlike the usually asymptomatic neurologic involvement of secondary syphilis, neurologic relapses may be fulminating, leading to death.

O. STS is positive in almost all cases. Skin and mucous membrane lesions often will show the T. pallidum spirochete on dark-field exam.

A. Secondary syphilis. Differential diagnosis: Infectious exanthems, pityriasis rosea, and drug eruptions. Visceral lesions may suggest nephritis or hepatitis from other causes. Red throat may mimic other forms of pharyngitis.

P. Same treatment as primary syphilis.

c. Latent syphilis (lasts from months to lifetime).

S. No physical signs; total diagnosis is on history.

O. Positive STS.

A. Latent syphilis.

P. Give 2.4 million units benzathine penicillin G IM once a week x 3 weeks.

d. Tertiary (late) syphilis may occur anytime after secondary syphilis, even after years of latency.

S. Essentially a vascular disease that may attack any tissue or organ. Signs and symptoms may mimic almost any disease. Called the "Great Imitator" because of this. A good in-depth history is required, looking for history of primary chancre and secondary syphilis untreated or inadaquately treated.

O. STS usually positive; T. pallidum might possibly be found in skin or mucous lesions.

A. Tertiary syphilis.

P. Same as latent syphilis, but there is no known method for reliable eradication of the treponeme from humans in the late stages of syphilis. There is also no confirmed cases where the treponeme left after treatment are capable of causing progressive disease.

e. Congenital syphilis transmitted through the placenta to the fetus.

S. May have minimal to no signs for 6-8 weeks after birth. Most common findings are on skin and mucous membranes - serous nasal discharge, mucous membrane patches, maculopapular rash, and/or condylomas (broad flat wartlike growths usually seen on genitals or near anus). These lesions are infectious. Lesions heal by themselves and if left untreated child develops defects: interstitial keratitis, Hutchinson's teeth, saddle nose, saber skins, deafness, and/or C.N.S. involvement.

O. Smears taken from lesion and checked under dark field show T. pallidum. STS is not conclusive as it is complicated by transplacental acquisition of maternal antibodies. Baby must be checked every 2-3 weeks for 4 months.

A. Congenital syphilis.

P. Aqueous penicillin G 50,000 units/kg. IM or IV in 2 divided doses daily x 10 days. Antibiotics other than Pen are not recommended.

2-60. CHANCROID. An acute localized usually self-limiting venereal disease with an incubation period of 3-5 days.

S. Initial lesion is vesicopustular with a necrotic base, surrounding erythema, and undermined edges. Multiple lesions started by autoinoculation and inguinal adenitis often develop. The adenitis is usually unilateral and consists of tender matted nodes of moderate size with overlying erythema. The nodal mass softens, becomes fluctuant, and may rupture spontaneously. With lymph node involvement, chills, fever, and malaise may develop; balanitis (inflammation of glans penis) and phimosis (tightening of the foreskin) are frequent complications. These signs usually occur in men; women frequently have no external signs.

O. Smear from lesion gram-stained shows short gram-negative bacillus (Hemophilus ducreyi). There is a skin test for chancroid; once it becomes positive, like tine test, it remains positive for life.

A. Chancroid. Differential diagnosis: Other veneral diseases and pyogenic lesions.

P. Gantrisin 500 mg. q.i.d. x 10-14 days; 0.5 gm tetracycline q.i.d. x 10-14 days; clean ulcer with soap and water b.i.d.; aspirate fluctuant buboes.

2-61. GRANULOMA INGUINALE. A chronic, relapsing granulomatous anogenital infection with an incubation period of from 1-12 weeks.

S. The initial lesion may be a vesicle, papule, or nodule usually on the penis or labia minora. The onset is insidious. This lesion becomes eroded and superficially ulcerated. The ulcer is shallow, sharply demarcated with a beefy-red friable base of granulation tissue with new nodule formation at the edge as the lesion extends. The advancing border has a characteristic rolled edge of granulation tissue. Large ulcerations may advance up onto the lower adbomen and thighs. Scar formation and healing may occur along one border while the other advances. The process may become indolent and stationary.

O. Gram-negative rod-shaped microorganisms found in mononuclear phagocytes from smears made from tissue scraping or secretions from the ulcers.

A. Granuloma inguinale.

P. Tetracycline 500 mg. q.i.d. x 2 weeks or streptomycin 1 gm q.i.d. x 7 days IM or ampicillin 500 mg. q.i.d. x 2 weeks.

2-62. LYMPHOGRANULOMA VENEREUM. An acute and chronic sexually transmitted disease with a 5-21 day incubation period.

S. The primary lesion that is seldom seen is a transitory small papule, vesicle, or ulcer that vanishes in a week to 10 days. In the male, it is usually found on the penis and in the female, on the vaginal wall or cervix. From there, invasion of the lymphatics occur. In the male, the inguinal nodes are involved with further extension into the deep iliac nodes. At first the nodes are discrete, later becoming enlarged, matted, adherent to the skin and finally fluid filled. The overlying skin becomes discolored and ultimately sinus formation with drainage occurs, which may continue for months. Healing is accompanied by extensive scarring, which may lead to elephantiasis of the genitals and rectal strictures. In the female, inguinal involvement is rare. It usually affects the rectovaginal septum, often with no localizing symptoms, until sinuses open and drain into the rectum, and blood and pus appears in the stool; this may be accompanied by malaise, anorexia, headache, and fever. This may last for many weeks. Later, chronic proctitis occurs and occasionally rectovaginal fistulas and perirectal abscesses. Extensive scarring often leads to rectal strictures and elephantiasis of the genitals.

O. Causative organism is a large virus and requires special tests for antibodies; tests are not totally reliable.

A. Lymphogranuloma venereum. Differential diagnosis: Early lesions; syphilis, genital herpes, and chancroid. Lymph node involvement; tularemia, tuberculosis, plague, neoplasm, or pyogenic infection. Rectal strictures; neoplasm, and ulcerative colitis.

P. Tetracycline 500 mg. q.i.d. x 2-3 weeks, gentamicin 40 mg. IM b.i.d. x 2 weeks, bed rest, warm compresses for buboes, and analgesics p.r.n.; aspirate fluid-filled nodes.

2-63. HERPES GENITALIS. Caused by herpes virus type 2 (herpes simplex). Can be sexually transmitted and is increasing in frequency and seriousness. Infection during pregnancy can cause spontaneous abortion, stillbirth, and neonatal death.

S. A 4-7 day incubation period. Starts with reddened area with itching; progresses into blister that breaks and becomes painful like a burn. All of this is usually recurrent. In severe cases there may be fever, malaise, anorexia, local genital pain, dysuria, leukorrhea (white or yellowish mucous discharge), and even vaginal bleeding.

O. Typical genital lesions are multiple shallow ulcerations, vesicles, and erythematous papules. Painful bilateral inguinal adenopathy is usually present. Scrapings and biopsies may show characteristic "ground glass" appearance of cellular nuclei with numerous small intranuclear vacuoles and small scattered basophilic particles.

A. Herpes genitalis. Differential diagnosis: Other venereal diseases.

P. Symptomatic treatment. There is no known cure but there is a control being tested that appears to be effective but only as long as taken. Amino acid (al-lysine) comes in tablet form; give 1,500 mg. daily in 2 doses. When lesions disappear, 1 tab a day as a maintenance dosage. A paste can be made by crushing a tablet, making into a paste, and applying directly onto the lesion. This usually clears the lesions within 24-48 hours; so far this appears to be very effective but only as a control, not a cure. This is the only venereal disease that does not as yet have a cure.

2-64. Other diseases that are considered venereal in nature include Pediculosis pubis (crabs), scabies, hepatitis B infections, vulvovaginal candidiasis, trichomoniasis, and nongonococcal urethritis. These diseases will be covered in other sections.

2-65. Treatment of venereal diseases by itself is not enough. Control and prevention must be stressed.

a. Prevention includes classes on VD and VD prevention measures plus insuring prophylactic devices are made available.

b. Control involves early detection and treatment of infected personnel and their contacts. Every patient diagnosed as having VD should be interviewed to determine with whom he has had sexual contact during the course of his illness and from whom he might have contracted the disease. If the patient does not want to give out the names and addresses of his contacts, you can establish and use a card system. With this system you have colored 3 x 5 cards, a different color for each type VD You can hand out a number of cards to the patient and tell him to give one card to each person with whom he had sex. Have him tell them to take the card to the medic. In that way you can examine and treat prophylactically each person who brings in a card and give them cards for their sexual contacts. In this way you should be able to eliminate the majority of the VD problem.

CHAPTER 3

CLEARING AIRWAY OBSTRUCTIONS AND CPR

3-1. CLEARING AN OBSTRUCTED AIRWAY.

a. Signs of obstruction in a conscious patient:

(1) Heimlich sign; hand to throat, as illustrated below.

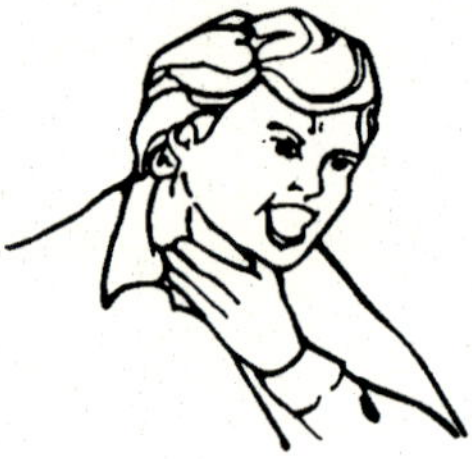

Universal distress signal for choking.

(2) Inability to speak.

(3) Wheezing sounds and an effort to breath.

(4) Cyanosis appearing.

b. Signs in an unconscious patient:

(1) Chest not rising.

(2) Cyanosis.

c. Treatment:

(1) With your fingers sweep mouth and throat of foreign material.

(2) With the heal of the hand deliver four sharp backblows between the patient's shoulder blades, as illustrated below.

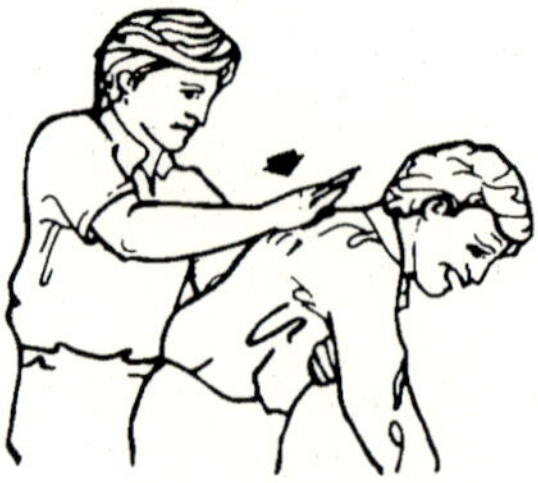

Back blow, standing.

(3) Perform abdominal thrusts:

(a) Stand behind the patient and wrap your arms around his waist.

(b) Place the thumb side of your hand against the patient's abdomen slightly above the navel and below the rib cage, as illustrated below.

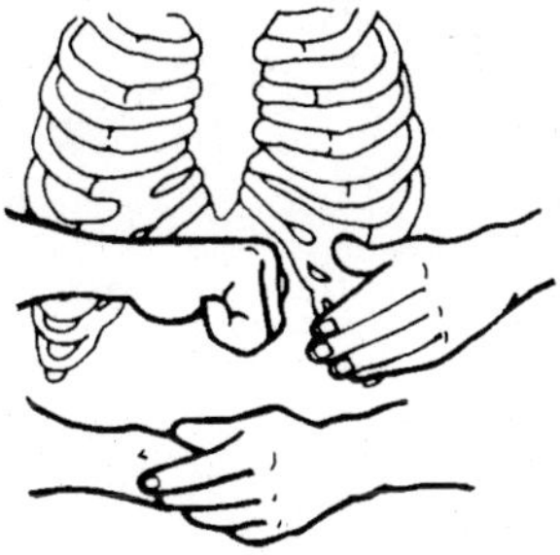

Hand placement for abdominal thrust.

(c) Grasp your fist with the other hand and press into the patient's abdomen with a quick upward thrust; repeat this four times.

(4) Repeat the backblows and abdominal thrusts until airway is clear.

(5) For a prone patient:

(a) Position patient on his back.

(b) Kneel astride patient's hips facing his head.

(c) Place one hand on top of the other and position the heel of your bottom hand on the patient's abdomen, slightly above the navel and below the ribcage.

(d) Press into the patient's abdomen with four quick upward thrusts.

(6) If the obstruction is not dislodged within a few minutes, perform an emergency cricothyroidotomy.

3-2. CARDIOPULMONARY RESUSCITATION.

a. Procedure for CPR with one or two rescuers.

(1) Establish unresponsiveness by gently shaking the patient and shouting "Are you OK?" If there is no response, turn the patient flat on his back and call out for help.

(2) Establish breathlessness by kneeling beside the patient;

hyperextend his neck. Place your ear over the patient's mouth and observe for chest rise (look, listen, and feel) x 5 seconds.

(3) If patient is not breathing, give four quick ventilations, not allowing all the air to escape between each ventilation in order to give a stairstep effect and maximum aeration of the lungs.

(4) Check for a carotid pulse.

(a) If a pulse is present, continue with mouth-to-mouth resuscitation at 12 ventilations per minute. Check for pulse and for return of spontaneous breathing after each cycle of 12 ventilations.

(b) If pulse is absent, rescuer begins CPR.

1. Initiate CPR by locating the notch where the sternum and the bottom of the ribcage meet. Place the middle finger of the lower hand on the notch and the index finger on the lower end of the sternum. Then place the heel of the other hand on the lower half of the sternum next to the index finger, as illustrated below.

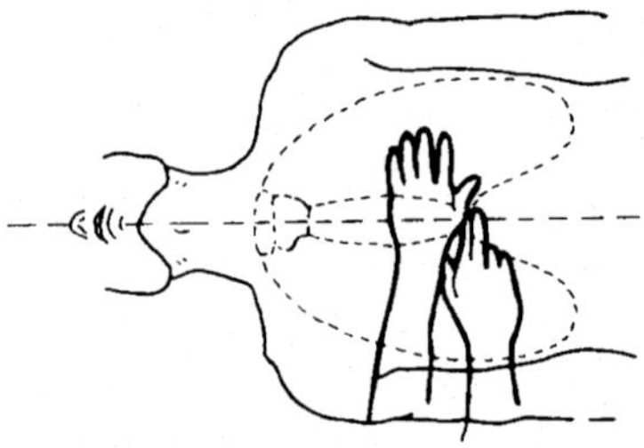

Hand placement.

2. Performance standards for CPR should be in accordance with the following chart.

CARDIOPULMONARY RESUSCITATION

COMMENTS	ADULT (ONE-MAN)	ADULT (TWO-MAN)
Rate of compression	80/min	60/min
Use of hands	2 hands	2 hands
Depth of compression	1 1/2-2 inches	1 1/2-2 inches
Resuscitation only	1 per 5 sec 12/min	1 per 5 sec 12/min
CPR	15 comp 2 vent	5 comp 1 vent
Checking pulse	carotid	carotid
Breaths	full-double size	full-double size
Mouth placement	mouth-to-mouth (nose)	mouth-to-mouth (nose)
Head tilt	hyperextension	hyperextension

COMMENTS	CHILDREN	INFANTS
Rate of compression	100/min	100-120/min
Use of hands	1 hand	2 fingers
Depth of compression	3/4-1 1/2 inches	1/2-3/4 inches
Resuscitation only	1 per 5 sec 12/min	1 per 3 sec 20/min
CPR	5 comp 1 vent	5 comp 1 vent
Checking pulse	carotid	over left nipple
Breaths	regular	puffs of air
Mouth placement	mouth-to-mouth (nose)	mouth-to-mouth and nose (both)
Head tilt	hyperextension	tilt (no hyperextension)

CHAPTER 4

MENTAL DISORDERS

4-1. Many different forms of mental disorders have been named and described, and each may vary greatly in signs and symptoms. Even psychiatrists may have difficulty in diagnosing a particular case. The nervous system section is important to review and consider when evaluating and treating mental disorders. Organic factors may be responsible.

a. Terminology.

(1) Anxiety: Feeling of tension due to real or imagined danger.

(2) Compulsion: An irresistible urge to act against one's better judgment and will.

(3) Delusion: A false fixed idea that cannot be erased by reason or evidence.

(4) Hallucination: Imaginary sensory perception without actual stimulus, either visual and/or auditory.

(5) Insight: Awareness and acceptance of oneself and one's problems.

(6) Illusion: A false interpretation of a real sensory stimulus.

(7) Mental hygiene: The development of healthy mental and emotional reactions and habits.

(8) Neurosis: A functional mental disorder with feelings of anxiety in which the personality remains intact and contact with reality is maintained.

(9) Obsession: An irresistible urge to think thoughts one does not wish to think.

(10) Paranoid: Characterized by suspiciousness, ideas of persecution.

(11) Phobia: An exaggerated or morbid fear of something or situation.

(12) Psychiatry: Branch of medicine that deals with disorders of the mind, behavior, and personality.

(13) Psychosis: A mental disorder in which the personality is very seriously disorganized, and the patient is often out of contact with reality. A "major" mental illness.

b. In many cases treatment is long term and requires special facilities. We cannot hope to cover all mental problems and their treatments in one chapter. Of more importance to us is the ability to recognize approaching trouble and what to do about it.

(1) Types of individuals who are more likely to get into

trouble:

(a) The shy, retiring, withdrawn individual, who has little to do with others. He may have insufficient emotional expression that leads to the accumulation of strong feelings.

(b) The braggart who talks too long and loud of his abilities at home, at work, sexually, and socially. He is usually insecure and wants the admiration of others.

(c) The perfectionist who wants everything just so and becomes very anxious when things are wrong.

(d) The sick bay commando who translates his insecurity, worry, and anxiety into somatic complaints.

(e) The man who depreciates himself and is always apologizing is usually becoming depressed.

(2) Changes denoting approaching mental difficulty:

(a) Any persistent changes in mood in a man's behavior.

(b) Tension, anxiety, apprehensive facial expression, excessive perspiration, tremulousness.

(c) Irritability, short temper, abruptness, complaining, and faultfinding.

(d) Frequent accidents or mistakes.

(e) Depression, self-blame, self-degradation.

(f) Withdrawal, escape from others.

(g) Somatic complaints of sleeplessness, nightmares, anorexia, nausea, stomachache, headache, muscle cramps, diarrhea.

(h) Loss of contact, loss of attention, doesn't make good sense, poor thought associations, strange or unexplained behavior, difficulty thinking, memory lapses, lack of correlation between thought and emotional expression.

4-2. PSYCHOSIS. A severe, major mental disorder characterized by various degrees of personality disintegration and failure to test and evaluate external reality correctly. These men are usually without clearly defined physical cause or structural brain changes. The basic types of psychoses are:

a. Manic-depressive reaction: Marked by major mood swings and emotional instability typified by "lows" and "highs."

b. Schizophrenic reaction: Disorientation and separation of personality.

c. Paranoid reaction: Marked by suspiciousness and delusions of persecution and/or grandeur.

d. Alcoholic: Marked by alcoholism and bouts of delirium tremens.

e. Toxic (drugs): Induced by toxic agents such as drugs.

S. and O. Each psychosis is a separate case affecting a separate human being. Not all cases have all the major symptoms. Below is a generally accepted group of symptoms:

(1) Deep depression with feelings of worthlessness. One of the foremost causes of self-destruction.

(2) Abnormal and inappropriate cheerfulness, out of keeping with surroundings or reality.

(3) Loss of contact with reality with strange, bizarre behavior. May be berserk, assaultive, totally withdrawn, etc.

(4) Total withdrawal from a group to such a degree that the patient actually lives in a "world of fantasy."

(5) Delusions and hallucinations.

A. Psychosis.

P. Close supervision of the patient since his condition is characterized by rapid and major mood swings. Establish communication as soon as possible. Fear is often largely responsible for his behavior. Reassure him and appeal to the "well" aspects of his personality. Force and restraints must be used when there is no other way to protect the patient or those around him. Restraints should not be placed over chest and abdomen and should be removed as soon as possible. Tranquilization for the violent or assaultive patient is often necessary. Use antipsychotics for psychotic behavior. Use the following in priority of order:

(1) Haldol (haloperidol) 2-5 mg. IM can be given every hour if needed. The drug of choice for severe psychotic, aggressive, or other uncontrollable behavior problems.

(2) Thorazine 100 mg IM. A greater sedative than (1). Blood pressure must be monitored since it may produce hypotension.

(3) Librium 100 mg IM to relieve anxiety. Especially useful in alcohol or drug abuse.

4-3. PSYCHONEUROSIS. A relatively benign group of personality disorders that arise from an effort to deal with specific, private, internal, and or psychological problems and stressful situations that the patient is unable to master without tension or disturbing psychological devices. The symptoms are numerous and varied. The chief characteristic is anxiety; however, there is good contact with reality. The confusion or symptoms make it difficult to assign a given case to a definite type. The essential consideration is recognition of the condition and the need for treatment. It must be remembered that one neurotic symptom is not a neurosis. All of us occasionally develop one, or even several, under special duress.

S. and O. Anxiety is the chief characteristic and is the most intolerable item to the patient. This anxiety may be free and unbound, such as crying, talking, etc., or expressed as various somatic complaints.

There is good contact with reality. May function effectively until encountering a stressful situation that he is unable to cope with. Often he controls this by various psychological defense mechanism such as repression, etc. Other symptoms may be fatigue, insomnia, lowered work output, inability to concentrate and even paralyzing indecision, feelings of inferiority and inadequacy.

P. Remove the stress situation if possible. Listen to him. Often simple ventilation of his problems is all that is required. Reassure and support him but be cautious with advice. Let him work out his own solutions. Antianxiety drugs are drugs of choice and follow in order of preference.

(1) Librium 10 mg. q.i.d.

(2) Valium 5 mg. t.i.d. (Use IV if anxiety is extreme.)

(3) Phenobarbital 1 gr. tab. q.i.d. P.O.

(4) Noludar 300 to 600 mg. h.s.

4-4. PERSONALITY OR CHARACTER BEHAVIOR DISORDERS. Characterized by defects in the development or structure of the personality, rather than by mental, somatic, or emotional symptoms. These include the antisocial and amoral personality and the sexual deviate. We find this kind of disturbance the most difficult to accept as an illness. These persons seem unable to learn from experience, are incapable of conforming to ordinary rules of society, and are often the "troublemakers" and/or "wise guys." The basic types of personality or character behavior disorders are inadequate or immature personality, emotionally unstable personality, passive-aggressive personality, compulsive personality, and the schizoid personality.

S. and O. (1) Symptoms of inadequate or immature personality are: Failure in emotional, economic, and occupational adjustments. Often good natured and easy going, but inept, ineffective, and unconcerned. Egocentric with childish mannerisms such as temper tantrums, bedwetting, sleepwalking, etc. Difficulty adjusting to new situations, accepting new responsibilities, or in getting along with fellow workers. Often AWOL. Functional somatic complaints with no organic cause such as headache, pain in chest, G.I. disturbance. Often presents self at sick call as an "unwilling warrior." A young man, first enlistment, unwilling to work, etc. He tries to manipulate his environment and those about him to achieve his own ends.

(2) Symptoms of emotionally unstable personality are: Marked tendency to swing and act with his own emotional mood. Exercises little or no restraint. Euphoric, talkative, and "having a ball" with no regard to the consequences of his actions. Anger, temper tantrums, and "mad at the world." A gesture of suicide. This is an attempt to gain some goal, gain concern, show of affection, or removal from a situation. This is not planned to end fatally, but sometimes does.

(3) Symptom of passive aggressive personality are: Antagonistic and subjective to pouting. May be destructive. Stubborn with cynical "biting wit." Shrewd, knows just how far he can go and does. May be manifested by helplessness, a tendency to cling to others as "mama's boy."

(4) Others have such variable range of symptoms that they defy a specific listing.

A. Personality or character behavior disorder.

P. The most important factor is recognizing a person has psychiatric problems and referring him for prompt treatment; do not waste time attempting to diagnose his illness. Try to understand yourself and be aware of your feelings toward the patient. Sometimes it is hard to remember he is sick when his behavior is unreasonable. Try to understand the patient by being an expert observer. What does he tell you by his behavior? "All behavior has meaning." Be an interested and sympathetic listener. This is one of the most effective tools in working with disturbed patients. Giving advice is rarely of any help. Paraldehyde is the drug of choice for any disturbed patient. Opiates are contraindicated. When restraining a combatant patient, be careful that you do not get injured. Keep accurate, comprehensive reports regarding all aspects of the case. These must be kept confidential and it is best for the patient that they are kept from him. Let the psychiatrist decide how much, if any, to tell him.

4-5. ORGANIC BRAIN SYNDROMES. Caused by organic impairment of the brain due to trauma, tumors, circulatory disturbances, metabolic disturbances, convulsive disorders, toxic or intoxicated states.

S. and O. Defects in memory (most recent events). Disorientation as to time, place, person. Sudden personality change with irritability most notable. Hallucinations and delusions. Convulsions to coma.

A. Organic brain syndromes.

P. Depends on the severity of the problem; treat according to the primary presenting symptom. Avoid an aggressive dictatorial attitude. Be calm and treat patient with kindness and understanding. Never argue with a mentally disturbed patient of any kind. If restraint or a treatment is in his best interest, then perform that treatment with a minimum of fuss. Get help as necessary. Even severely disturbed patients tend to respond much better to the calm, straightforward, businesslike approach.

4-6. DISASTER REACTIONS. In this case a disaster does not necessarily involve groups of people; a disaster can pertain to one individual.

a. Emotional injuries are not as visible as a wound or a broken leg, but severe fear, excessive worry, guilt, depression, or overexcitement is evidence that emotional damage has occurred.

b. It is normal for an injured person to feel upset. The more severe the injury, the more insecure and fearful he becomes, especially if the injury is to a highly valued body part. For example, an injury to the eyes or genitals, even if relatively minor, is likely to be severely upsetting. An injury to some other part of the body may be especially disturbing to an individual for his own particular reason. For example, an injury to the hand may be terrifying to a baseball pitcher or pianist, and a facial disfigurement may be especially threatening to some men and most women.

b. Fear, insecurity, anxiety, or guilt may cause the patient to be irritable, stubborn, or unreasonable; he may seem uncooperative, unnecessarily difficult, or even emotionally irrational.

c. The goals in treatment of disaster reactions are to return the individual to work as soon as possible. Minimize his immediate disability even if prompt return to work is not possible, decrease the intensity of his emotional reaction until more complete care (if needed) can be arranged, and prevent actions harmful to him and to efforts of others.

d. Disaster reactions and helpful measures.

(1) Normal reactions are trembling, muscular tension, perspiration, nausea, mild diarrhea, urinary frequency, pounding heart, rapid breathing, and anxiety.

(2) Underactive reactions (slowed down, numbed) are the most common reaction to disaster. Symptoms are vacant expression, standing or sitting without moving or talking, and individual appears to be without emotion.

Helpful measures include: Establish contact gently--offer a cup of coffee, drink of water, or a smoke, use his name, encourage him to talk and be a good listener. Try to get him to tell you in his own words what actually happened. Show empathy but don't overwhelm him with pity. Find him a simple routine job to do.

(3) Overactive reactions. The individual is argumentative, talks rapidly, jumps right into jobs, and works hard but doesn't complete one thing before starting something else (jumps from job to job), and he usually makes endless suggestions.

Help measures include: Let them talk about it (don't argue with them, and be aware of your own feelings), give them something warm to eat or drink or a smoke, and give them jobs requiring physical activity (make sure they are supervised on the job).

(4) Individual panic (blind flight) is not a common reaction. Symptoms include wild running about, unreasoning attempt to flee, loss of judgment, and uncontrolled weeping.

Helpful measures include: Trying kindly firmness first (don't use brutal restraint, strike them, or douse them with water), use sedatives only as last resort, get help (if necessary) to isolate, and show empathy for their problem.

(5) Physical reactions are severe nausea and vomiting and conversion hysteria (can't use some part of the body).

Helpful measures include: Show them you are interested, try to get them to talk about what happened, make them comfortable, don't call attention to their disability, and try to find them some small job to keep them busy and help make them forget their problem.

4-7. DEPRESSION. May occur in reaction to some outside adverse life situation, usually the loss of a loved one through death, divorce, etc.; financial disaster; or loss of an established role. Neurotic depression differs from episodes of normal sadness in that the patient cannot "shake off" the feeling of dejection and the effect is disproportionately intense and enduring. Any illness, severe or mild, can cause significant depression. Corticosteroids, oral contraceptives, antihypertensive medications such as alpha methyldopa, guanethidine, clondine, and propranolol have been associated with the development of depressive syndromes. The appetite-suppressing drugs, while acting initially as stimulants, often result in a depressive syndrome when withdrawn. Alcohol, sedatives, opiates, and most of the psychedelic drugs are depressants. Depression accounts for over half of all attempted suicides. The risk of suicide must always be considered when dealing with a severely depressed patient. Suicidal thought should be inquired after, and any suicidal gesture taken seriously.

S. Somatic complaints such as headache, disrupted or excessive sleep, libido, and anxiety are common in most depressive states. With severe depression there may be delusions of a hypochondriacal or persecutory (paranoid) nature.

O. Lowered mood, varying from sadness to intense feelings of guilt and hopelessness. Difficulty in thinking, inability to concentrate or make decisions is usually present in most depression. In severe depression there may be evidence of psychomotor retardation that may progress into a stuporous condition whereas the patient may lie awake in bed but do nothing of his own accord. Responses to external stimuli may be retarded or absent. In agitated depression the patient may be restless, sad, fearful, and apprehensive. They may pace the floor and wring their hands. They may repeat over and over in an explosive manner such words as "damn." Hallucinations are rare; however, they may complain of bizarre symptoms such as "a rotting brain" or "plugged intestines." They may be destructive to property and attempt self-injury or suicide.

A. Depression due to ___________. Differential diagnosis: Depression secondary to illness or injury (e.g., brain trauma, tumor, etc.) or drug intake.

P. Show empathy. Observe patient without making them feel they are being watched. Try to get the patient to ventilate. NOTE: Do this by making it obvious that you are sincerely interested in the patient's problems and by being a good listener. Don't interrogate. If the patient is agitated, sedate with either antipsychotic or anxiety drugs (see paragraph 4-3, 4-4). If agitation is extreme or medication is refused, give Valium IM or IV. Be constantly alert for a suicide attempt and evacuate when feasible.

4-8. ALCOHOLISM. There are as many explanations for the cause of alcoholism as there are alcoholics. Professional investigators even disagree on many points. Our society is oriented around an alcohol-serving social environment such as beer ball games, initiation rites, wetting down parties, rating parties, retirement parties, and almost any other excuse that 2 or more people can come up with. Alcohol is a C.N.S. depressant, in any amount, even though the sense of euphoria caused by depression of the inhibitions leads the uninitiated to claim that it is a stimulant. A practical working definition of alcoholism is: When the intake of alcohol interferes in any way with a person's job, family, physical condition, or interpersonal relationships, that person can be considered an alcoholic. It does not matter whether the person drinks all the time, rare binges, or only one drink if the above criteria are met.

a. Alcoholism is classified as:

(1) Episodic excessive drinking: Characterized by becoming intoxicated as often as 4 times per year.

(2) Habitual excessive drinking: The person becomes intoxicated more than 12 times per year or is recognizably under the influence of alcohol more than once per week.

(3) Alcohol dependence or addiction: Determined by direct evidence such as withdrawal symptoms or by strong presumptive evidence such as inability to go 1 day without drinking or continued heavy drinking in excess of three months.

b. There are many problems associated with alcoholism but the most common is delirium tremens (DTs) or alcohol withdrawal syndrome. DTs are caused by withdrawal from drinking after a period of heavy continuous drinking. Usually occurs about 48 to 72 hours after the last drinking bout.

S. and O. Attacks begin with an aversion to food, anorexia, nausea, vomiting and abdominal cramps, anxiety, restlessness, apprehension and irritability, diaphoresis, tremors, talking or mumbling continuously. Picks at imaginary objects in the air, on self, on the bed, etc. Progresses to hallucinations and nocturnal illusions, fleeting at first then becoming constant. These are primarily visual and often are animal in nature with tigers, elephants, bugs, rats, and snakes all being imagined. These hallucinations often incite terror. Patient is suggestive to sensory stimuli, especially to objects seen in dim light. Vestibular disturbances are a common complaint. He complains that the bed is rocking, the room is rotating, and even that the world is "spinning and he is afraid of flying off." The patient may have a grand mal seizure known as "Rum Fit."

A. DTs or alcohol withdrawal syndrome.

P. Place patient on bedrest in a well-lighted space. Avoid loud noises and do not leave him alone. Someone should be present to talk to him and reassure him at all times. Restraints are to be used only when absolutely necessary and then removed as soon as possible. Mylanta or Amphojel may be given to settle G.I. distress. IV therapy with vitamin supplement diet. Maintain sufficient hydration to ensure an output of 25 to 40 cc. per hour of urine. Keep input and output chart. Medications to sedate man should be used with caution since alcohol and tranquilizers do not mix. Sedate with 15 to 20 ml. paraldehyde IM.

Prophylaxis: When a heavy or binge drinker gets a severe case of the "shakes" 2 to 3 days after he has had a drink, the following measures may be used.

a. Valium for acute alcohol withdrawal 10 mg. IM or IV initially then 5 to 10 mg. q.3-4h. if necessary. Continue for 3-4 days as needed then give Valium 5-10 mg. P.O. q.i.d. as necessary.

b. Force fluids and diet balanced with vitamin supplements including B complex.

4-9. DRUG ABUSE.

a. LSD, marihuana, alcohol, and barbituate intoxication are covered in Chapter 14, NBC.

b. Stimulants (amphetamines and cocaine).

S. and O. Acute amphetamine intoxication includes sweating, tachycardia, elevated blood pressure, hyperactivity, dilation of the pupils, and acute brain syndrome with confusion and disorientation.

A. Stimulants.

P. Stimulants can be withdrawn abruptly and withdrawal usually results in lassitude, prolonged sleep, increased hunger and eating, and depression lasting several days to several weeks. Occasionally 3-10 days after discontinuing amphetamines, an abstinence syndrome develops with delirium, sleeplessness, and increased motor activity.

c. Opiate dependency. (opium, heroin, methadone, morphine, meperidine and codeine). Sudden withdrawal from narcotics is not dangerous.

S. and O. (1) Mild intoxication: Analgesia, feeling of euphoria and carefree relaxation, drowsiness, mood changes, mental clouding, occasional anxiety, frequent nausea, occasional vomiting, contracted pupils, and decreased G.I. function.

(2) Overdosage causes respiratory depression up to and including respiratory arrest, nausea and vomiting, deep sleep to coma, pinpoint pupils, peripheral vasodilation, and massive pulmonary edema.

(3) Withdrawal causes craving and anxiety within 4 hours. Yawning, tearing, runny nose, and sweating in 8 hours. Plus pupil dilation, piloerection, tremors, hot and cold flashes, aching bones and muscles, and anorexia in 12 hours. Increased intensity of the above plus insomnia restlessness and nausea, increased B.P., temperature, pulse, and respiration in 18-24 hours. Increased intensity of the above plus curled up position, vomiting, diarrhea, weight loss (about 5 lbs a day), spontaneous ejaculation or orgasm, hemoconcentration, leukocytosis, eosinopenia, and hyperglycemia in 24-36 hours.

A. Opiates. Differential diagnosis: Mild intoxication and overdose are difficult to distinguish from other drug reactions without track marks and fairly reliable history.

P. Overdose. Give antagonist such as Narcan (naloxone).4 mg. IV can be repeated at 5-10 minutes intervals. Results are dramatic. Supportive care and treat complications. Close observation x 24 hours.

CHAPTER 5

NUTRITIONAL DISEASES AND DEFICIENCIES

5-1. GENERAL. Nutritional diseases and deficiencies are usually related directly to ignorance of sound nutritional practice and to poverty. Many people exist on a diet based almost exclusively on one principal starchy staple food--rice, millet, or corn for example. Another factor is parasitic and infectious diseases. These contribute to decreased intestinal absorption, sometimes to increased requirements, and usually to some degree of anorexia. These create a vicious progressive spiral where a diet deficiency is compounded. In most cases where you find evidence of a marked deficiency of one particular substance or group of substances, other deficiencies also exist. The single most important thing in the treatment of nutritional diseases is starting a completely adequate diet.

5-2. PELLAGRA (mal de la rosa, psilosis pigmentosa, Alpine scurvy, or chichism). The principal manifestation of a severe deficiency of niacin, usually complicated by deficiencies of other B vitamins. It is found worldwide and is usually associated with diets high in corn and containing little or no meat, milk, fish, or other good sources of protein. The disease is more prevalent during the spring.

S. Onset is gradual with loss of strength, loss of weight, and sore, red tongue. Dermatitis may occur. Diarrhea or alternating periods of diarrhea and constipation may occur.

O. Look for red tongue, gastrointestinal disturbances, psychic disturbances, and dermatitis. The tongue is swollen, denuded of its papillae (glossitis), and often painful and extremely sensitive. The dermatitis, characteristically, is symmetrically distributed. In most instances it is restricted to parts exposed to the sun. In the early stages the rash resembles a sunburn. This may be followed by vesiculation and bulla formation. The skin becomes thickened and roughened, and as the acute inflammation subsides, the brownish pigmentation remains. Repeated attacks lead to marked atrophy of the skin. The psychic disturbances in the early stages are that of neurasthenia, which increases in severity with progression of the disease. In advanced and long-standing cases, true psychoses occur. In these cases, spastic gait, peripheral neuritis, and other indications of organic involvement are not uncommon.

A. Pellagra (lack of nicotinic acid and tryptophan in the diet).

P. High protein, high vitamin diet. Nicotinic acid or niacinamide 50-500 mg. daily oral or injection. Give therapeutic doses of thiamine, riboflavin, and pyridoxine daily.

5-3. BERIBERI. Caused by a deficiency in vitamin B1 (thiamine hydrochloride) and other vitamins, and is found in areas where the diet consists primarily of polished rice, white flour, and other nonvitamin bearing foods. Increased need for vitamin B1; fever, high carbohydrate intake, or alcoholism may lead to deficiency.

S. Onset is usually gradual with progressive weakness of the most used muscle groups (most commonly in extensor muscles of the thigh). In many instances, patient is unable to rise from squatting position.

O. Atrophy of the muscles most used. Sensory disturbances

(hyperesthesia or hypoesthesia) usually appear at the same time but are usually less prominent. In severe cases many muscle groups may be affected and you see flaccid paralysis, muscular atrophy, with or without evidence of cardiac enlargement, and tachycardia.

With a more serious form (wet beriberi), the clinical picture is predominantly that of acute congestive heart failure with relatively little evidence of nervous system involvement. The onset is frequently rapid and acute, and the marked edema may mask the presence of muscle atrophy. Sudden collapse occurs frequently.

A. Vitamin B1 (thiamine) deficiency (beriberi). Differential diagnosis: Tabes dorsalis, post diphtheritic paralysis, and acute heart failure resulting from other causes.

P. Thiamine hydrochloride 20-50 mg. orally IV or IM in divided doses daily x 2 weeks then 10 mg. daily orally. Alternative: Dried yeast tablets (brewer's yeast) 30 gm. t.i.d. Well balanced diet of 2,500-4,500 calories a day when tolerated.

Prognosis: Recovery is rapid and complete in infants and small children. Recovery is slow in adults and there may be permanent disability, such as muscle weakness or flaccid paralysis, due to nerve cell degeneration. In the acute form of wet beriberi, deaths are frequent.

5-4. SPRUE (psilosis, Ceylon sore mouth, malabsorption syndrome). Sprue syndromes are diseases of disturbed small intestine function characterized by impaired absorption, particularly of fats, and motor abnormalities. It is not associated with any particular diet or dietary deficiency. Characteristically affects white upper-class individuals of long residence in endemic areas. Occurs in Far East, Puerto Rico, sporadically in U.S., and rarely in Africa.

S. Main symptom is diarrhea, explosive and watery at first, later stools are fewer, more solid, and characteristically pale, frothy, foul-smelling, and greasy. Patient has sore tongue and mouth and flatulent indigestion. Abdominal cramps, weight loss (often marked), pallor, irritability, muscle cramps, and weakness may occur.

O. Paresthesia (abnormal sensation from numbness to heightened sensitivity), asthenia (lack or loss of strength), abdominal distention, and mild tenderness are present. At first there are small painful ulcers on the tongue and buccal mucosa. Later the tongue becomes acutely inflamed and denuded. The ulcers can extend into the pharynx and esophagus and may cause dysphagia. Signs and symptoms of multiple vitamin deficiencies will be found in severe cases.

A. Sprue (malabsorption syndrome). Differential diagnosis: Anatomic abnormalities (fistulas, blind loops, jejunal diverticulosis) or regional enteritis.

P. Folic acid 10-20 mg. daily orally or IM for 2-4 weeks until remission of symptoms, then 5 mg. folic acid daily, tetracycline 250 mg. q.i.d. x 10 days. High calorie, high protein, low fat diet. Multiple vitamins should be given daily.

5-5. PROTEIN AND CALORIE MALNUTRITION.

a. Kwashiorkor (malignant malnutrition). Caused by inadequate proteins with adequate calories. Usually occurs in infants after weaning but may occur in children of any age and even in adults. Occurs wherever people subsist on starchy staple foods without adequate protein supplements.

S. Irritability, apathy, skin changes (rash, desquamation, depigmentation or hyperpigmentation, ulceration), inflammation of lips and mouth, conjunctivitis, sparse or depigmented hair, anorexia, vomiting, and diarrhea.

O. Growth and maturation are retarded, muscular wasting, edema (usually starts in the feet and lower legs but may affect any part of the body including the face). Liver enlargement also occurs and may or may not be palpable. R.B.C. nearly always shows moderate anemia.

A. Kwashiorkor.

P. Restore and maintain fluid and electrolyte balance. All but the most severely ill respond to a diet based on milk; dilute milk feeding can usually be introducted after 24 h. Sufficient milk should be given to supply 2-5 gm of protein/kg./day. At this stage, more calories in the form of sugar and cereal may be added to the diet to provide 150-250 k cal/kg./day. Correct remaining vitamin and mineral deficiencies. Small frequent feeding around the clock are tolerated best in early stages of recovery. Antibiotics may be indicated, but treatment of malaria and other parasitic infections should be delayed until patient is clinically improved. Whole blood is contraindicated unless Hb is < 4 gm%.

b. Marasmus. Total starvation, a protein and calorie malnutrition.

S. Constant hunger; thin, emaciated body but protuberant abdomen.

O. Retarded growth; atrophy of muscle tissue; skin is loose and wrinkled, especially around the buttocks, and when pinched between thumb and forefinger, shows almost a complete absence of subcutaneous fat. No edema; face is drawn and monkeylike. Diarrhea and anemia are frequent but not always present.

A. Marasmus.

P. Initial feedings should be slow and increased gradually There must be adaquate intake of calories and protein; same treatment as for kwashiorkor.

5-6. SIMPLE GOITER (endemic goiter). An enlargement of the thyroid gland without either hyper- or hypothyroidism due to lack of iodine in the diet. Can be due to excess intake of goitrogenic vegetables (rutabagas, turnips, cabbage, mustard seeds).

S. In the majority of cases there are no symptoms or symptoms resulting from compression of the structures in the neck and chest (wheezing, dysphagia, respiratory embarrassment).

O. Swelling of neck, palpable thyroid gland often extremely large.

A. Simple goiter. Differential diagnosis: Toxic, diffuse, or modular goiter.

P. Iodine therapy 5 gtt. daily S.S.K.I. (saturated solution of potassium iodine) or 5-10 gtt. of a strong iodine solution in a glass of water. Continue until gland returns to normal size, then place patient on maintainance dose 1-2 gtt. daily or use iodized table salt.

5-7. OSTEOMALACIA (rickets). A calcium-phosphorus deficiency primarily of women, particularly during pregnancy and lactation; can be secondary to disorders in fat absorption (sprue, diarrhea, pancreatitis) or due to prolonged use of aluminum hydroxide gels, causing chronic phosphate depletion.

S. Usually mild aching of the bones, particularly long bones and ribs, muscular weakness, and listlessness.

O. Bony tenderness is common and severe tetany may occur. Bones become soft and flexible; deformities are more frequently caused by bones bending (bowing) rather than fractures, particularly in the legs, thorax, and spine.

A. Rickets. Differential diagnosis: Arthritis, osteoporosis, osteogenesis imperfecta.

P. Treatment can only protect against further deformities. Diet high in calcium and phosphorus, 25-100 thousand units vitamin D daily. Treat contributing disease if present.

5-8. SCURVY. Due to inadequate intake of vitamin C, but may occur with increased metabolic needs or decreased absorption. Frequently seen in formula-fed infants, elderly bachelors, and food fadists.

S. Mild or early manifestations are edema and bleeding of the gums. Severe or late manifestations are swelling of the joints, marked bleeding tendency, loosening or loss of teeth, poor wound healing, or in severe cases old scar tissue breaking down and reopening of healed wounds.

O. Mild or early manifestations are porosity of dentine and hyperkeratotic hair follicles. In severe or late cases, patient bruises easily, severe muscle changes, and anemia.

A. Vitamin C deficiency (scurvy).

P. a. Ascorbic acid 50 mg. q.i.d. x 1 wk in infantile scurvy then 50 mg. t.i.d. x 1 mo with prophylactic doses (25-30 mg./day) supplemented by orange or tomato juice. In vomiting or diarrhea, give one-half oral dose IM or IV as sodium ascorbate.

b. For adult scurvy, 250 mg q.i.d. until asymptomatic. When parenteral therapy is required, give sodium ascorbate at the same dosage. Ascorbic acid 300-500 mg./day P.O. in divided doses should be given for several months in chronic scurvy with gingivitis, repeated hemorrhagic manifestation, or joint symptoms.

5-9. VITAMIN A DEFICIENCY. Fat-soluble vitamin necessary for normal function and structure of all epithelial cells and for synthesis of visual purple in retinal rods (night vision). Toxic if too much is ingested (e.g., seal and polar bear liver).

S. Mild or early manifestations are dryness of skin and night blindness.

O. Mild or early manifestation of follicular hyperkeratosis. In late or severe cases, softening of cornea, dryness of conjunctiva, atrophy and keratinization of the skin.

A. Vitamin A deficiency usually in conjunction with other deficiencies.

P. Oleovitamin A, 15-25 thousand units once or twice a day orally. If absorption defect is present, give same dosage IM. Care must be used as minimum toxic dose in adults is about 75-100 thousand units daily.

S and S for hypervitaminosis A are anorexia, loss of weight, dry and fissured skin, brittle nails, hair loss, gingivitis, splenomegaly, anemia, and C.N.S. manifestations.

CHAPTER 6

PEDIATRICS

6-1. The pediatric patient may mean the neonate (up to 4 weeks), the infant (1 month to 1 year), the child (1 year to 6 years), or the preadolescent (6 years to 12 years). The treatment and drug dosage of a 9-pound infant may be vastly different from an 11-year-old preadolescent. The adolescent will be treated generally as an adult (over 12 years old). For purposes of identification, specify the age and the approximate weight of the pediatric patient. In assessing the seriousness or chronicity of a disease in the pediatric patient, steadily increasing height and weight is not the sign of a very sick patient. A fat child who remains fat is generally not very sick or at least not chronically sick. A child with good appetite is rarely very sick.

a. History is the most important single factor in making a proper assessment for many pediatric problems. It should be obtained from the mother or guardian. If the child is old enough to talk, you can obtain much valuable information from him or her. Allow the informants to present the problem as they see it, then fill in the necessary past and family history and pertinent information.

b. Examination of pediatric patients, except newborn and infant, follows the same procedures as the examination of adult patients.

(1) Newborn examination.

(a) General appearance. The prime concern in the first few minutes of life is respiration. A crying baby has a good respiration.

(b) Skin color. Definite jaundice in the first 24 hours is pathologic and means infection, erythroblastosis (Rh factor), or prematurity.

(c) Extremities. All should move erratically.

(d) Reflexes. Sucking reflex should be present at birth.

(e) Digits. The fingers and toes may be cyanotic, but the trunk should be pink. A baby depressed from too much anesthesia at birth, prematurity, or difficult labor will lack some of the above. Try mildly painful stimulation (pinch); it may bring the baby out of its depression.

(2) Infant examination. Every child should receive a complete systematic examination <u>periodically</u>.

(a) Child should be observed from the time he or she is first brought into the room and during the entire examination.

(b) A friendly manner, quiet voice, and a slow and easy approach will usually help in the examination; if not, proceed as gently as possible in an orderly and systematic manner.

(c) Holding for examination. Before 6 months of age an infant will usually tolerate an examination table. From 6 months to 3 or 4 years of age most examinations can be performed best while the child is held in the parent's lap or over the shoulder.

(d) Parents should remove their child's clothing. If you must remove the child's clothing, do it gradually to prevent chilling or alarming the child.

(e) It is usually best to begin by examining an area unlikely to be associated with pain or discomfort. Painful/uncomfortable areas should be examined last.

(f) Take and record height, weight, and head circumference at each examination. These measurements give information regarding patterns of growth when compared with previous examination measurements.

c. The newborn generally weighs 7-1/2 pounds (3.4 kg.) in modern countries; in deprived countries, weight will probably be less than 7-1/2 pounds. Any newborn less than 5-1/2 pounds (2,500 gm or 2.5 kg.) is by definition "premature" regardless of the length of pregnancy and will require more care, have less chance of survival, and will grow and mature slower. A normal term infant's birth weight should at least double in 5 months and triple in 12 months.

d. Vital signs:

	Pulse/min	Respiration/min	B.P. (Systolic)
(1) Birth	140	40	60-80
(2) Six months	110	30	90
(3) One year	100	28	90
(4) Three to four years	95	25	100
(5) Five to ten years	90	24	100

e. Laboratory norms for infant and child:

	Birth	Three months	One year	Five years
(1) Hb	16-20	10-11	12-13	12.5 - 13.5
(2) W.B.C.	10-20,000	5-9,000	6-10,000	6-10,000
(3) HCT	50-60	30-33	35-36	38-41
(4) Neutrophils	45-55%	30-40%	35-45%	40-50%
(5) Lymphs	30-45%	50-60%	50-60%	45-55%

f. Calculating drug dosages (Young's Rule):

For children over 2: $$\text{Child dose} = \frac{\text{age (years)} \times \text{adult dose}}{\text{age} + 12}$$

For children under 2: $$\text{Child dose} = \frac{\text{age in months} \times \text{adult dose}}{150}$$

g. Feeding. The child must be fed by frequent intake of fluid and calories. A schedule of feeding is not necessary. A sick child must be encouraged to eat or drink.

(1) Breast feeding. This is usually superior to bottle feeding. Make sure the mother has no breast infection, she has milk, and the infant can suck properly. The infant receives all the vitamins and nutriments that are required if the mother is healthy and is receiving proper nutrition (it never hurts to give supplemental daily multivitamins to a breast-feeding mother).

(2) Bottle feeding. The infant may be fed by breast alternating with bottle or with bottle alone. If milk formula is not available, one will have to be improvised.

(3) Nutritional requirements:

(a) Calories per day. First year, 50 calories per pound (about 1,000 calories per day at age one year).

(b) Fluid. Two to three ounces per pound per day. Feedings may be given as often as possible to the sick child if the child will take it, unless some medical contraindication exists. The healthy child may eat from three to eight times daily.

(c) Caloric content:

1. Cow milk = 20 calories per ounce.

2. Evaporated milk = 40 calories per ounce.

3. Sugar = 120 calories per ounce or 60 calories per tablespoon.

(d) Milk will provide enough sodium, potassium, calcium, etc. to nourish any child temporarily, but if it is not fortified, it must be supplemented with iron and vitamin C and D. Be sure the milk is pasteurized. If there is a doubt, boil (15 seconds at a rolling boil is required).

(4) Improvising a formula. The formula should be about as thick or viscous as cow's milk. It should be reasonably palatable. Taste it yourself; if it tastes bad to you, the child may not take it. It should be comfortably warm. The bottles should be sterilized. If bottles are not available, spoon feed or drip the milk in with syringe or tubing. A good oral solution can be made using 5 percent dextrose, 1 tablespoon of sugar, and 1/2 teaspoon of salt per liter and is especially useful in a dehydrated patient who is not vomiting. It provides fluid, calories, and salt, but if it is to be used for extended periods, it must be fortified with vitamins.

6-2. THE DEHYDRATED CHILD. Newborns and infants can become dehydrated fairly rapidly due to illness or lack of fluid intake.

S. Fever; dry skin, mucous membranes, and tongue; sunken eyeballs; poor skin turgor, and depressed fontanelles.

O. Decreased or no urine output; urine dark and concentrated with a high specific gravity and a high hematocrit.

A. Dehydrated child.

P. Fluid replacement is of prime importance. If the dehydration is not severe and the patient can take fluids by mouth, then fluids should be forced. If the dehydration is severe or the patient cannot take fluids by mouth, then fluids must be replaced IV. Do not try to replace all the fluid deficit in a short period as it may throw the child into shock. Estimate the fluid deficit. Figure the daily requirement.

Maintenance fluid requirement:

0 - 10 kg. 100 cc./kg.

11 - 20 kg. $\frac{100 \text{ cc./kg.}}{10}$ + 50 cc./kg.

21 kg. and over $\frac{100 \text{ cc./kg.}}{20}$ + 50 cc./kg. + 25 cc.

Then give the daily requirement plus 1/2 of the deficit over the first 24 hours. (A good replacement fluid is 1/4 strength normal saline in 50% D5W.)

Patient should be catheterized and urine output monitored closely. You are looking for a return to good skin turgor, moist mucous membranes and tongue, and lightening of the urine. Lowering of urine specific gravity is your most important sign. Treat the cause, e.g., fever, throat infection, etc.

6-3. FEVER OF UNDETERMINED ORIGIN (FUO).

a. Fever is generally a sign of infection, but infants can spike fever for almost any reason (e.g., cutting teeth, constipation, reaction to diet, allergy, diaper rash, etc.). Fevers due to infections are usually low-grade in adults but may be much higher in infants and young children. Children often convulse with temperatures over 104o F. (occasionally at lower temperatures).

b. Treatment. Initially, lowering the temperature (if it is 104o F. or above) is of primary importance. Give Tylenol (Tempra, acetaminophen) 10 mg./kg. q.4h. if child is less than 1 year old; give aspirin 65 mg./yr of age q.6h. first if child is 1 year or older. Then give a sponge bath or alcohol bath to cool the body. The patient must be monitored closely and baths repeated as needed to keep the temperature down. If unexplained fever has been present over 24 hours, a white count and differential should be done. Ideally, the patient should be treated for the specific disease; however, if a diagnosis can't be made, broad spectrum antibiotics will often cure the infection. Tetracycline should not be used in the premature and can stain teeth in children even if used for short periods. Additional treatment consists of nursing care and maintaining fluid and caloric intake.

6-4. DIAPER RASH. A form of primary irritant contact dermatitis due to prolonged contact of the skin to a combination of urine and feces.

S. and O. Erythema; thickening on the skin in the perineal area; beefy red, sharply marginated lesions with satellites; and a history of skin contact with urine and feces.

A. Diaper rash. Differential diagnosis: Other forms of primary irritant contact dermatitis.

P. Frequent diaper changes. Avoid rubber or plastic pants. Talcum powder can be used as an absorbent. Corn starch should not be used as it is a media in which C. albicans flourishes (80 percent of cases lasting more than 4 days are caused by C. albicans). Apply Mycostatin (nystatin, Mycolog) cream or Silvadine ointment with each diaper change. In extremely inflammatory diaper rash, 1% hydrocortisone cream can be alternated with Mycostatin at every other diaper change.

6-5. CHICKEN POX (VARICELLA). Primarily a disease of childhood, but in large areas of the tropics it is principally an adult disease. Varicella and herpes zoster are caused by the same virus, with varicella being the primary infection and herpes zoster being a recurrent infection. Varicella is highly contagious (80-90 percent of exposed susceptibles are infected).

S. History of contact 10-20 days (average 12-13 days) prior to onset. Usually no prodrome, but a mild fever with itchy and runny nose is sometimes seen 1-3 days before rash appears. Onset is usually abrupt with the appearance of the rash. Systemic symptoms, if any, are mild.

O. Rash appears in crops, with faint erythematous macules rapidly developing into papules and vesicles. The vesicles are thin-walled and superficially located on the skin with distinct areolas (dewdrop on red base) that rupture easily and rapidly encrust. Successive crops (usually 3) appear in the next 2-5 days, giving rise to lesions in all stages being seen at one time. Rash is heaviest on the trunk and lighter on the extremities. If a secondary bacterial infection does not develop, the crusts fall off in 1-3 weeks, leaving no scars. Varicella can vary from a mild disease with few vesicles to a severe disease with as many as 5 crops of lesions covering most of the skin. Systemic symptoms, which are usually mild or absent, may be severe and generally parallel the extent of skin involvement. Usually laboratory tests are of little aid, although sepsis may be accompanied by an abrupt rise of neutrophilia in the W.B.C.

A. Chicken Pox. Differential diagnosis: Severe forms--smallpox, impetigo, multiple insect bites, papular urticaria, rickettsialpox, and dermatitis herpetiformis.

P. Symptomatic. Fluids, control of itching with antihistamines, attention to cleanliness (handwashing, bathing), antipyretics as needed. Treat secondary infections.

6-6. SCARLET FEVER. A formerly common ailment that is rarely seen today, probably because antibiotic therapy prevents the opportunity for the streptococcus to progress in individual patients or to create massive epidemics. Scarlet fever is associated with Group A streptococcal strains that produce an erythrogenic toxin, leading to a diffuse pink-red cutaneous blush that blanches on pressure. The rash, an additional feature of an illness that otherwise resembles streptococcal pharyngitis, is best seen on the abdomen, on the lateral chest, and in the cutaneous folds.

S. and O. Along with the characteristic manifestations of the rash are circumoral pallor surrounded by a flushed face, a "strawberry tongue" (inflamed beefy red papillae protruding through a white coating), and Pastia's lines (dark red lines in the creases of skin folds). The upper layer of the previously reddened skin often desquamates after the fever subsides.

A. Scarlet fever due to Group A streptococcus.

P. The course and management of scarlet fever are essentially the same as for other clinically evident Group A infections.

6-7. MUMPS (PAROTITIS). A common childhood disease that is asymptomatic in 30-40 percent of cases. Most children are infected and develop lifetime immunity but a few remain susceptible throughout adolescence and adult life.

S. and O. History of contact 14-21 days prior. Bilateral or unilateral painful swelling of the parotid gland is usually the only manifestation. Systemic symptoms may consist of high fever and headache or mild respiratory symptoms or occasionally C.N.S. symptoms that appear prior to or in the absence of parotid gland involvement, or symptoms may be absent. (Mumps virus is the most common cause of meningitis in childhood.) Mild to moderate abdominal pain may be present.

The gonads may be involved (orchitis or oophoritis) in postpubertal individuals with sudden onset of fever, chills, systemic symptoms, and lower abdominal pain in females or extreme testicular pain and testicular swelling in males. Contrary to common belief, mumps, orchitis, and oophoritis do not result in sterility. Symptoms subside in 3-14 days. Mumps usually last approximately 1 week.

A. Mumps. Differential diagnosis: Cervical lymphadenitis of pharynx, tonsillar or skin infection, other parotides, acute lymphoma, or lymphosarcoma.

P. Symptomatic. Control fever, pain, and discomfort. Treat orchitis or oophoritis conservatively with rest, testicular support, and analgesics. Corticosteroids may result in more rapid subsidence of testicular swelling.

6-8. VIRAL CROUP. Most commonly affects children between 3 months and 3 years of age. Characteristically occurs during late fall or early winter and is usually caused by the parainfluenza virus. It can also be caused by respiratory syncytial virus, influenza virus, rubeola virus, or adenoviruses. The major cause of symptoms is inflammation and edema in the subglottic area that can cause significant narrowing of the airway at the level of the cricoid cartilage.

S. Gradual onset, with history of several days upper respiratory tract infection prior to the onset of barking cough and harsh, high-pitched sound during inspiration (inspiratory stridor). If the lower respiratory tract is significantly involved, there may be wheezing. The child may become anxious and restless as hypoxemia and hypercapnia develop.

O. Mild temperature. Possible decreased breath sounds on ausculation. Cyanosis is a late sign and may herald complete airway obstruction. W.B.C. seldom increases to more than 15,000 with no significant leftward shift.

A. Viral Croup. Differential diagnosis: Bacterial croup (epiglottitis).

P. Cool mist therapy. (If vaporizer is not available, improvise by using steam in an enclosed room. Do not let steam go directly on patient as it may cause burns.) Monitor urine specific gravity to insure adequate hydration. Observe patient closely for signs of increasing hypoxia and impending respiratory failure. Keep patient calm and at bed rest. Do not use sedation unless an artificial airway is in place. The most effective method of keeping a child calm is having the mother or some other familiar person present. About 25-30% oxygen can be administered to relieve hypoxia. Patients starting O_2 therapy often have a marked decrease in respiratory effort and should be monitored closely for the first few minutes of oxygen administration.

Bronchial dilators (such as Bronchaid or Primatene Mist) often provide temporary relief of respiratory distress. If commercial preparations are not available, you can make a preparation of 0.5 cc. of epinephrine to 3.5 cc. of sterile water in a spray bottle.

If respiratory distress continues and there is progressively increasing cyanosis and decreasing air entry, an artificial airway must be provided. Generally, endotracheal intubation with a small endotracheal tube is used to reduce trauma to the glottis and subglottic area. (A particularly traumatic tracheal intubation can convert a reversible subglottic narrowing into a fixed nonreversible subglottic narrowing.) The best endotracheal tube care is mandatory and consists of careful tube stabilization and suctioning, postural drainage, chest percussion and humidification of inspired air. If all else fails, a tracheostomy is necessary.

6-9. EPIGLOTTITIS (BACTERIAL CROUP). The most serious form of croup syndrome. It generally affects children 3-7 years old, with no particular seasonal distribution. The most common pathogen is Hemophilus influenzae type B, but beta-hemolytic streptococci and pneumococci have been implicated in rare cases.

S. Abrupt onset over a period of only a few hours. Young children often present with high fever and respiratory distress. Older children may appear toxic and complain of difficulty in swallowing and severe sore throat. Child may have a muffled voice but usually it is not hoarse.

O. Pooling of secretions in the posterior pharynx and drooling are signs caused by extreme dysphagia (inability or difficulty in swallowing). The child, within a few hours, may be in marked respiratory distress with severe inspiratory stridor (harsh, high-pitched sound during inspiration) and retractions. The pharynx is likely to be inflamed. Diagnosis is made by markedly enlarged, friable (easily cracked or broken), "cherry-red" epiglottis. Direct visualization using a tongue blade or laryngoscope is extremely dangerous, as stimulation of the epiglottis has produced laryngeal obstruction and death. No throat cultures should be obtained until epiglottitis has been ruled out or an artificial airway is in place as this may also cause laryngospasm that causes laryngeal obstruction.

Lab findings: W.B.C. of more than 15,000 and a leftward shift is usually present.

P. Once the diagnosis is made, an artificial airway should be introduced. Because of the marked swelling and friability of the tissue, intubation is extremely difficult. A smaller than usual endotracheal tube should be used and a tracheostomy set should be available. An IV should be initiated prior to the intubation and antibiotic therapy can be started by that route. Ampicillin 300 mg./kg./day in 6 divided doses or ampicillin and chloramphenicol are the drugs of choice.

The endotracheal tube should remain in place until the patient is able to breath around the tube easily and when there is a marked decrease in the epiglottic swellings, usually after 24-72 hours. Mortality rate may be as high as 90 without intubation and antibiotic therapy.

6-10. MENINGITIS. See Chapter 2, Section III, Bacterial.

6-11. MEASLES AND GERMAN MEASLES. See Chapter 2, Section IV, Viral.

6-12. DIPHTHERIA. An acute infection of the upper respiratory tract or skin caused by Corynebacterium diphtheriae. A toxin-producing, gram-positive rod with irregular swellings at one end giving it a club-shaped appearance. Irregularly distributed within the rods are granules that stain dark giving them a beaded appearance. The incubation period is 1-6 days.

S. and O. Pharyngeal diphtheria: Mild sore throat, moderate fever, and malaise followed fairly rapidly by severe prostration and circulatory collapse. Pulse is more rapid than temperature would seem to justify. A tenacious and gray membrane, surrounded by a narrow zone of erythema and a broader zone of edema forms in the throat and may spread into the nasopharynx or trachea, producing respiratory obstruction. High fever, prostration, difficulty in swallowing, and noisy breathing develops even without laryngeal obstruction. Cervical lymph nodes become swollen, and swelling is associated with brawny edema of the neck ("bullneck"); palatal paralysis may occur. Bleeding from the nose and mouth are common and petechiae may appear on the skin and mucous membranes.

Nasal diphtheria: Occurs in 2 percent of cases. Serosanguineous (containing serum and blood) nasal discharge and excoriation of the upper lip are characteristic and may be the only symptoms.

Laryngeal diptheria: Occurs in 25 percent of cases, and occasionally may be the only manifestation. Stridor (harsh, high-pitched sound during respiration) is apparent. The progressive laryngeal obstruction can lead to cyanosis and suffocation.

Other forms: Cutaneous, vaginal, or wound diphtheria composes less than 2 percent of all cases and are characterized by ulcerative lesions with membrane formation. They may be very hard to identify in burns or wounds.

Lab findings: W.B.C. is usually normal or slightly elevated. Urinalysis may show proteinuria of a transient nature.

A. Diphtheria. Differential diagnosis: Acute streptococcal pharyngitis, mononucleosis, occasionally other viral pharyngitis, purulent sinusitis, epiglottitis, and viral croup.

P. As the toxin causes the main damage, antitoxin should be administered ASAP. Delay beyond 48 hours must be avoided because antitoxin administered beyond that point may have little effect in altering the incidence or severity of complication. These include myocarditis, toxic polyneuritis, and bronchopneumonia. Sensitivity to horse serum should always be skin tested for before administering the antitoxin. If positive and the diphtheria is severe, give 50 mg. Benadryl IM initially, start an IV of Ringer's lactate or $D_{5}W$ to be used for treatment of anaphylactic shock if necessary, then and only then start an IV to administer the required antitoxin. The patient must be closely monitored for signs of reaction to the antitoxin.

Mild pharyngeal diphtheria or when the membrane is small or confined to the anterior nares or tonsils, 40,000 units. Moderate pharyngeal diphtheria, 80,000 units. Severe pharyngeal or laryngeal diphtheria, 120,000 units regardless of child's weight infused in 200 ml. of isotonic saline over a 30-minute period.

Penicillin V is the drug of choice to eliminate the organism and stop toxin production 250 mg. q.i.d. x 10 days or 600,000 units of procaine Penicillin G IM b.i.d. x 10 days. Alternate is erythromycin 25-50 mg./kg./d. in 4 divided doses orally x 10 days.

Bed rest for 10-14 days is usually required. Strict isolation until antibiotic therapy has made respiratory secretions noninfectious is also required (usually 1-7 days). IV therapy may be necessary. Warm salt water gargles or irrigation are helpful and codeine phosphate 3 mg./kg./d. in 6 divided doses may also help with the discomfort.

Prevention: Routine DPT (diphtheria, pertussis, and tetanus) immunization should be given to all infants and children.

All children exposed to diphtheria should be examined and treated if any signs of early diphtheria show.

All asymptomatic individuals, even if previously immunized, should receive diphtheria toxoid and either erythromycin 20-30 mg./kg./d. in 4 divided doses orally x 10 days or 25,000 U./kg. of benzathine penicillin G.

CHAPTER 7

GYNECOLOGY

7-1. Gynecology encompasses those diseases that are peculiar to women. History and physical examination have certain features that separate them from general ones.

a. History.

(1) Age, gravidity (number of times pregnant), parity (number of live deliveries). Medical records list these, for example, as G3P2Ab1 (three pregnancies; two deliveries; one abortion, either spontaneous or induced).

(2) Chief complaints, in the patient's words, in order of severity.

(3) Present illness. A chronological order of symptoms with details.

(4) Past medical/surgical history in chronological order from childhood through the present, with the complications and treatments for each. All operations and injuries with dates and outcomes.

(5) Obstetrical history. Number of pregnancies, duration of pregnancies and labor details, weight and sex of infants, stillbirths and abortions.

(6) Family history. Age and health of parents and siblings. Family history of any tuberculosis, diabetes, hypertension, bleeding disorders, heart disease, cancer.

(7) Marital and/or cohabitation history. Duration and compatibility of past and present relationships, ages and causes of deaths, if any, and ages and health of children, if any.

(8) Social history. Occupation, hazards, alcohol and tobacco consumption habits, drug usage, sleep and exercise habits, and general activities.

(9) Review of systems. Same as a general history, except for genitourinary. Menarche (age at onset of menstruation), last menstrual period, regularity, duration, amount and character of flow, spotting, discharges, and pain.

b. Examination. Same as the general examination except for:

(1) Breasts. Size, shape equality of both sides, masses, tenderness, scars, or nipple discharge. Breast examination is performed by gentle palpation in a circular fashion from the nipple to the outside, also covering the nodes under the arms. Attempt to express a discharge from the breast nipple as well. Perform this maneuver with the patient's arms down at the sides and over her head, in the supine position.

(2) Pelvic examination.

(a) Drape a sheet over the patient in the supine position

with her legs flexed and spread open. Have a female assistant at your side or at the patient's side for support. Obtain a good direct light source, a water-base lubricant such as KY jelly, and surgically clean gloves.

(b) Genitalia. Look for inflamed, hypertrophied, atrophied, ulcerated, or any other abnormal areas; vaginal discharge; clitoral abnormalities; skin changes over the perineum, thighs, pubis, or perianal region. Check the urethral meatus for redness, exudates from the labial gland ducts, etc.

(c) If pathological study assistance is available, obtain vaginal mucus from the posterior of the vagina for cell studies.

(d) Insert a comfortably warm speculum into the vagina. Ask the patient to relax and bear down. Carefully spread the labia with a gloved hand, insert the speculum blades slowly downward and inward, watching the insert closely. As the cervix is approached, slowly open the blades and allow the blades to straddle the cervix between them. Lock the screw lock.

(e) Inspect the cervix. Obtain cervical mucus from the cervical entrance and from any irregular lesions or sites. Insure the cervical size is not excessively large or small in proportion to the vagina. The cervix should be smooth with no large lacerations, no wide opening, of a pink color, and without blood or discharge.

(f) Unlock blades and slowly withdraw them. Watch for pink folds of the vaginal walls without blood or discharge or lesions. Leaving the blades at the introitus, or vaginal opening, ask the patient to again bear down. A drooping of the cervix indicates decensus, or loss of support, of the uterus itself. Drooping of the vaginal roof may indicate cystocele; protrusion of the vaginal floor upward may indicate rectocele. These will be explained. Take smears of any questionable exudates.

(g) Bimanual palpation.

1. Place one palm down on the abdomen as you stand between the patient's legs. Slightly flex the fingers. Press down firmly. Have the patient take shallow, rapid breaths to aid in relaxation.

2. With the other hand, gloved and coated with a small amount of lubricating jelly, slowly part the labia with the index and middle fingers. Hug the floor of the vagina with the fingers and touch the cervix with the fingertips. "Trap" the uterus between the hands and, without letting it loose, run the outside hand fingertips over the entire front and side surfaces of the uterus. It should be in the midline, be firm and smooth just above the pubis, and be somewhat movable with relatively little pain. Feel behind the cervix for any masses, fullness, or tenderness.

3. With the uterus still trapped between the hands, sweep the outside hand over to the side of the uterus to meet the fingertips of the vaginal hand. "Trap" the fallopian tube and ovary. You should not be able to feel the tube. The ovary is an almond-size, slightly tender organ attached to the side of the uterus. Feel for size, consistency, position, and contour (firm, just lateral to the uterus, smooth). Document all masses noted.

4. With the index finger of the internal hand still in the vagina, gently insert the middle finger into the rectum very slowly but firmly. Palpate as you did for the vaginal exam. This exam will aid in diagnosis of a vaginal stricture, is used in virgins, for tender masses and to explore the back of the uterus and rectal strength.

(3) Laboratory studies.

(a) Collections of Bartholin's, Skene's discharges, vaginal walls, posterior vaginal fornix, or rear pouch, or cervical opening, or os, are taken with a clean cotton applicator and treated as for a simple Gram stain unless you feel a need for culturing and these facilities are available.

(b) Wet preps. These are for vaginal discharges. Moisten a slide with a drop of sterile saline. Transfer a drop of discharge on a wooden applicator to the drop of saline on the slide. Read under a microscope immediately.

1. Trichomonas vaginalis. Look for the typical trichomonads with a whipping tail. See the laboratory plates for an example.

2. Hemophilus vaginalis. Vaginal cells may be dusted with small dark particles. These are called "clue cells." See the laboratory plates.

(c) KOH preps. Add a drop or two of 10% potassium hydroxide to a slide. Transfer a drop of discharge with a wooden applicator. The solution will dissolve R.B.C.'s, inflammatory, and epithelial cells. Candida albicans mycelia will display as hyphae and spores. Any whitish plaques in the vagina are to be scraped for this test.

(d) Pap smears. These smears of cervical cells are invaluable as a cancer screen when pathology facilities are available. With the vaginal speculum in place without lubricant other than sterile saline, transfer a specimen scraped from the center of the opening of the cervix to a slide. Smear the drops lightly across the slide. Repeat the procedure with a drop of fluid from the back of the vagina. Fix both slides immediately with 97% ethanol, Aqua-Net hair spray, or Pro-Fixx cytology fixative by spraying lightly across the slides. Be sure to have the patient's name on each slide. Pap smear readings are very difficult during active bleed.

(4) Procedures. Dilatation and curettage (D&C). This procedure involves opening of the cervix and scraping away of the endometrium or inner lining of the uterus. This procedure requires supervised practice prior to attempting the procedure yourself. Never forcefully perform this procedure. Uterine perforation can easily result. D&C is indicated for abnormal or postmenarchal questional bleeding and for spontaneous (incomplete) abortion. Contraindications include normal intrauterine pregnancy, acute cervicitis, endometritis, or pelvic inflammatory disease. The procedure may be performed under general anaesthesia, spinal (level of L3-L4 spine, inject 10-15 cc. of 0.25% Marcaine carefully), paracervical block (0.25% Marcaine injected just inside the vaginal mucosa next to the cervix on each side, 5 cc.), or 50-75 mg. Demerol IV <u>slow</u> while monitoring carefully.

(a) Explain the procedure to the patient.

(b) Palpate the uterine size and position. Attempt now and when "sounding" the uterus to rule out any lesions or growths that may bleed.

(c) Insert and lock down a speculum. Glove and wipe in a circular fashion outward the entire cervical stump with antiseptic sponges on transfer forceps three times. Discard the swabs and forceps. Bend the uterine sound to the estimated angle of the uterine position. Grasp the cervix with a tenaculum forcep at the six o'clock position and gently insert the sound until resistance is met. Here you will again try to note any lesions or growths as you insert the sound. Read the depth of the uterine cavity by noting the level of the mucous or blood on the sound as you would the oil level on a dipstick. Make a mental note of the depth of the uterine cavity. Starting with the smallest Hegar dilator, insert the dilator into the cervix to the dilator lip. Proceed to the next larger size until the cervix is at least as open as the loop of the largest curette, probably a #8 Hegar. Start with a small sharp curette by scraping in and out the entire diameter of the cervical canal. Fix the tissue obtained in 10% formalin. Repeat the four-quadrant scraping of the uterus by going to the depth of the uterus and scraping outward all along the uterine walls, in deep even gentle strokes to obtain long strips of endometrium. Curette the top of the uterus in an up-and-down fashion. Fix these specimens as before in formalin. If questionable specimens are obtained, fix and identify them separately. Insert a dry sterile sponge on a uterine forcep and swap the cavity with a twisting motion as you withdraw. Reinsert uterine polyp forceps and grasp for masses. Withdraw the forceps and observe for bleeding. Replace the uterus by removing the tenaculum and speculum and pushing the uterus gently but firmly upward bimanually. Place patient on bed rest for three days and limit activity for at least seven days. Excessive bleeding may require packing the uterine cavity with long continuous sterile roller gauze and shock care until out of danger and hemostasis is achieved.

7-2. THE BREAST. A modified sweat gland of duct tissue secreting nutritive fluid during the first several weeks after delivery (postpartum).

a. Postpartum mastitis (pyogenic cellulitis) generally occurs after several weeks of nursing. The infection occurs through the nipple and into the ducts. About 75 percent of all patients have unilateral involvement.

S. Chills, fever, malaise, regional pain, tenderness, and induration (hardening).

O. Gram stain of any discharge usually shows Staphylococcus aureus. A notable fluctuant mass can be palpated in the later stages. Axillary lymphadenopathy may be noted. An abscess may form in most cases.

A. Diagnosis is generally unmistakable.

P. Prevent by good hygiene. Suppress lactation (milk production) by wearing a tight binder for 72 hours, apply ice packs one hour on and one hour off. Give analgesics as needed. Broad-spectrum antibiotics such as Keflex, 250 mg. P.O. q.i.d. x 10-14 d. Incise and drain abscesses and pack with iodoform gauze.

b. Mammary dysplasia (cystic breast disease) is the most common single breast disorder encountered.

S. Painful masses in breast, perhaps a discharge.

O. Multiple tender masses in a patient that is often 30-50 years old, often worse during menstrual periods. Sizes may go up or down. No skin retraction should be present.

A. Differential diagnosis includes breast carcinoma and adenofibroma, which require biopsy to diagnose.

P. Biopsy is needed if at all possible. If symptoms and history are classical for this disorder, infiltrate the breast locally with lidocaine 1% or procaine 1%, insert a 20-gage needle into the cyst and withdraw the watery fluid that should be straw-colored to black. Reexamine every 2-4 weeks for 3 months, then every 6-12 months. If no fluid is obtained or a persistent lump is noted, a biopsy is indicated.

7-3. VULVITIS. The vulva is subject to the same diseases as the skin elsewhere on the body. Vaginitis (covered later) is secondarily induced.

a. Eczema is a common pruritic moist dermatitis often from contact with an irritant in soap, bath oils, deodorants, clothing, dyes, etc.

S. Pruritus, occasionally a discharge, and the lesion are presented.

O. An excoriated (ulcerated) crusted lesion is noted.

A. Differential diagnosis: Includes seborrhea, psoriasis, and intertrigo.

P. Eliminate any irritant. Burow's solution b.i.d. for three days. Local application of a steroid cream (hydrocortisone, Valisone, etc.) b.i.d. until the lesion resolves. Antihistamines for itching as needed (Benadryl 25-50 mg. h.s. to q.i.d.).

b. Psoriasis is of unknown etiology.

S. Pruritus and a lesion are presented. History may be long term.

O. Erythematous, slightly elevated, flattened lesions without the typical silvery appearance of scaling seen elsewhere on the body.

A. Differential diagnosis: Includes seborrhea, eczema, and intertrigo.

P. Improved hygiene is important. Apply hydrocortisone cream 1% b.i.d. If no improvement occurs, try Valisone in the same dosage.

c. Seborrhea is based on a genetic predisposition involving hormones, nutrition, infection, and emotional stress.

S. Pruritus may present, along with a lesion that may be infected.

O. A dry, scaling lesion with underlying erythema will present.

A. Rule out fungal involvement with a KOH prep. Differential diagnosis: Includes eczema, psoriasis, and intertrigo.

P. No greasy ointments. Potassium permanganate dressings b.i.d. (soak dressing in 100 mg. of permanganate in 1 liter of water). Ammoniated mercury ointment after soaks: 5% ammoniated mercury, 3% liquid petrolatum and petrolatum q.s. ad 100%.

d. Intertrigo is caused by the macerating effect of heat, moisture, and friction. It is worse in hot humid climates and in obese patients.

S. Itching, stinging, burning sensation in a noticeable irritation.

O. Possible fissures, erythema, denuded appearance. Urinalysis may show an indication of diabetes, KOH prep may show candida, direct smear may even show many cocci.

A. Differential diagnosis: Includes eczema, psoriasis, and seborrhea which may preclude intertrigo itself.

P. Dust well with talc b.i.d. Potassium permanganate dressings prepared as above or Domeboro dressings in a 1:20 mixed ratio.

7-4. BARTHOLIN'S CYST AND ABSCESS.

S. Periodic painful swelling on either side of the introitus (vaginal opening) and dyspareunia (painful intercourse).

O. Swelling at mid to lower third of labia, usually 1-4 cm. in size, and tender and fluctuant (wavelike sensation on palpation indicating a fluid-filled sac). Rule out gonorrheal involvement by direct smear of exudate.

A. Differential diagnosis: Includes inclusion cysts, sebaceous cysts, and congenital abnormalities (these are not usually tender).

P. Local heat to the lesion. Ampicillin or erythromycin 250-500 mg. q.i.d. for 10 days. After the infection subsides, open the lesion and excise or exteriorize. If an abscess develops, incise and drain, pack with iodoform gauze.

7-5. CONDYLOMA ACUMINATA. A viral infection that does not affect a fetus.

S. Small masses on the vulva, vagina, or perineum will present with itching.

O. Pink clusters of soft narrow-based lesions that are pointed and elongated, with or without a profuse irritating discharge.

A. Rule out condyloma latum (the primary lesion of syphilis).

P. Culture any discharge for gonorrhea. Perform a darkfield exam to rule out spirochetes. Treat any secondary infection that may exist. A 25% podophyllin in benzoin tincture may be applied to the lesions only and is to be washed off in 2 hours. Do not touch the normal tissue with the podophyllin. Isolate the lesions by surrounding the lesions with mineral oil.

7-6. MOLLUSCUM CONTAGIOSUM. A virus that incubates in 1-4 weeks.

S. Asymptomatic small skin tumors will present.

O. Pink to gray, discrete, umbilicated epithelial skin tumors generally less than 1 cm. in diameter on primarily the vulva introitus.

A. Diagnosis is generally unmistakable.

P. Biopsy is indicated if the diagnosis is in question. Lightly curette away the lesions. Apply Neosporin-G cream to the curette sites and dress.

7-7. HERPES GENITALIS. A herpes type II viral infection.

S. Painful clear little "bumps" on the labia and introitus, perhaps with tender "knots" in the groin.

O. Occasional inguinal lymphadenopathy and a group of vesicles with surrounding erythema and edema. Often a history of lesions coming and going.

A. Herpes zoster is similar, but generally doesn't recur. Erythema multiforme is a larger vesicle often found on plantar surfaces that sometimes looks like tiny "targets" of concentric circles and becomes purplish as the lesions enlarge; fever is concurrent.

P. (1) Rule out concurrent gonorrhea and syphilis.

(2) Virus culture for herpes species.

(3) Caesarean section patients with active lesions.

(4) Pap smear (herpes has been linked with cervical carcinoma).

(5) A 2% lidocaine ointment for pain q.i.d. for less than 2 weeks.

(6) No occlusive dressings or medications except lidocaine ointment.

7 8. VAGINITIS. An inflammation and/or infection of the vagina.

a. Atrophic vaginitis.

S. Tender, itching vagina generally in an older, postmenopausal or even a castrated patient.

O. Occasionally a clear vaginal discharge with an atrophied, erythematous, sometimes dryer appearance to the vagina.

A. Rule out other forms of vaginitis with saline and KOH preps of discharge.

P. Apply Premarin cream, 2-4 gm p.v. q.d. Use this medication cautiously with full knowledge of side effects, contraindications, etc. Use the smallest amount necessary to control the symptoms.

b. Trichomonal vaginitis. Caused by trichomonas vaginalis.

S. Vaginal symptoms of burning, itching, and tenderness with discharge.

O. Petechial spotting with erythema of the vaginal wall (with a strawberrylike appearance), usually with a thicker yellow to green frothy discharge. A stat. saline prep reading shows trichomonads.

A. Wet prep rules out other organisms.

P. Rule out other organisms including gonorrhea. Flagyl 250 mg. t.i.d. for 7-10 days. Treat the patient's sex partner at the same time.

c. Candidal vaginitis. Caused by Candida albicans, also known as Monilia.

S. Vaginal symptoms as above.

O. Erythema with a generally thick, white cheesy curdlike discharge. Thrush (whitish) patches may exist on the vaginal walls. KOH preps should show mycelia and hyphae.

A. Rule out other organisms including gonococci.

P. Nystatin vaginal suppositories 100,000 unit, 1 supp p.v. daily x 14 days.

d. Nonspecific vaginitis. Generally caused by Hemophilus vaginalis.

S. Vaginal symptoms as above.

O. Acrid, viscous, or thin watery milky discharge. Wet preps will show some epithelial cells coated with bacteria, giving a dusty appearance.

A. Rule out other organisms, including gonococci.

P. Sultrin cream, 1 applicatorful p.v. b.i.d. for 6 days, then 1 q.d. h.s. for 8 days.

7-9. CYSTOCELE. A herniation of the posterior bladder wall into the vagina.

S. Sensation of retained urine after urinating and of vaginal "looseness."

O. Presents as a reducible nontender mass that is soft and located in the anterior vaginal wall. As the patient strains, the bladder can sag downward.

A. Differential diagnosis: Includes bladder tumors and stones, both of which are firm and easily outlined. Rarely is a small bowel hernia differentiated.

P. This disorder may be alleviated by the patient manually reducing the bladder by pressing it upward from the vagina. Intermittent use of a Menge pessary placed just inside the introitus may help. Surgery, an anterior vaginal colporrhaphy, is often the only near-permanent cure.

7-10. RECTOCELE. A herniation of the rectal pouch into the vagina.

S. Constant urge for a bowel movement and a vaginal/rectal sense of fullness.

O. A finger can be inserted rectally and cause posterior pouching of the rectum. Straining down worsens the pouching. A soft posterior vaginal fullness. Defecation may be painful.

A. Differential diagnosis: Includes enterocele (a similar disorder occurring further back in the vagina from intestinal herniation), prolapsed cervix (seen on speculum-assisted vaginal examination), and rarely a tumor, which would be firmer and more easily delineated.

P. Stool softeners or laxatives (only for short periods). Avoid straining, coughing, or lifting. Get good exercise and bowel habits, as well as good dietary habits to facilitate elimination. Surgery (colpoperineorrhaphy) is generally curative.

7-11. CERVICITIS. An inflammation/infection of the cervix. This is the most common gynecological disorder generally encountered.

S. Discharge, low back pain, dyspareunia, dysmenorrhea (painful menstruation), urinary frequency and urgency, and/or dysuria.

O. Thin, mucuslike leukorrhea (discharge); an erythematous, petechial cervix and posterior fornix (back pouch of vagina) with a discharge from the cervical os (opening). Smears show W.B.C.'s. Cervical erosion and eversion may be noticeable.

A. Rule out infectious organisms by wet preps, KOH preps, and smears.

P. Pap smear first. If no organisms present, give AVC cream, 1-2 applicatorsful p.v. h.s. or b.i.d. for 28 days, through the entire menstrual cycle. Treat specific organisms as in the forms of vaginitis. Cryosurgery (with a CO_2 wand) may be necessary in intractable cases.

7-12. CERVICAL POLYPS. Small pedicled growths on the cervix.

S. Discharge, abnormal vaginal bleeding.

O. Flesh- to red-colored rounded or flame-shaped tissue on a pedicle or strand of tissue on the cervix or, if redder, coming from the endocervix.

A. Differential diagnosis (based on pathologic studies): Includes endometrial neoplasm or growth, small submucous myoma, endometrial polyp, and products of conception from an incomplete spontaneous abortion.

P. Work up and treat any associated cervicitis. Remove at the base of the lesion. Cervical dilatation may be necessary for polyps located high up in the endocervix. Send lesion to lab for pathologic studies. Full D&C if other polyps are suspected. Warm vinegar douche q.d. for 3-7 days to reduce inflammation.

7-13. ENDOMETRITIS. An inflammation/infection of the uterine lining, generally postpartum, post-D&C, or post incomplete abortion.

S. Fever, pain in the lower abdomen in the centerline, and low back pain.

O. Occasionally a discharge from the cervical os; history of recent delivery, abortion, or D&C. W.B.C. count may be mildly elevated.

A. Rule out masses by palpation; rule out carcinoma by D&C and study of samples obtained, or by a simpler endometrial biopsy done in like fashion.

P. Endometrial biopsy and smear as indicated. Specific antibiotics for organisms (Vibramycin 200 mg. for 1 day, then 100 mg. q.d. for 9 days is useful). D&C if abortion has been suspected. This must be done in a less vigorous fashion than normally. If moderately severe systemic symptoms are present, consider a slight delay, using antibiotics first. Monitor for any systemic infection until after all symptoms subside.

7-14. UTERINE MYOMA (fibroid). The most common gynecological neoplasm. It is a round, firm, benign uterine tumor composed of smooth muscle and dense connective tissue.

S. Lower adbominal pain, bleeding, dysmenorrhea, discharge, dyspareunia, urinary frequency, sensation of pressure, and constipation.

O. Palpable enlargement of the uterus, feeling firm and rounded.

A. D&C may help confirm, as no abnormal specimens may be found. Differential diagnosis: Includes other neoplasms and benign hypertrophy; sarcoma and adherent adnexa. Surgical sections are the principal diagnostic tool.

P. Defer surgery until postpartum, if patient is pregnant, unless the uterus feels to be over two months larger than the EDC (estimated date of confinement) computes to. Watch for signs of distress. A torsioned pedicle of a myoma or intestinal obstruction may necessitate emergency surgery and blood transfusion. Excision with perhaps hysterectomy (uterus removal) is indicated if the disorder is extensive.

7-15. SALPINGITIS (pelvic inflammatory disease). An infection of the fallopian tubes, usually bilaterally, with a rapid spread to the rest of the pelvis.

S. Severe, nonradiating cramping lower abdominal pain, chills, fever, abnormal menses, leukorrhea, dyspareunia, and dysmenorrhea.

O. Thickening of the adnexal structures and palpation of the tubes (not normally paplable) on pelvic exam. Adynamic ileus (stoppage of fecal passage) may present. History of nausea and pain since last period. Discharge. Stable hematocrit and W.B.C. count to 15,000-20,000. The erythrocyte sedimentation rate will be increased.

A. Differential diagnosis: Includes appendicitis (lower fever and W.B.C. count, localized RLQ pain, nausea, and vomiting) and ectopic pregnancy (a sudden RLQ or LLQ pain, with bleeding, soft tender mass and recent irregular menses).

P. Culture discharge (rule out tuberculosis and gonorrhea). Treat organisms appropriately (ampicillin, 500 mg. P.O. q.i.d. for 7-10 days). Control pain with analgesics and suppress menstruation with Enovid (10-15 mg. P.O. q.d. for 28 days). Treat fever and malaise symptomatically. Observe, as this disorder is potentially very dangerous. RULE OUT MASSES. Since this can be an emergency, ruling out masses helps to reduce the chance that it becomes a surgical emergency.

7-16. TUBO-OVARIAN ABSCESS. A formed abscess of the tubes that may spread to the ovaries.

S. Spikes of fever, malaise, bilateral lower quadrant pain with an acute onset, sudden and pronounced. Metrorrhagia and hypermenorrhea (later section).

O. Palpable mass, tender. Possible history of disappearing mass with softening of the abdomen, suggesting rupture of the abscess. Increased W.B.C. count and sed. rate (erythrocyte sedimentation rate). Biocept-G negative.

A. The Biocept-G rules out pregnancy and thus ectopic pregnancy. If pain is unilateral, rule out appendicitis by history and lower W.B.C. count and sed. rate. Endometriosis (endometrium growing outside the uterine cavity in its normal position) is ruled out by the cyclic nature of the pain.

P. Vibramycin 200 mg. P.O. b.i.d. for 10 days. Constant monitoring for abdominal softening. Local heat and analgesics. Surgery is indicated if rupture is suspected. If access via the cul-de-sac is possible, aspiration of abscess contents for temporary alleviation of the mass by large-bore needle may be of value.

7-17. OOPHORITIS. An infection of the ovaries, generally secondary to another infection but clinically significant from a potential infertility standpoint, since healing of ovarian tissue is not well accomplished.

S. Pain, fever, and menstrual abnormalities. Evidence of other infection as the complaints are noted.

O. Enlargement of the ovary and excessive tenderness to palpation. Anemia and increased W.B.C. count and sed rate are noted.

A. Other adnexal infections may coexist.

P. Analgesics such as codeine sulfate 30-60 mg. every 4-6 hours. Observe for systemic signs. Vibramycin 200 mg. stat., then 100 mg. q.d. for 13 days. Local heat, rest, fluids. Drain abscesses (if pointing down to the cul-de-sac, by large-bore needle aspiration). If chronic in nature, and if the patient is older, removal of the ovaries and tubes (salpingo-oophorectomy) bilaterally may be needed.

7-18. OVARIAN CYSTS AND TUMORS. Many varieties of cysts and tumors may be noted on pelvic examination and palpation of the ovaries. Rule out the known disorders in this chapter, wait one full menstrual cycle, and recheck the size and, of course, the nature of palpable adnexal masses; obtain specialist assistance if the mass has not regressed during the trial period. If it has, make a note of all findings and recheck the patient periodically to watch for recurrence.

7-19. PREMENSTRUAL TENSION. A cyclical disorder.

S. Anxiety, agitation, insomnia, inability to concentrate fully, feelings of inadequacy, depression, and weight gain.

O. Document the symptoms. Lab and pelvic exams are inconclusive.

A. Rule out hyperthyroidism (if lab facilities permit, increased T3 and decreased T4 with perhaps a palpable thyroid), hyperaldosteronism (decreased serum potassium, increased serum sodium, alkalosis, and increased plasma aldosterone), and hyperinsulinism (decreased blood sugar). Also note any clinical symptoms. Psychoneurosis and psychosis are also to be considered, but they are not cyclical.

P. Reassurance is very important. Diuretics, such as Aldactone 2 mg./kg./d. in divided doses under supervision. Antidepressants as needed. Psychiatric help as needed, or assistance with differentiated disorders.

7-20. DYSMENORRHEA. Pain with menstrual periods. Secondary dysmenorrhea is a term applied to dysmenorrhea from organic causes (chronic pelvic inflammatory disease, endometriosis, etc.). This generally occurs over five years after menarche or at the beginning of having menstrual periods.

S. Pain with menstruation, abdominal bloating, breast tenderness, and a sensation of pelvic heaviness around the time for the patient's period.

O. History of intermittent premenstrual cramping through the period in the lower abdominal midline.

A. Diagnosis is based on history and absence of other pelvic exam findings.

P Analgesics as needed. Local heat and reassurance. Motrin 400 mg. P.O. q.i.d. from the onset of cramps to the end of the period.

7-21. AMENORRHEA. Failure to menstruate at the appropriate time. Primary amenorrhea is when the patient has never menstruated, while secondary amenorrhea is when over 90 days pass with no menstrual flow.

S. and O. All hinge on the absence of menstrual flow.

A. Assessment is usually unmistakable.

P. Work up the patient as follows:

(1) Perform the most accurate pregnancy test possible (the Biocept-G, if available to be done).

(2) If pregnancy test is negative, give Provera 10 mg. P.O. q.d. for 5 days.

(3) If patient bleeds, anovulation (no ovulation) occurred.

Nothing further.

(4) If the patient doesn't bleed, and if possible, draw a serum FSH and LH (follicle-stimulating hormone and luteinizing hormone). Then give Premarin 1.25 mg. P.O. q.d. for 21 days, then Provera as above.

(5) If no bleeding, trace the tract through to the uterus to target organ or outflow tract failure.

(6) If patient bleeds, get serum FSH and LH results. If they are low, then C.N.S. or pituitary failure is suspected. Refer the patient out for the C.N.S. or pituitary tumor workups.

(7) If the FSH and LH are high, then ovarian failure is suspected, dictating referral for karyotyping (chromosome studies) for genetic deficiencies.

(8) Remember, amenorrhea is complex and elusive. If at any time the disorder or its workup exceeds the practitioner's expertise or facilities, the case should be referred to a specialist with the means to work up and manage the case.

7-22. ABNORMAL UTERINE BLEEDING. A symptom of atypical menstrual flow in amount or timing. Hypermenorrhea (excessive flow) or menorrhagia; polymenorrhea (flow less than every 24 days); and metrorrhagia (flow at times other than regular time for the period) are examples.

Subjective and objective findings are as above.

A. Based on history, examination, and appropriate lab testing.

P. (1) Take a careful history and perform a careful exam. Take vaginal smears for cytology and bacteriology (fix first then add 1% HCl, which hemolyzes the red blood cells, if the bleeding is active. HCl is hydrochloric acid).

(2) Run a urinalysis, hematocrit, STS, W.B.C. count with differential, sed. rate, bleeding time, clotting time, clot retraction time, and platelets.

(3) Cervical biopsy and D&C may be critical.

(4) Hypermenorrhea. D&C, support hypovolemia, Provera 5-10 mg. q.d. for 4 days starting with the 21st day of the cycle. First day of bleeding is the first day of the cycle.

(5) Metrorrhagia. Give Enovid 10 mg. P.O. q.d. on days 5-20.

(6) Unknown or unresponsive entities should be referred for further study.

7-23. MENOPAUSE/CLIMACTERIC. Climacteric is the onset of menopausal symptoms, while menopause itself is the cessation of menses for over one year. These can of course occur due to removal or major dysfunction of the ovaries.

S. The climacteric begins at ages 40-55 with hot flushes,

diaphoresis, and depression or agitation.

O. Vaginal atrophy with dyspareunia and pruritus may exist.

A. If bleeding suddenly recurs, rule out neoplasms by pelvic exam palpation.

P. (1) Reassurance and understanding are essential.

(2) Mild sedatives as needed.

(3) If symptoms are severe or patient is fairly young, Premarin should be given low dose (0.3-2.5 mg. ranges) and adjust upward to control the symptoms that are presented to you.

7-24. CONTRACEPTION.

a. Rhythm uses basal body temperature to figure the period of ovulation. It is the only method allowed in Catholic areas.

(1) Take the temperature immediately upon awakening and before arising. Be sure to chart this reading daily.

(2) One to 1 1/2 days before ovulation, the temperature drops; 1-2 days after ovulation, the temperature rises about 0.7 degrees F. Wait 3 days after the temperature rises before allowing intercourse. The BBT thermometer is best and most accurate of all when utilizing this method.

b. Oral contraceptives. Selection is important. These medications generally work by artificial suppression of FSH secretion by the posterior pituitary. Young girls (16-20) must avoid oversuppression of the pituitary hormones, while older women must avoid thromboembolism.

(1) Ask about nausea and vomiting in previous pregnancies, fluid retention, weight gain, acne, history of varicose veins, etc.

(2) If menstrual flow is heavy and long, use more progestin (Norinyl 2 mg., or Norlestrin 2.5 mg.) to avoid breakthrough bleeding.

(3) If flow is shorter than normal, consider more estrogen and less progestin (Ovulen, Ortho-Novum, Enovid).

(4) If menstrual or other side effects are noted, increase estrogen and decrease progestin to increase the menstrual flow, or vice versa to decrease the flow. Watch the dosages of each hormone in the pills to adjust the flow in this manner.

(5) Give 1 tab P.O. q.d. If 1 day is missed, take two tabs the next day. If two or more days are missed, discontinue the tablets until the start of the next month and use another form of contraception until then.

(6) If women are very regular in timing, amount of flow, and duration of flow, try norethindrone acetate 0.2 mg. q.d. It has fewer side effects.

(7) Know the pills before prescribing, read the information, rule out any contraindications before prescribing.

c. Diaphragm and spermicidal jelly. Fitted to proper size to snugly cover the cervix and covered with jelly, this method works well when left in place after intercourse for at least 8 hours.

d. Condoms. Help prevent VD and work well with immediate postcoital withdrawal of the penis to prevent leakage of semen.

e. Foam. Spermicidal foam such as Delfen given as 1-2 applicatorsful p.v. before intercourse works well. Irritation and messiness may be noted.

f. Intrauterine devices (IUDs). The Cu-7 and Tatum-T work well when properly monitored after careful installation. Prep the cervix as for the D&C. Sound the uterus and measure the inserter to the noted depth. Turn the IUD to a position lateral so as to make it open when inserted to either side. Insert the device, pull back the inserter and withdraw the inserter. Cut the string to a couple of inches outside the cervix. Have the patient feel for the string regularly and after each period.

NOTE: This chapter is not all-inclusive and much of the data is for information only. Many of the tests cannot be performed with existing facilities. This information is useful to the practitioner becoming aware of the possibilities of disease entities and treatments in a basic way. Practice under close supervision is essential to learn properly these techniques. Be sure to refer patients to the specialists if ever in doubt or if inadequate facilities exist.

CHAPTER 8

OBSTETRICS

8-1. Obstetrics is that branch of surgery that deals with the management of women during pregnancy, labor, and the puerperium (42 days following childbirth and expulsion of the placenta; the generative organs usually return to normal during this time).

8-2. DIAGNOSIS OF PREGNANCY. In about one-third of cases it is difficult to make a definitive diagnosis before the second missed period because the variability of physical changes induced by pregnancy, possibility of tumors, obesity, and poor patient relaxation often interfere with the examination. If in doubt, schedule a reexamination in 3-4 weeks. If available the Early Pregnancy Test (E.P.T.) or in Europe, the Predictor Test, an anti-HCG test for pregnancy, can be used at least 9 days after her last period was due. This test claims a 97 percent accuracy rate.

a. The following symptoms and signs are usually due to pregnancy, but even two or more are not diagnostic. A record or history of time and frequency of coitus may be of considerable help.

(1) Symptoms. Amenorrhea (missed period), nausea and vomiting, urinary frequency and urgency (first trimester), breast tenderness and tingling (after 1-2 weeks), "quickening" (first movement of the fetus felt in the uterus; may appear about 16th week), weight gain.

(2) Signs. Skin pigmentation (after 16th week), epulis (hypertrophic gingival papillae often seen after first trimester), breast changes (enlargement, vascular engorgement, colostrum), abdominal enlargement, cyanosis of vagina and cervical portio (about the 6th week), softening of cervix (4th or 5th week), softening of cervicouterine junction (5th or 6th week), irregular softening and slight enlargement of the fundus (about 5th week), generalized enlargement and diffuse softening of corpus (after 8th week).

b. Positive manifestations. Not usually present until the 4th month, but is undeniable proof of pregnancy: Ausculation of fetal heart, palpation of fetal outline, recognition of fetal movement.

c. Differential diagnosis. All the presumptive signs and symptoms of pregnancy can be caused by other conditions and all tests for pregnancy can be positive in the absence of conception. Some examples for missed period are psychic factors (fear of pregnancy, venereal disease, emotional shock); endocrine factors (thyroid, adrenal, or ovarian dysfunctions); metabolic factors (anemia, diabetes, systemic disease); nausea and vomiting factor (acute infections, G.I. disorders, emotional disorders); urinary frequency, GU infection, pelvic tumor, emotional tension. These are just a few examples, there are many more factors that may cause a false diagnosis of pregnancy.

8-3. MINOR DISCOMFORTS OF NORMAL PREGNANCY.

a. Backache.

b. Syncope (lightheadedness and fainting).

c. Dyspnea (difficulty in breathing).

d. Urinary symptoms (frequency, urgency, and stress incontinence).

e. Heartburn.

f. Constipation (avoid enemas as they may induce labor).

g. Hemorrhoids.

h. Breast soreness.

i. Ankle swelling (restrict salt).

j. Varicose veins (provide elastic support).

k. Leg cramps (discontinue medications containing large amounts of phosphorus. Reduce dietary phosphorus intake by limiting meat to 1 meal a day and milk to 1 pint a day).

l. Abdominal pain due to pressure, round ligament tension, flatulence, distention, bowel cramping, and uterine contractions. Intra-abdominal disorders and uterine or adnexal disease can also cause abdominal pain and must be considered and treated as required.

m. Morning sickness occurs in one-half of pregnant women usually starting during 5th or 6th week and persisting until the 14th-16th week. Most severe in the morning upon rising. Treatment: Reassurance and dietary restriction; restrict fats, odorous foods, and spiced dishes. In general, dry foods at frequent intervals are indicated.

8-4. HYPEREMESIS GRAVIDARUM. Persistent severe vomiting; can be fatal if not controlled. Only about 0.2 percent of pregnant women develop hyperemesis gravidarum and cause is not known.

S. Persistent severe vomiting.

O. Acidosis, weight loss, avitaminosis, and jaundice.

A. Hyperemesis gravidarum. Differential diagnosis: Any of the diseases with which vomiting is associated, e.g., infections, poisoning, neoplastic disease, hyperthyroidism, gastric disorders, gallbladder disease, intestinal obstruction, hiatal hernia, and diabetic acidosis.

P. Hospitalize patient in a private room at complete bed rest without bathroom privileges. Allow no visitors (not even husband) until vomiting stops and patient is eating. Place patient N.P.O. x 48 hours. Maintain normal nutrition and electrolyte balance by IV therapy with vitamin and protein supplements as required. Give chlorpromazine IM or suppositories. If no response after 48 hours, institute nasogastric tube feeding of a well-balanced liquid baby formula by slow drip. As soon as possible, place patient on a dry diet of 6 small feedings daily with clear liquids 1 hour after eating. If the situation continues to deteriorate in spite of therapy, therapeutic abortion may be required. Urgent indications are delirium, blindness, tachycardia at rest, jaundice, anuria, and hemorrhage.

8-5. ECTOPIC PREGNANCY. Pregnancy outside the cavity of the uterus. Occurs in 0.5 percent of pregnancies. About 98 percent of ectopic pregnancies occur in the fallopian tubes.

S. Amenorrhea or disordered menstrual pattern followed by uterine bleeding, pelvic pain, and pelvic mass formation. May be acute or chronic. Acute (about 40 percent of cases): Sudden onset of sharp or cutting, intermittent severe lower quadrant pain that does not radiate, with backache during the attack. Scant but persistent uterine bleeding is present in approximately 80 percent of cases. At least two-thirds of patients give history of abnormal menstruation; most have been infertile. Chronic (about 60 percent of cases): Increasing pelvic discomfort, slight but persistent vaginal spotting.

O. Acute: Palpable pelvic mass in 70 percent of cases. Collapse and shock occur in about 10 percent of cases, often after pelvic examination. Chronic: Palpable pelvic mass. Lab findings: CBC shows anemia with slight leukocytosis. Urine urobilinogen elevated in ectopic pregnancy with internal bleeding. Pregnancy tests are of little value in diagnosis.

A. Ectopic pregnancy. Differential diagnosis: Many acute abdominal illnesses, e.g., appendicitis, salpingitis, uterine abortion.

P. Hospitalize patient if there is a reasonable likelihood of ectopic pregnancy. Treat for shock. If possible, type and cross match blood. A transfusion should be started before surgery is begun. Surgical treatment is imperative. Besides normal debridement, generally a salpingectomy will be required. Iron therapy for anemia may be necessary during convalescence.

8-6. PREECLAMPSIA-ECLAMPSIA. Usually occurs in last trimester or early in the puerperium. Preeclampsia denotes the nonconvulsive form; with the development of convulsion and coma the disorder is termed eclampsia. About 10 percent of pregnancies develop preeclampsia-eclampsia and about 5 percent of cases progress to eclampsia. Ten to 15 percent of the women with eclampsia die. Cause is unknown. Predisposing factors are vascular and renal disease, sodium retention, and multiple pregnancy.

S. Preeclampsia: Headache, vertigo, malaise, irritability (due in part to cerebral edema); scintillating scotomas (irregular luminous patches in the visual field after physical or mental labor), visual impairment, epigastric nausea, liver tenderness, and generalized edema.

Eclampsia: Severe preeclampsia symptoms plus generalized tonic-clonic convulsions, coma followed by amnesia and confusion, laborious breathing, frothing at the mouth, twitching of muscle groups (e.g., face, arms), nystagmus (constant involuntary movement of the eyeball), and oliguria or anuria.

O. Preeclampsia: Persistent hypertension or a sudden rise of blood pressure, generalized edema, and proteinuria during the last 4 months of pregnancy. Opthalmoscopic examination in severe preeclampsia and eclampsia reveals variable arteriolar spasm, edema of optic disc, and with increasing severity, cotton-wool exudates and even retinal detachment.

Eclampsia: Marked hypertension preceding a convulsion, and hypotension thereafter (during coma or vascular collapse), and 3-4 + proteinuria. Opthalmoscopic examination reveals papilledema, retinal edema, retinal detachment, vascular spasm, arteriovenous "nicking," and hemorrhages. Repeated opthalmoscopic examination is helpful in judging the success of treatment.

A. Preeclampsia-eclampsia. Differential diagnosis: Primary hypertension, renal and neurologic disease.

P. Preeclampsia: Objectives are to prevent eclampsia, permanent cardiovascular and renal damage, ocular or vascular accidents, and to deliver a normal baby. Delivery should be delayed, if possible, until disease is under control or improvement is marked.

Bed rest with sedation under alert supervision, including frequent B.P. readings and urine protein determination, and careful recording of fluid intake and output. Try to achieve a zero water balance between intake and output. Give diuretics and hypertensive drugs as needed. Place patient on a low-fat, high carbohydrate, with moderate protein, salt-poor (less than 1 gm a day) diet. Opthalmoscopic examination should be done daily.

Eclampsia: Same as preeclampsia plus give magnesium sulfate 10 ml. of 25% aqueous solution IV or IM initially, then 5 ml. IV or IM q.6h. to prevent or control convulsions, lower B.P., and encourage diuresis. (Do not repeat magnesium sulfate if urinary output is less than 100 ml./h., respiration is less than 16/min, or knee jerk reflex is absent.) In case of overdose, give calcium gluconate (or equivalent) 20 ml. of 10% solution IV slowly, repeat every hour until urinary, respiratory, and neurologic depression have cleared (do not give more than 8 injections in 24 hours).

Place patient at absolute bed rest in darkened quiet room. No visitors. Use indwelling catheter, leave B.P. cuff on her arm. Do not disturb patient with unnecessary procedure (e.g., bath, enemas, douches, etc.). Patients with eclampsia often develop premature separation of the placenta with hemorrhage and are susceptible to shock.

Because severe hypertensive disease, renal disease, and preeclampsia-eclampsia are usually aggravated by continuing pregnancy, the best method of treatment is termination of pregnancy. Control eclampsia before attempting induction of labor. Labor can usually be induced by rupturing the fetal membrane. Use oxytocin (Pitocin) to stimulate labor if necessary. If the patient is not at term, if labor is not inducible, if she is bleeding, or if there is a possible disproportion, a cesarean section may be necessary. Most patients improve dramatically in 24-48 hours, but early termination of pregnancy is usually required.

8-7. ANEMIA DURING PREGNANCY. Iron deficiency anemia and folic acid deficiency anemia can be prevented and treated by administering prophylactic multivitamin plus iron capsules to all pregnant women during pregnancy and for 1 month following delivery.

8-8. ABORTION (MISCARRIAGE). At least 12 percent of all pregnancies terminate in spontaneous abortion; of these, three-fourths occur before the 16th week of gestation.

S-O. Abortion is broken down into four classifications:

Inevitable abortion: The passage of some or all of the products of conception is momentarily impending. Bleeding and cramps do not subside.

Complete abortion: All of the conceptus is expelled. When complete abortion is impending, the symptoms of pregnancy often disappear;

sudden bleeding begins, followed by cramping. The fetus and placenta may be expelled separately. When the entire conceptus has been expelled, pain ceases but slight spotting persists.

Incomplete abortion: A significant portion of the conceptus (usually placental fragments) remains in the uterus. Only mild cramps, but bleeding is persistent and often excessive.

Missed abortion: Pregnancy has been terminated for at least 1 month, but the conceptus has not been expelled. Symptoms of pregnancy disappear and body temperature is not elevated. Brownish vaginal discharge but no free bleeding. Pain does not develop. Cervix is semifirm and slightly patulous (open, distended, spread apart); uterus becomes smaller and irregularly softened.

Lab finding: Pregnancy tests are negative or positive. Blood and urine findings are those usually found in infection or anemia if these complications have occurred.

A. Abortion. Differential diagnosis: Bleeding must be differentiated from bleeding from aborting ectopic pregnancy, anovulatory bleeding in nonpregnant women, and membranous dysmenorrhea.

P. If abortion has occurred after 1st trimester, the patient should be hospitalized. In all cases, uterine contractions should be induced with oxytocin (not ergot preparations) to limit blood loss and aid in expulsion of clots and tissues. Ergotrate should only be given if complete abortion is certain. Treat for shock. If there are any signs of infection, give antibiotics. D&C is indicated to remove possibly retained tissue.

8-8. HYDATIDIFORM MOLE AND CHORIOCARCINOMA. A degenerative disorder of the chorion (develops into placenta); occurs in 1 out of 1,500 pregnancies; is five times more prevalent in the Orient than in Western countries; and more common in women over 40. Malignant change occurs in about 4 percent (higher in Asia) of cases and is often fatal when it does occur.

S. Excessive nausea and vomiting in over one-third of cases. Uterine bleeding beginning at 6-8 weeks is observed in virtually all cases and is indicative of threatened or incomplete abortion.

Choriocarcinoma may manifest itself by continued or recurrent uterine bleeding after evacuation of a mole or by presence of an ulcerative vaginal tumor, pelvic mass, or evidence of distant metastatic tumor. Diagnosis is established by pathologic examination of curettage or biopsy.

O. Uterus larger than would be expected in normal pregnancy of the same duration in one-fifth of cases. Intact or collapsed vesicles may be passed through vagina. Preeclampsia-eclampsia, frequently of the fulminating type, may develop during the second trimester, but is unusual. Vaginal smear reveals heavy cell groupings and a predominance of superficial cells.

A. Hydatidiform mole. Differential diagnosis: Hyperemesis gravidarum, multiple pregnancy (extra enlarged uterus), threatening or incomplete abortion.

P. Hospitalize, treat symptoms, evacuate the uterus; probably will require D&C. If the uterus is larger than a 5-month pregnancy, a hysterectomy is preferred. If malignant tissue is discovered, chemotherapy is necessary.

8-9. CHILDBIRTH.

a. Signs and symptoms of impending childbirth:

(1) Nausea and vomiting.

(2) Mother displays intense anxiety.

(3) Heavy show of blood/bloody mucous.

(4) Intense desire to defecate.

(5) Rapidly occurring contractions with increasing intensity and desire to bear down.

(6) Bulging of membranes from vulva and/or spontaneous rupture.

(7) Dilation of anus with expulsion of feces.

(8) Crowning of the fetal head (figure 1).

b. Delivery of the infant: NOTE: Maintain sterile technique whenever possible, but do not endanger the mother or infant with undue delay.

(1) Place mother in dorsal position, with legs bent and hands grasping knees. Assign an assistant to stand at head of bed to monitor vital signs and offer verbal support and encouragement to the mother.

(2) Attempt to gain mother's confidence and cooperation by explaining what you are doing and what you expect of her.

(3) If time permits, put on sterile gloves and drape perineal area with sterile towels.

(4) As birth approaches, the head distends the perineum more and more with each contraction. When two to three inches of fetal scalp show, an episiotomy may be necessary to prevent serious laceration. Cut the episiotomy 1 to 1 1/2 inches long. (See figure 2.)

(5) Apply gentle pressure with palm of hand to crowning head and perineal area to prevent rapid expulsion of the head. NEVER TRY TO STOP DELIVERY BY PUSHING FORCEFULLY AGAINST THE HEAD.

(6) Encourage mother to pant during contractions to allow for slow, gentle delivery.

(7) As head is delivered, provide support with both hands and allow the head to rotate naturally to the side.

(8) Immediately slip finger around infant's neck and feel for cord that may be wrapped around the neck and choking the infant. If present, attempt to gently slip it off over the head. If it is not possible to remove the cord, clamp and cut the cord at once. (See (14)

below.)

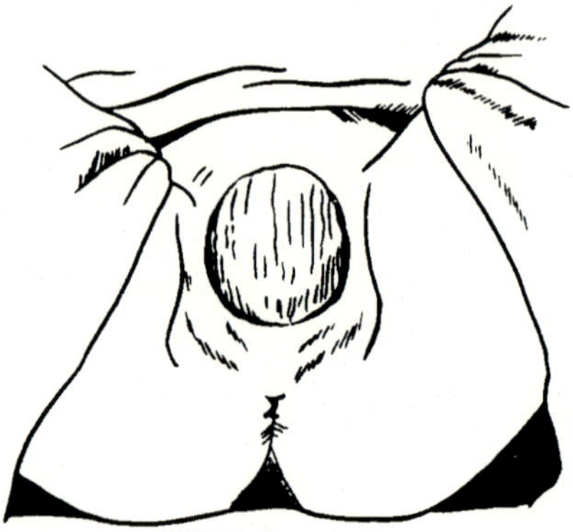

FIGURE 1

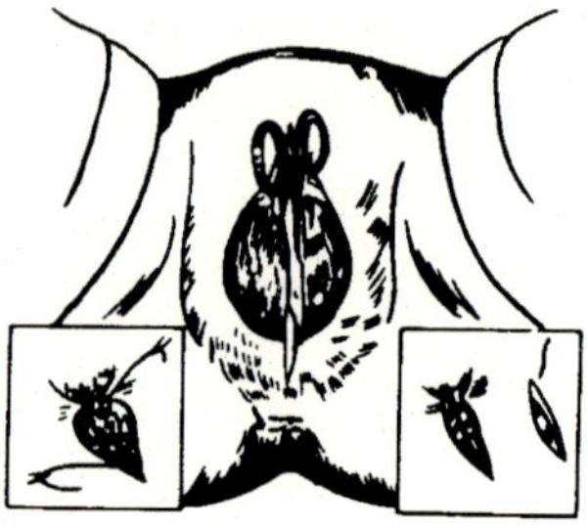

FIGURE 2

(9) If membranes are still intact over the infants face, remove by snipping them at the nape of the neck and pulling away from face and airway at once.

(10) Suction nose then mouth gently with bulb syringe to insure adequate airway. (Newborns are obligate nose breathers.) (See figure 3.)

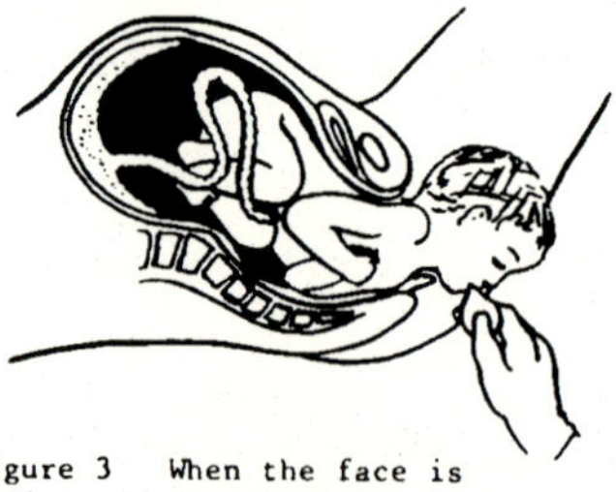

Figure 3 When the face is delivered, the shoulders reside under the pubis; the mouth and oropharynx should be aspirated.

(11) After insuring patient airway, proceed to deliver the shoulders. Place hands on either side of head and exert gentle downward pressure (toward the floor) to deliver the anterior shoulder. Then exert

gentle upward pull to permit delivery of the posterior shoulder. Support the rest of the body as it is born. (See figures 4 and 5.)

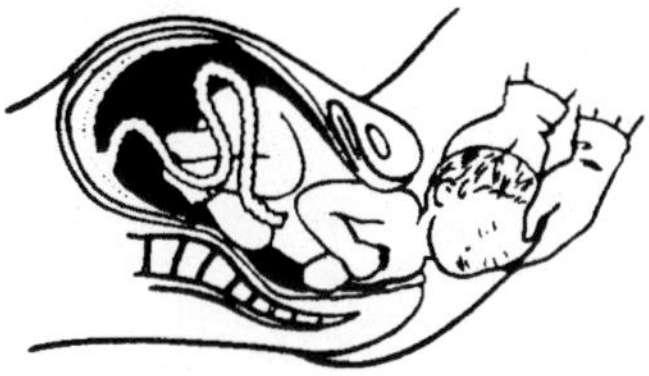

Figure 4 The head rotates to accommodate the shoulders during passage through the birth canal.

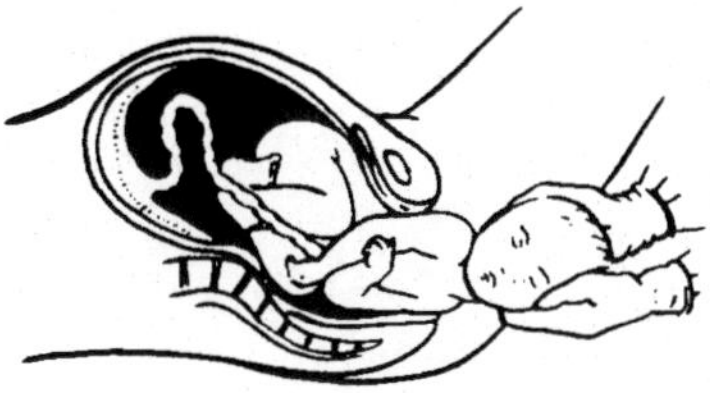

Figure 5 Following rotation, the shoulders are delivered.

(12) With firm grip on body, hold infant along length of arm, with head lower than feet and again suction the nose and mouth. Keep the infant below or equal to the level of the mother until the cord stops pulsating. DO NOT HANG INFANT BY THE FEET.

(13) If infant does not cry spontaneously, apply gentle stimulus to back and soles of feet by rubbing and gently patting.

(14) Wait for cord to stop pulsating, then tie off cord several inches apart and cut between the two ties. Apply first tie several inches from infant's body. Observe for evidence of excessive bleeding from ends of cord.

(15) Wrap infant in blanket, then place on mother's abdomen.

c. Delivery of placenta.

(1) Signs of separation of the placenta.

(a) Large gush of blood from the vagina.

(b) Umbilical cord protrudes 2 to 3 inches farther out of the vagina.

(c) Fundus rises upward in the abdomen.

(d) Uterus firming and becoming more globular.

(2) Expulsion.

(a) Ask mother to "bear down" to expel the placenta. Avoid excessive massage of the uterus.

(b) Apply GENTLE downward pressure on fundus to aid delivery, but do not apply excessive pressure or force.

(c) Check the placenta for evidence of missing portions; any section missing can mean continued uterine bleeding.

d. Care of the newborn.

(1) Maintain patient airway.

(2) Administer eye care (silver nitrate or penicillin prophylaxis).

(3) Observe cord stump for evidence of bleeding.

(4) Provide artificial respiration and cardiac support as needed.

e. Care of the mother.

(1) Observe for signs of excessive bleeding and shock.

(2) Prevent relaxation of the uterine muscles by frequent massage and close observation.

(3) Be prepared to administer IV fluid therapy as needed.

(4) Suture any lacerations and the episiotomy with chromic gut, 00 or 000. Start above apex of vaginal incision and close the vaginal mucosa with a running stitch. Suture the perineal portion as any other wound, making sure that anatomic structures are approximated. (See figure 2.) If the anal sphincter muscle or rectal wall is torn, these are repaired first. Try to get patient evacuated if lacerations are severe.

(5) Take mother's temperature 4-5 times a day. Any elevation above 100.4°F. present on successive days is evidence of infection.

(6) If membranes are ruptured more than 12 hours prior to delivery, assume infection to be present and start antibiotic therapy. If infection occurs after delivery, as evidenced by fever, foul smelling discharge, and tender uterus, start antibiotic therapy.

f. BREECH DELIVERY. (See figures 6-8.)

(1) Let baby be expelled spontaneously to the umbilicus.

(2) Cut a generous episiotomy.

(3) Deliver buttocks by gently pulling upward.

(4) Pull gently until an axilla is visible. Do not exert pressure above the iliac crests upon the abdomen (of the infant) to avoid injury to the abdominal organs.

(5) Have an assistant press downward on the fundus gently.

(6) Deliver the anterior or posterior shoulder, whichever is easier.

(7) Deliver the other arm.

(8) Deliver the head as follows:

(a) With baby lying face down on your arm, put your index finger in baby's mouth.

(b) Hook two fingers of the other hand over each of the baby's shoulders, palm on baby's back.

(c) Pull downward until occiput is under the symphisis.

(d) Bring head out by raising the baby's body up toward the mother's abdomen.

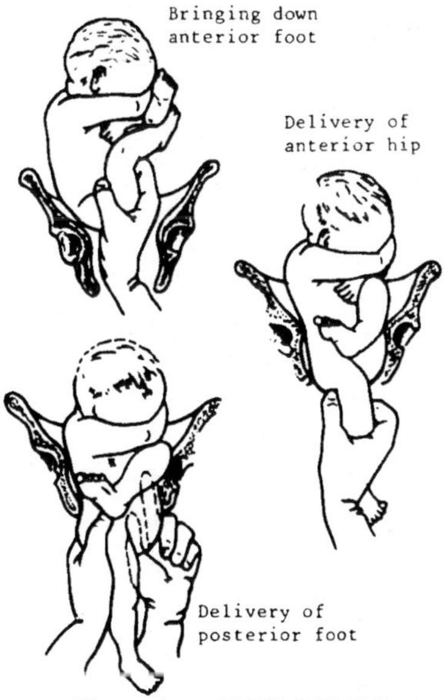

Figure 6 BREECH DELIVERY

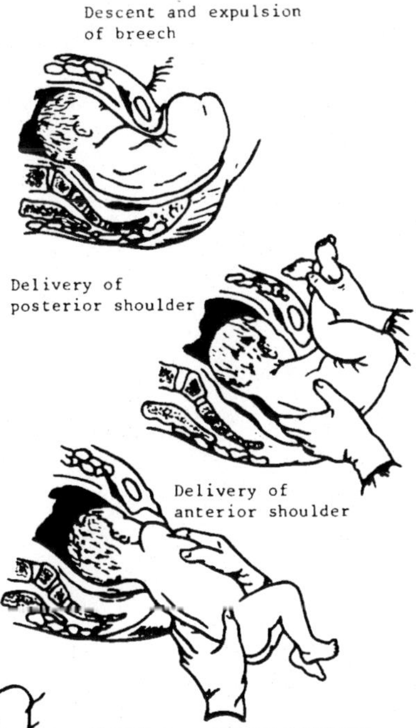

FIGURE 7 BREECH DELIVERY

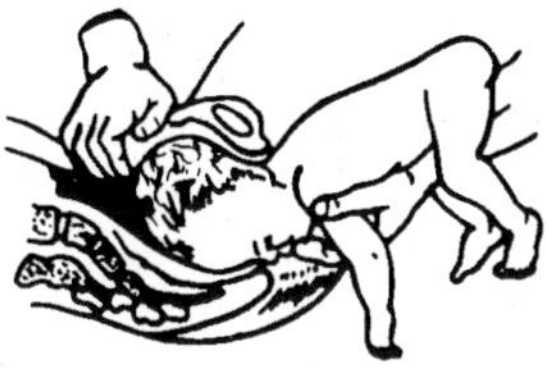

Figure 8 Wigand maneuver for delivery of head. Fingers of left hand inserted into infant's mouth or over mandible; right hand exerting pressure on head from above.

CHAPTER 9

ORTHOPEDICS

9-1. FRACTURES.

a. A fracture is a break in a bone. The break does not need to be complete to be considered a fracture; the bone may only be cracked, or in the case of stress fractures the bone tissue itself may only be torn.

b. To diagnose a fracture without X rays requires the utmost use of history and physical examination. If there is any doubt, treat as a fracture. Fractures may be suspected by one or more of the following:

(1) The patient feels or hears the bone break.

(2) Partial or complete loss of motion.

(3) Crepitus or grating.

(4) Deformity.

(5) Swelling and discoloration.

(6) Abnormal motion at fracture site (arm bending but not at the elbow).

(7) Point tenderness.

(8) Muscle spasm.

c. The main objective in fracture treatment is to prevent broken bones from moving, thus preventing further damage to tissue, nerves, and blood vessels. The basic principles of treating fractures are:

(1) Check and maintain airway (if appropriate).

(2) Determine extent of injury.

(3) Control hemorrhage.

(4) Start IV (if appropriate):

(a) Massive tissue damage.

(b) Fracture of femur.

(c) Any open fracture.

(5) Dress wounds.

(6) Immobilize (splint) fractures.

(a) Splint them where they lie. (Gross deformities may be gently corrected to alleviate circulatory inhibition if present.)

(b) Immobilize the joint above and the joint below the fracture.

(c) Pad the splint to prevent further injury or discomfort. Add extra padding over bony prominences.

(d) Traction is required on most fractures of long bones to overcome muscle contractions.

(7) Under conditions where patient cannot be evacuated, reduce fractures as soon as possible.

(a) Use anesthetics for reduction p.r.n. Fracture reduction can usually be accomplished by injecting local anesthesia into the hematoma of the fracture. An adjunct (e.g., morphine, Demerol) can be used for very painful procedures.

(b) Pad areas of pressure.

(c) Cast or splint in position of function.

(d) Bivalve all casts to allow for swelling and hold in place with ace wrap until swelling subsides (about 3 days), then replace with plaster wrap.

(e) Elevate and cool fractured extremities.

(f) Check extremities frequently for circulation loss.

d. Spinal column injuries. Any injury to the spinal column is potentially dangerous. Although a patient may have no apparent injury, moving him without proper precautions may result in spinal cord injury, causing paralysis.

(1) Fractured lower spine.

(a) Pain, tenderness, muscle spasm, deformity, paralysis, loss of bladder and/or bowel control may be present.

(b) If patient is conscious, place the patient in a swayback position (illustrated below) to avoid flexing the spine. (Flexing the spine can cause bone fragments to lacerate or compress the spinal cord.) If patient is unconscious transport in prone position with head rotated to side (be certain patient does not also have a neck injury).

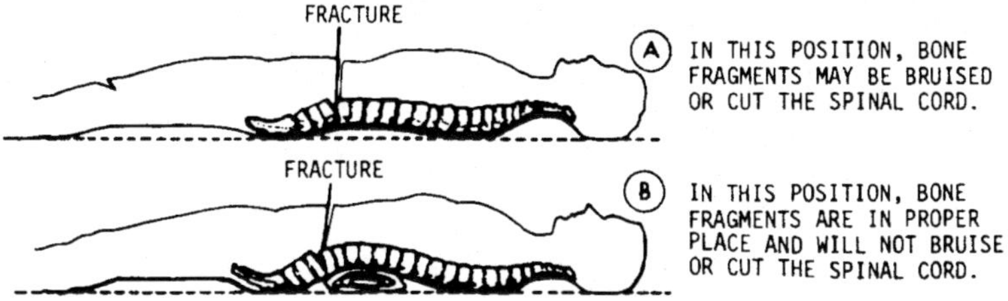

PATIENT PLACED IN A SWAYBACK POSITION.

If the patient is lying in a face-up position, place a folded blanket under the small of his back. If the patient is lying face down, place a folded blanket under his chest. This will keep the spinal column properly aligned and in a swayback position.

(c) Always move the entire vertebral column as a nonflexible unit.

(d) Use rigid litter or board longer than the patient is tall for transportation.

(e) Improvise some type of reversible bed so that the patient can be turned every 2 hours to prevent bed sores. (See illustration below.)

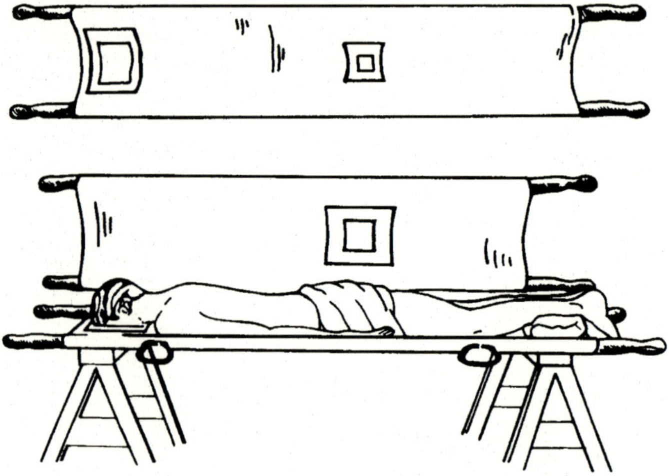

(f) An indwelling catheter must be used, and the patient should receive an enema daily.

(g) Patient must remain immobilized for 8-10 weeks.

(2) Fractured cervical spine.

(a) Signs and symptoms are similar to lower spinal column injury, but paralysis may include arms and upper body, even making the patient unable to breath. Any movement can cause further permanent damage.

(b) Make a thorough examination of the patient without moving his head.

(c) If patient is conscious, the first question should be, "Where do you hurt?" Suspect cervical spine injury if patient complains of severe occipital, shoulder, and arm pain, motor weakness, and numbness in arms and legs.

(d) To transport the patient. With the help of another person--

1. Hold the patient so his head and body are aligned.

2. Place the patient onto a firm surface (door or rigid stretcher). (If he is lying on his face, roll him onto the surface so he is lying on his back.) Be careful to hold the head in a neutral position.

3. Place a small rolled towel or sheet under the neck.

4. Place sandbags or boots filled with sand or dirt on either side of the head to stabilize it, or have someone hold the head in a neutral position while transporting the patient.

(e) Definitive treatment.

1. Fit into a head halter with padding to chin and apply traction in a straight line using a 10-15 lb weight. (A head halter can be improvised, but remember the patient will be in traction for at least 3 weeks. Think of his comfort when improvising.)

2. If there is no evidence of damage to the cord, place the patient on a foam mattress or a firm air mattress.

3. Patients with spinal cord damage must be placed on a turning frame (as with lower back injuries).

4. Commonly with cervical spine injuries, some sensory loss or paralysis may appear due to swelling, transection, or compression of spinal cord. Some or all of this paralysis may disappear as the swelling goes down.

5. Meticulous skin care must be maintained to prevent pressure sores.

6. Place patient N.P.O., giving only IV fluids for the first few days until there is evidence of audible peristalsis.

7. Catheterize patient using indwelling Foley catheter.

8. Usually after 3 weeks of traction, a cervical collar can be applied in cases where there is no cord damage (a collar can be made using a very well padded wire ladder splint). This should be worn for 8-12 weeks.

e. Craniocerebral injuries.

(1) Head injuries result either from penetration or impact. The damage may result from direct injury or may be secondary to compression, tension, or shearing forces caused by the injury. Note illustrations below.

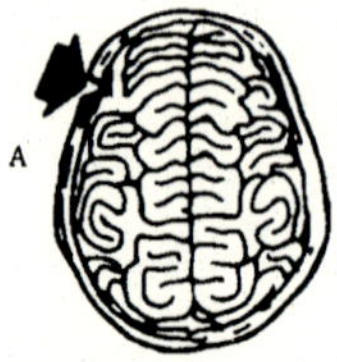

A blow to the skull (direct injury) may result in fracture (A)

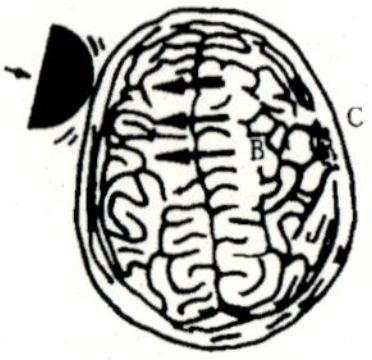

Or, in the absence of fracture, it may cause sufficient movement of the brain (B) to result in tearing some of the veins bridging from the cortical surface to the dura (C) with consequent development of subdural hematoma

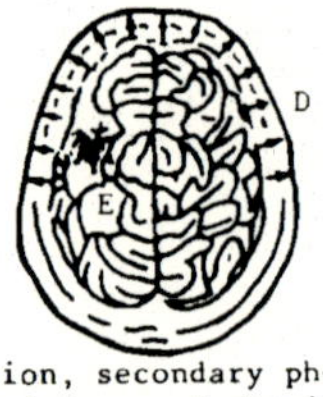

In addition, secondary phenomena may result from the injury. Ischemia and particularly cerebral edema may ensue. Elevation of intracranial pressure secondary to ischemia cerebral edema (D), a mass lesion (E), or combination of these processes may occur and affect the outcome.

(2) Head injuries are classified as either closed or open.

(a) Closed injuries. Except for a possible bruise or contusion, there is no obvious external damage. Injury may be to the brain itself or to the pia or arachnoid meninges. Rupture of the blood vessels of the pia is particularly important in closed injuries. Blood spilled onto brain cells is a foreign substance and disturbs the functioning of these tissues. Blood collecting within the cranium exerts pressure against the brain. If there is no fracture of the skull, or if skull fracture is such that the integrity of the dura is not disturbed, the cranium is unyielding. If the skull is depressed or displaced inwardly, it may exert direct pressure on the brain even without formation of a hematoma (blood pool).

(b) Open wound. In an open wound there is obvious external damage. Open wounds of the head are subclassified according to whether or not the integrity of the dural is disturbed.

1. Nonperforated dura mater. The wound may be no more than a laceration of the scalp that, although not to be taken lightly, may not be serious. There may be one or more fractures of the skull, but the dura is not perforated. In either case, the possible internal damage is likely to be or become more serious than that of the scalp and skull. If the skull is fractured, it will hold in the same manner as a closed injury against the pressure of any hemorrhage that may occur within the cranium.

2. Perforated dura mater. With the skull and dura opened, the meninges are exposed to the open air and to pathogenic invasion. If the delicate meninges are opened, the brain itself is exposed. If the skull is fractured in such a way that it is no longer a

closed vault, part of it may be torn away, and brain tissue may be extruding through the opening.

(3) All head injuries are potentially dangerous, not only because of the immediate tissue damage and increased susceptibility to infection, but also because of the probability that some vital area or special sense is or will become involved. For these reasons, it is extremely important that all signs and symptoms referable to the nervous system be carefully noted and recorded with the time of their occurrence or observation.

(a) State of consciousness. The following descriptive adjectives should be used, as appropriate, to define the state of consciousness observed.

Conscious. Patient is alert and oriented in time and space.

Confused. Patient is alert but disoriented and excited. (For purposes of taking fluids by mouth, patient is conscious.) The disorientation and excitement, which are not in keeping with the total situation, may be temporary and have a psychological basis in addition to or instead of brain injury.

Somnolent. Patient is excessively drowsy or sleepy, but responds to stimulation.

Semicomatose. Patient responds to painful stimuli but makes no spontaneous movements. (For purposes of taking fluid by mouth, patient is considered unconscious.)

Comatose. Patient does not respond to any applied stimulus; he is unconscious in the usual sense.

(b) Pupil size. Normally, pupils of the eyes tend to become very small in the presence of strong light and to dilate as the light fades. Dilation in the presence of strong light indicates central nervous system impairment. Normally, the pupils are equal in size. When neither eye is obviously injured and the pupils are of unequal size, brain impairment should be assumed and is an ominous sign.

(c) Muscles. The musculature on one or both sides of the face may droop due to lack of stimulation from the brain through the cranial nerves serving the facial muscles. There may be loss or impairment of speech. Paralysis and lack of tone in the muscle mass of any part of the body when there is no damage to the area nor suspicion of spinal cord damage is presumptive evidence of impairment of the brain area controlling movement of those muscles.

(d) Vital signs. The vital signs--temperature, blood pressure, respiration--are especially important in head injuries since changes in these indices frequently indicate the onset of complications.

(e) Headache, nausea, dizziness, and loss of consciousness (which may be brief, intermittent, or extended) may accompany a closed head injury, depending upon the particular injury and its severity. If injury is from impact with a blunt surface, an elevated contusion (bruise) forms when blood and other fluids collect in a pocket in the subcutaneous tissue between the dermis and the skull; there may be fracture in which part of the skull is displaced inwardly. In the more severe injuries, vomiting and paralysis of some muscle group may occur. The patient may bleed from the nose, mouth, or ears in the absence of obvious injury to these parts. Cerebrospinal fluid coming from the nose or ears indicates a grave injury. Normally a clear liquid, cerebrospinal fluid becomes cloudy when mixed with small quantities of blood. Signs of increasing intracranial pressure include: elevated blood pressure, slow pulse, restlessness, dilation of one or both pupils, decreased respiration, cyanosis, delirium or irritability, and paralysis. Unless a qualified person is available to relieve the pressure by opening the skull, increased respiratory failure, heart failure, and death may be expected.

(4) Closed head injuries may be difficult to diagnose. What may initially appear to be a minor injury with no complications may develop. (within 24 hours to 2 weeks or longer) into a life threatening problem due to gradually increasing intracranial pressure. It is important in head injuries to get a good history at the time of injury and do a complete neurological exam (see Chapter 1, Section VII, Nervous System). If there was any period of unconsciousness, the patient should be placed under observation for at least 24 hours with frequent neurological examinations. You should compare these examinations to determine if there is any deterioration in the neurologic findings.

(5) Emergency medical treatment of head wound.

(a) Assure an open airway. Clear the air passage of any vomitus, mucus, or debris as necessary; place the patient in coma position; turn the semicomatose or comatose patient from one side to the other every 20 minutes. As the patient's condition stabilizes, turning him every hour may be sufficient. Maintaining an open airway is usually not a problem for patients who have only scalp lacerations; the first consideration with these patients is to control the profuse bleeding.

(b) Control bleeding and protect wound. Place a sterile pressure dressing over the wound; do not remove or disturb any foreign material that may be in the wound; leave any protruding brain tissue as it is, and apply the dressing over this tissue.

(c) Prevent or treat shock. Apply measures for prevention or treatment of shock, with the following exceptions and modifications:

Do not put patient in head-low position.

Do not give morphine.

Give necessary fluids by mouth if possible (patient must be conscious and not nauseated). If required, give them very slowly.

(d) Observe patient. Observe the seriously injured patient for hours or until he can be transported to surgery. Take and record vital signs (which include pulse, respiration, and blood pressure) periodically. When possible, seek help from professional medical personnel if symptoms indicating intracranial injury or increased intracranial pressure appear.

f. Fracture of the femur.

(1) Usually there is a marked displacement of the fragments due to contraction of the large muscles in the thigh. This usually carries

varying degrees of shock due to trauma to the bone and soft tissue and loss of blood.

(2) First treat the patient as a whole; restore lost blood and fluid, treat for shock, relieve pain, and always make a search for associated injuries.

(3) If the fracture is an open one, it should be cleaned, debrided, and converted to a closed fracture as soon as the patient's condition permits.

(4) Traction must be used along with immobilization for all fractures of the femur. Use Thomas leg splint or improvise a traction splint of some type.

(5) Union takes at least 12-14 weeks. If there is any doubt, continue the immobilization with reduced traction for 4-8 more weeks.

(6) When union is sound, remove traction and have patient exercise the limb and joints freely in bed for several days, then allow the patient to walk using crutches until you are sure the union is sound.

g. Fracture of the lower jaw (see Chapter 19, Dental Emergencies and Treatment).

h. Fracture of the clavicle.

(1) Pain in shoulder, injured shoulder usually lower than uninjured shoulder, patient cannot raise his arm above his shoulder, patient usually supports the elbow on the affected side with opposite hand, and the fractured ends can usually be felt under the skin.

(2) Pad axillae and over the shoulder.

(3) Use two belts, strips of cloth, cravats, or roller bandages in a figure eight fashion to bring the shoulders up and back.

(4) Support the forearm with a sling and secure it to the body to reduce movement.

(5) Figure eight bandage must remain in place for 4-6 weeks.

i. Rib fracture.

(1) Pain in breathing and coughing. Pain and tenderness at fracture site are produced by hand pressure on the sternum. Sometimes the fracture can be felt. Patient usually holds his hand tightly over the break. If lung is punctured, the patient may cough up bright red frothy blood.

(2) Treat any penetrating chest wounds, hemothorax or pneumothorax (see Chapter 16, Emergency War Surgery).

(3) Control pain and apprehension, but avoid drugs that depress the respiratory and cough reflex centers. Pain is best relieved by intercostal blocks (repeated as necessary).

(a) Injection of one rib may be effective, but usually the

ribs above and below must also be injected to attain relief.

(b) Inject at least 5 cc. of lidocaine a hand's width proximal (toward the spine) under the margin of the rib after aspirating to insure you are not in a blood vessel.

(4) For fractures of upper ribs--

(a) Cleanse the skin and paint with tincture of benzoin.

(b) Have patient hold his breath following expiration while you apply two long 3" adhesive strips across the shoulder of the injured side. Strips should extend well down on the abdomen in the front and to the lower back in the rear (illustration below).

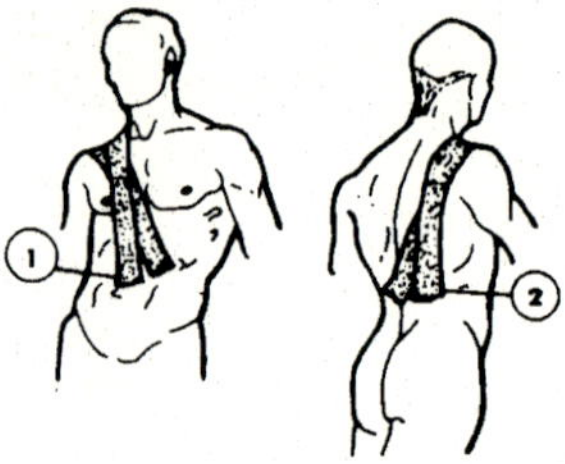

STRAPPING UPPER RIBS.

(5) For fractures of lower ribs--

(a) Apply a piece of felt or foam rubber 1-2" thick over the fracture.

(b) Have patient hold his breath following expiration while you apply 3" adhesive strips extending beyond the midline anteriorly and posteriorly (illustration below).

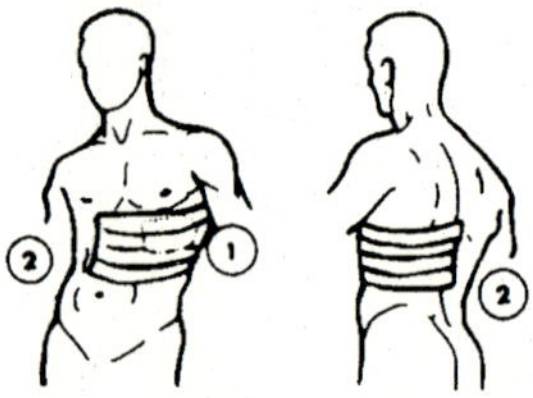

STRAPPING LOWER RIB FRACTURES.

(6) An alternate method for fractures of upper and lower ribs is to apply a 6-8" elastic bandage encircling the trunk from below the costal cage to just below the level of the nipples. (See illustration below.)

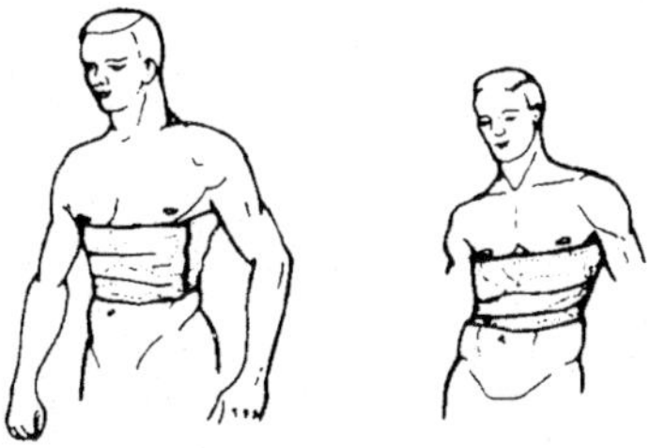

STRAPPING WITH ELASTIC BANDAGE OR MUSLIN DRESSING.

(7) Union takes 4-6 weeks.

j. Fractures of fingers or toes.

(1) Manually manipulate fracture into position.

(2) Tape fractured finger or toe to adjacent finger or toe.

(3) Union takes 2-6 weeks.

9-2. SPRAINS.

a. A sprain is caused when a joint is stretched beyond its normal range of motion causing a stretching of the joint capsule and the ligaments surrounding the capsule--some fibers tear but the continuity of the structure remains intact. The amount of tearing of the ligaments determines the severity of the sprain.

b. Symptoms are very sharp pain at the time of injury accompanied by a sensation of no support in that particular joint. In addition, there is rapid swelling and loss or decrease of function in the joint.

c. Treatment.

(1) Sprains should be immobilized either by cast or taping depending on their severity.

(a) Hematomas around the sprained joint usually denote a severe sprain and should be splinted or put in a cast for at least 3 weeks.

(b) Minor sprains should be taped to support the ligaments and give them time to heal.

(2) Keep the joint at rest and elevate the part if possible.

(3) Apply cold compresses immediately after the injury and for the first 24 hours, then apply heat to relieve pain and promote circulation.

9-3. DISLOCATION.

a. A dislocation starts the same as a sprain but continues until the ligaments are torn and the bone pulls out of the joint capsule. This displacement of bone may be either partial or complete. Dislocations are frequently accompanied by fractures, and structures such as blood vessels, nerves, and soft tissue surrounding the joint may be injured.

b. Symptoms are pain, deformity, swelling, discoloration, and usually a loss of motion. In severe cases, shock may be present.

c. Treatment.

(1) Dislocations should be reduced as soon as possible. Muscles surrounding the joint suffer a shock and you have a period of little or no pain, but as the muscles recover, they try to pull the bone back into the joint by contracting. The longer the bone is out of joint the stronger the contractions and the more damage is done to the surrounding tissue. By the same token, the stronger the contractions the more severe the pain and the harder it is to reduce the dislocation.

(a) Morphine or Demerol should be used in major dislocations to relieve pain and relax the muscles.

(b) The principle to follow in the reduction of dislocations is to pull the bone straight out and away from the joint and allow the muscles to pull the bone back into the joint by gradually releasing the pressure exerted.

(c) Once the dislocation has been reduced, the patient should feel immediate relief.

(d) Check distal capillary filling of the nail beds, blanching, pulse (pulse may or may not be present), color (look for cyanosis or pallor), and warmth of extremity to insure adequate peripheral circulation.

1. If circulation is insufficient, you will have severe pain in the flexor muscles, swelling, coldness, cyanosis or pallor, and paralysis and/or impairment of sensations.

2. Treatment should be started immediately. Treat symptomatically. Relieve anything that may cause circulatory impairment. Apply traction and ice packs (to relieve swelling). If after 2 hours circulatory impairment is not relieved, make S-shaped incision over the joint and extending distally. Incise the fascia and remove the hematoma. This may be sufficient to allow the collateral blood supply to relieve the circulatory insufficiency. (If it is necessary to repair arteries, see Chapter 16, Emergency War Surgery.)

(e) After dislocation has been reduced and blood supply is adaquate, immobilize the joint for at least 3 weeks.

9-4. STRAINS.

a. Strains are due to overstretching or overexerting a muscle or tendon, causing a tearing or rupture.

b. Symptoms are a sharp pain and cramps immediately upon injury, swelling, redness, heat, and loss of function.

c. Treatment.

(1) Place patient in a comfortable position that lessens tension and reduces pressure on the injured muscle or tendon.

(2) Apply heat.

(3) Strap injured area with adhesive tape to immobilize the area.

CHAPTER 10

BURNS AND BLAST INJURIES

10-1. BURNS.

a. How to manage situations causing burns.

(1) Patient with clothes on fire: Since flames ascend, get the patient flat on the floor, forcibly if necessary, with flames uppermost, then smother flames with coat, rug, or blanket.

(2) Scalds: Immediately rip off affected clothes so as to reduce time of application of hot fluid to skin.

(3) Patient in a burning room: Rescuer first hyperventilates, ties a wet cloth around his face and enters room, holding breath and staying low. Give oxygen to patient immediately upon rescue.

(4) Electrical: Push patient off the conductor with a nonconductor or pull him off by his belt. Do not touch his body while he is in contact with the conductor unless you are wearing insulated gloves. First check for heartbeat or pulse. If there is none, start CPR until heart resumes beating and patient is breathing on his own, or is pronounced dead or for a maximum of 3 hours.

b. Calculation of depth (degree) of burn.

(1) First degree:

(a) Examples: Sunburn, low intensity flash.

(b) Only the outer layer (epidermis) is burned.

(c) Symptoms: Tingling, painful, hyperesthetic (extremely sensitive to touch).

(d) Signs: Reddened, blanches with pressure, minimal or no edema.

(e) Course: Peeling and complete recovery within seven days.

(f) Treatment: Noxzema cream or mild analgesics.

(2) Second degree:

(a) Examples: Scalds, flash flame.

(b) Most but not all of the thickness of the skin is burned. Capillary walls are damaged with leakage of plasma into the tissues.

(c) Symptoms: Very painful; sensation to pin prick normal or slightly decreased.

(d) Signs: Blisters either intact or broken; weeping surface; mild edema.

(e) Course: Heals with no scarring or minimal scarring in 2-3 weeks. Infection may convert to third degree.

(3) Third degree:

(a) Example: Fire burns.

(b) The full thickness of the skin is destroyed. Edema is greatest.

(c) Symptoms: Painless to pin prick. Symptoms of shock may appear if edema is great enough.

(d) Signs: Skin is dry, pale white, or charred. Edema is present.

(e) Course: A scab will form and slough in about three weeks. Skin grafting will be necessary since scar, not skin, will cover the burn.

c. Treatment.

(1) First aid for all burns involves the following items:

(a) Relieve pain. (Morphine is the most active way to reach pain in severe burns. IV injection 8 to 10 mg. may bring relief).

(b) Prevent or treat shock.

(c) Prevent infection through strict asepsis.

(d) In burns due to electricity or severely swollen membranes in mouth and throat, the burn may have to be ignored while resuscitative measures are carried out, or CPR instituted to restore the heartbeat.

(2) Remove all clothing except that which is stuck.

(3) Treat chemical burns: Local treatment of chemical burns varies with the burning agents. Wash the burn with large quantities of water; acid burns should be neutralized by washing with a dilute sodium bicarbonate solution, and alkali burns with vinegar or dilute acetic solution. Otherwise the treatment is the same as for thermal burns.

(4) Examination of patient: Make careful initial evaluation combined with an accurate diagnosis.

(a) History and type of burning agent.

(b) Duration of exposure to heat.

(c) Careful examination of the depth of burn. Although burns are classified in degrees, the important factor from a therapeutic and prognostic viewpoint is whether the full thickness of the skin is affected. This may be checked in the following manner:

1. Areas of full thickness of skin loss show insensitivity to pin prick and loss of light touch.

2. If hair can be picked out with little resistance or no pain, the burn is a deep one.

(d) Careful evaluation of the extent of the burn (percent of the body surface area burned). This may be accomplished by the "Rule of Nines" method.

d. Calculating the area of the burn.

(1) No one can treat a burn intelligently unless he is able to correctly observe and record the area of the burn expressed in percent of total body surface.

(2) RULE OF NINES:

Each upper extremity	9%
Head and neck	9%
Anterior trunk	18%
Posterior trunk	18%
Each thigh	9%
Each lower leg	9%
Perineum	1%

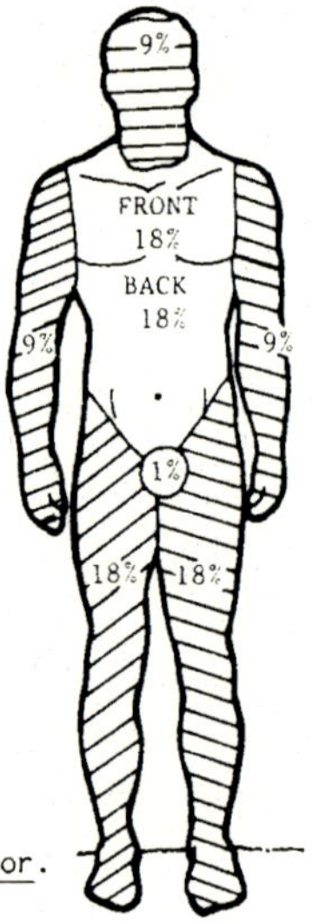

CAUTION: Do not overestimate percentage. Common error.

e. Classification of burns by severity.

(1) Critical burns.

(a) Second degree over 30% area.

(b) Third degree over 10% area.

(c) Third degree of hands, feet, or face.

(d) Any burn complicated by respiratory injury or other injury such as fractures or major soft tissue injury.

(2) Moderate burns.

(a) Second degree of 15-30% area.

(b) Third degree of 4-10% not involving hands, feet, or face.

(3) Minor burns.

(a) Second degree less than 15% area.

(b) Third degree less than 4% area not involving hands, feet, or face.

f. General principles of burn treatment.

(1) Cleansing: The cleaning of burned areas should be accomplished by gentle washing with pHisoHex and sterile saline when the burn is fresh. Wash away all trash, dirt, and bits of clothing. After danger of infection is past, burned area may be washed with ordinary soap and tap water.

(2) Blisters: What should be done about blisters? Leave intact blisters alone until they break themselves, then cut away with iris scissors. Any intact blister showing evidence of infection within it (purulent contents or surrounding lymphangitis) should be immediately opened and debrided in a sterile manner.

(3) All second degree or more burns should receive a tetanus booster.

(4) Ointments: There is no proven evidence that any antibiotic ointment applied to a burned surface is any more advantageous than plain vaseline or no ointment at all. However, it has been the personal experience of others that routine light application of Furacin ointment or Silvadene Cream to all second and third degree burns decreases the incidence of infection, and may prevent a deep second degree from going to a third degree burn. A very rare patient may exhibit a sensitivity to Furacin ointment or Silvadene Cream, but the benefit far outweighs the risk.

(5) Bandaging: Numerous papers variously supporting the "open method" and the "closed method" exist. You cannot go wrong by following this rule:

(a) All burns of the head, neck, and perineum should be left open.

(b) All burns of the hands, joints, and circumferential burns of the trunk and extremities should be bandaged.

(c) For burns involving a single aspect of the trunk or extremity, either method is fine.

Use own judgment, depending on the circumstances. If in doubt, bandage.

CAUTION: Extensive bandaging of a patient hospitalized in a warm room may cause hyperpyrexia.

(d) When bandaging, a nonadherent material should be placed next to the burn to prevent granulation tissue growing into the gauze only to be ripped off at the next dressing change. An ideal such material is parachute nylon obtained from a surplus parachute. Cut it up in small pieces, package and autoclave it, and that will make an ideal nonadherent material to place next to the burn. If such is not available, use the finest mesh gauze that is available.

(e) Burns of the hand should be bandaged using a bulky dressing with the hand in the position of function (slight extension at the wrist and all fingers moderately flexed). If the fingers are burned, place bandaging between the fingers. The tips of the fingers should be exposed to allow for circulation to be checked and to preserve the patient's sense of touch.

(f) Burn bandages should be bulky so as to absorb exudate. Change the original burn bandage at 5 to 7 days if there are no complications. Change the dressing earlier if it is stained from the inside out, if there is malodor, if there is an increased pain or unexplained elevation of the patient's temperature.

(6) Burn over joints: Immobilize the joint to allow healing.

(7) Antibiotics: No systemic antibiotics are indicated for burns less than 15%. For second or third degree burns over 15%, give procaine penicillin 1.8 million units and streptomycin 1.0 gram daily in divided doses for 5 days. Thereafter, rely on sensitivity disc if infection is apparent in the wound.

(8) Pain: Small second degree burns can usually be managed with oral codeine, 1/2 grains from 1 to every 3 hours. Second degree burns over 20% usually require parenteral narcotic analgesics. The drug of choice is morphine; the second choice is Demerol.

NOTE: If hypotension or shock exist, which is possible if the burn is over 20%, give the analgesic intravenously in 1/3 to 1/2 of the IM doses. The reason for this is that subcutaneous or IM medications are not picked up by the patient in shock because of decreased blood flow. Therefore, the medications will not give pain relief even if repeated and will accumulate in the extravascular spaces until such time as the shock is corrected. Then they will pick medication up into the circulation all at once and constitute an overdose.

(9) Environmental temperature: The ideal environmental temperature for treatment of a large burn is 75 degrees to 80 degrees F.

(10) Burns of the genitalia: The urethra may close off from excessive edema in one-half hour, therefore place a Foley catheter as early as possible.

(11) Transportation of burned patients: If transportation to a hospital requires less than one-half hour, the only treatment required is about 1/8 grain morphine intravenously. If transportation is expected to require more than one-half hour, start an IV of Ringer's lactate or Saline. The patient does not tolerate prolonged transportation as well after 48 hours as he does before that time.

(12) Establishment of intravenous lifeline: All patients with burn over 20% must have an 18-gage needle (or preferably an intravenous catheter) placed and anchored securely in a vein as soon as the diagnosis is made because intravenous fluids and whole blood will be required. The

most practical site for a corpsman to do a cutdown is the greater saphenous vein just anterior to the medial malleolus of either ankle.

(13) Oral intake: Burned patients are usually quite thirsty and demand large quantities of water. Fluid replacement in burns less than 15% can usually be administered entirely by mouth. In more extensive burns, paralytic ileus and vomiting are quite common during the first few days. In an extensively burned patient, all oral intake is withheld and the entire replacement therapy is intravenous.

(14) Respiratory tract burns: A burn of the trachea or bronchi is a very serious complication of a burn injury. It is most apt to occur in flame burns about the face, or if the burn was sustained in a close-fire explosion, or if live steam is involved. Edema of any of the upper respiratory passages after such a burn may quickly cause death. As soon as the burned patient is seen, determine if respiratory tract damage has occurred.

(a) The symptoms of respiratory tract burns are hoarseness, coughing, rapid respiration, or cyanosis. Redness in the posterior pharynx may be present. Rales or rhonchi in the lung may be or may not be present. If a respiratory tract burn exists, a tracheostomy should be performed as soon as pain is relieved and replacement therapy has been started (fluids or whole blood). Give oxygen.

(b) Recent evidence clearly shows that a tracheotomy should not be done in burn patients unless there is a clear indication for it. The concept of "prophylactic tracheotomy" in the burned patient should be abandoned. If the tracheotomy is done, be sure it is done into the second or third tracheal rings, located just below the cricoid cartilage and above the isthmus of the thyroid gland. A "low" tracheotomy below the fourth ring is dangerous; the endotracheal cannula may rest on the carina or enter a main stem bronchus.

g. Treatment of pulmonary edema.

(1) Semi-Fowler position (sitting up).

(2) Morphine grains 1/6, IM or IV.

(3) Oxygen in high concentration (8-9 liters per minute).

(4) Aminophylline 250-500 mg. IV slowly.

(5) Reduction in the blood volume by venesection (300-500 ml.) or tourniquets on two of the four extremities applied with sufficient pressure to obstruct venous but not arterial flow. Rotate every 15 minutes.

h. Pathologic physiology.

(1) Edema inevitably follows burning. Heat causes capillary injury, resulting in vasodilation and increased capillary permeability.

(2) A burn is a three-dimensional wound consisting of length and width (area) and depth. Depth cannot be visualized and is difficult to determine accurately, but is an extremely important factor affecting the volume of edema that will occur. Examples: In a first degree burn,

vasodilation is the only change that occurs, and edema is minimal. A second degree burn, being deeper, involves a large volume of tissue plus more extensive capillary damage so that edema occurs. Although there is no edema in the charred eschar of a third degree burn, the volume of edema around and under it is greater than the volume of edema in a second degree burn of comparable area. Remember that the greatest fluid losses occur deep in the wound, hence appearance is misleading.

i. Edema time factors.

(1) The rate of edema formation (intravascular fluid loss) is greatest in the first 8 hours after burning. Edema continues to form, but at a less rapid rate, until about 36 to 48 hours after burning, at which time the total edema is maximal.

(2) Resorption of edema then occurs and proceeds slowly over 5 to 7 days, but burn edema may persist for 2 or 3 weeks.

(3) From the above statement it is apparent that the danger of shock is greatest in the first 24 hours after burning and is almost never a problem after 36 to 48 hours, if adequate fluid replacement therapy has been given. After the possibility of respiratory tract burn has been considered, all efforts in therapy are then directed towards proper fluid therapy to replace the fluid extravasated into the tissues as edema.

j. Fluid replacement in minor burns.

(1) In general, there is not a significant danger of shock in burns less than 20% and these can be handled with an oral fluid replacement therapy consisting of a solution of 1/2 teaspoon of salt and 1/2 teaspoon baking soda in one quart of water.

(2) The solution should be thoroughly chilled for optimal patient tolerance. If vomiting occurs, discontinue oral intake and use the intravenous route.

(3) In a disaster, when IV fluids may not be available, oral electrolyte replacement solution may be a lifesaving measure for all patients with burns up to 35%. The recommendation limiting the use of oral therapy to patients with less than 20% burns is conservative and assumes availability of IV fluids.

(4) If both IV and oral fluids are given, the oral intake must be included in the calculated 24-hour fluid replacement plan.

k. Calculation of fluid replacement therapy in moderate or serious burns.

(1) Fluid replacement requirements are governed by many complex variables and it is impossible to state in a formula exact replacement requirements. The burn formula below is a very practical and valuable as an initial rough estimate fluid replacement guide.

(2) Brooke formula:

(a) Ml. of fluid to be given in the first 24 hours = (% body burn) x (wt. in kilograms) x (0.5 cc.) colloid plus (% body burn) x (wt. in kilograms) x (1.5 ml.) Ringer's lactate solution plus 2,000 ml. 5%

dextrose in water.

(b) Expressed in terms of pounds instead of kilograms, the formula becomes: ml. first 24 hours = (% burn) x (wt. in pounds) x 0.23 ml. colloid + (% burn) x (wt. in pounds) x (0.67 ml.) Ringer's lactate solution plus 2,000 ml. of 5% dextrose in water.

(c) Give one-half of the total calculated 24-hour requirement in the first 8 hours after the burn, starting from the time the burn occurred. Give the remainder evenly over the remaining 16 hours.

(d) In applying the formula to burns over 50%, calculate as though only 50% had been burned.

(e) Do not count first degree burns in computing the fluid requirement.

(f) During the second 24 hours, give one-half of the volume of colloid and Ringer's lactate as calculated for the first 24 hours, plus 2,000 ml. of 5% dextrose in water.

Problem: A 150-lb man sustains a total body burn of 35% consisting of 20% first degree, 25% second degree, and 10% third degree. Plan fluid therapy. Assume you have dextran.

Ml. first 24 hours = 35 x 150 x 0.23 ml. colloid + 35 x 150 x 0.67 ml. Ringer's lactate plus 2,000 cc. 5% dextrose in water which equals 1,207 ml. dextran plus 3,517 ml. Ringer's lactate plus 2,000 ml. dextrose in water.

The total volume of fluids to be given in the first 24 hours after the burn is 6,724 ml. One half of this amount, or about 3,500 ml., should be given in the first 8 hours after the burn. Therefore, appropriate fluids for the first 8 hours after the burn would be 2,000 ml. of Ringer's lactate, then 500 ml. Dextran, then 1,000 ml. dextrose 5% in water. If IV fluids are started late and you are trying to catch up, you can give as much as 200 ml. in 1 hour (300 drops per minute) without overloading the circulation. Or if treatment has been delayed and the patient is already in shock, fluid administration by two separate veins may be necessary.

(g) By far the most accurate guide to adequacy of administered fluids is the rate of urinary output. Therefore, all patients receiving prolonged therapy should have a Foley catheter in place and urinary output measured at least hourly. A urinary output of 25 to 40 ml. per hour is adequate. A rate much over this indicates fluids are being given too rapidly.

1. Oliguria (very low rate of urine output).

(1) A special problem is posed by the severely burned patient who has oliguria or anuria even after fluid therapy has been started, since acute renal failure is a rare complication of severe burns. Should the case be considered one of renal failure or should it be assumed that fluid therapy has been insufficient? This question is crucial since the accepted method of treatment for renal failure is rigid fluid restriction, a plan that would be disastrous if in fact the oliguria is due to inadequate fluids. In this circumstance the correct course of action is intensive therapy with whatever fluid appears to be deficient on the assumption that oliguria is caused by inadequate fluids. If oliguria persists, then he has

a renal shutdown and you stop the flow of IV fluids after 1,000 ml. of colloid and 1,000 ml. of electrolyte solution have been given rapidly (150-300 drops per minute), then renal failure due to organic changes is likely to be present.

(2) Oliguria is often encountered in extensive second degree burns, while anuria is more commonly a complication of extensive third degree burns.

m. Other care in the first 24 hours.

(1) Record the urine output, pulse, and blood pressure at least hourly. It is preferable not to give anything by mouth for the first 48 hours in severely burned patients. If there is severe thirst, small amounts of water may be given, but the amount must be recorded and subtracted from the total allowance.

2. Since acute gastric dilation is a common complication, examine the abdomen frequently for distention. It may be necessary to pass a nasogastric tube.

n. The second 24-hour period.

(1) The fluid regimen consists of 1/2 of the colloid and electrolyte solutions given during the first 24 hours, plus 2,000 ml. 5% dextrose in water.

(2) Fever of 101-102°F. (orally) is not uncommon even in the absence of infection.

o. Treatment after 48 hours. By 48 hours, edema is maximal but its production has ceased. The physiology of electrolyte imbalance that may occur after 48 hours is too complicated to be considered in this manual. A general rule is to give only 5% dextrose and water in order to dilute the large amount of sodium being immobilized from the burn edema.

p. Outline of immediate treatment plan.

(1) Relieve pain.

(2) Obtain history, including weight of patient.

(3) Map area and degree of burn.

(4) Determine need for tracheotomy.

(5) Start Ringer's lactate of dextran, using a large-bore needle (an 18-gage is preferable).

(6) Do cut down if necessary.

(7) Insert Foley catheter.

(8) Initiate local care, like cleansing and dressing.

(9) Give penicillin and streptomycin if indicated.

(10) Give tetanus toxoid.

(11) Plan fluid replacement requirement.

10-2. BLAST INJURIES.

a. General information. The human body is not constructed to tolerate very marked or sudden increases in pressure. This is obvious from our past experiences in wars and from the experiences of deep-sea divers. The effects of a blast depend upon the wave length and the substance this blast or "shock" waves are transmitted by. Long slow waves are very low pitched and do very little damage since usually only one or two waves pass through the body. A sudden increase of 7 psi may rupture the tympanic membrane; however, it will take a sudden increase in excess of 30 psi to injure the hollow organs or cavities of the body.

b. Types of blast.

(1) Air. The waves travel slowest in air and do not do as much damage to the human body. Most injuries from an air blast are not true blast injuries but are caused by flying debris, etc.

(2) Water. Blast waves travel much faster in water than in air and will cause damage at greater distances. The human body has essentially the same density as sea water, which allows blast waves to pass through solid tissue without injury. Most of the damage from a water blast occurs to the hollow viscera, lungs, abdomen, and gas-filled cavities.

(3) Solid. Blast waves travel fastest through solid objects. The denser the substance, the faster they travel. These waves traveling through the deck of ships, etc., produce breaks in major blood vessels often without a break in the skin.

c. Classification of blast injuries.

(1) Primary. Injuries caused by the effect of blast waves on the body such as ruptured tympanic membranes, damage to hollow viscera, etc.

(2) Secondary. Injuries caused by flying debris such as shrapnel, bricks, chunks of plaster, etc. This classification also covers those who were trapped and injured in a building that was blown up around them.

(3) Tertiary. Injuries caused by the blast picking up the body and hurling it through the air striking some other object.

NOTE: It is frequently very hard to determine just which classification is proper and there are many times when more than one classification of injury will coexist in the same patient.

d. Common blast injuries. It is necessary to suspect blast injuries after any incident that would cause them. With no external marks or visible symptoms, the victim might be required to do something that could prove fatal to him. If there are no visible signs of injury and the patient is developing shock, it is a good indication of blast injury. Victims are often treated as "walking wounded" and only when shock, dyspnea, apprehension, tremulousness, and fear are apparent, is the correct diagnosis made.

(1) Ruptured tympanic membrane. As previously noted, this is the most common blast injury and occurs when there is as little as 7 psi sudden increase in pressure.

(a) Symptoms: A sudden, severe, lancinating pain in the ear. There may be bleeding from the affected ear and various degrees of hearing loss.

(b) Treatment: Clean the opening or meatus gently then "leave it alone." Do not pack, syringe, or instill any medication.

(2) Blast lung. When the symptoms of pain and clinical signs are first in and remain localized in the upper abdomen, the chances are very good that the blast injury is thoracic.

(a) Symptoms: In addition to the routine blast symptoms there is usually cyanosis, rapid pulse, and pain in the chest and upper abdomen with moderate abdominal rigidity. The patient may be coughing with ineffective expectoration of bloody, frothy mucous. There are usually multiple hematomas along the anterior costal lines.

(b) Treatment: Move as little as possible and it is best to stabilize patient for 48 hours before even evacuating him if possible. Administer oxygen for relief of cyanosis and dyspnea. Always suspect pulmonary edema from alveolar hemorrhage, and if it is mandatory to use IV fluids, use with extreme caution and run at slow rate. Atropine sulfate may be given in small doses to help diminish secretions. Avoid any ether or gaseous anesthetic agents. Antibiotics are useful for serious blast lung cases.

(3) Blast abdomen. Many persons describe the sudden onset of pain as a "kick in the belly," followed by a remission then by a recurrence. When clinical signs occur first in the upper abdomen then spread to the lower abdomen, then abdominal blast injury is most certain. When clinical signs remain from the onset in the lower abdomen, there is little doubt of intraperitoneal damage.

(a) Symptoms: Sudden occurrence of abdominal pain, a brief period of remission, then reoccurrence of severe, unremitting, and most of all increasing pain. Frequent bowel evacuations with difficulty in urination. Melena or frank passage of bright red blood in the stool.

(b) Treatment: The serious cases can be treated only with surgery. Place them high on the evacuation list. If hemorrhage or perforation is suspected with good reason, then request advice on dosage of antibiotics to sterilize the bowel. Keep N.P.O., insert nasogastric (NG) tube, catheterize with indwelling catheter, and consider pain relief. Withhold morphine until a careful assessment is made of the injury and treatment schedule. For example, do not give morphine if he will be on anesthesia and surgery within the following 1 to 2 hours.

(4) Other blast injuries. For fractures and other tissue trauma, treat the same as at any other time. Contusions of the scrotum and testicular pain are common; treat with adequate support. The transient paresis of the limbs that has been described in association with blast injuries is probably due to minor vascular disturbances in the spinal cord.

CHAPTER 11

HEAT AND COLD INJURIES

11-1. HEAT INJURIES.

a. Factors that govern heat injuries.

(1) Water.

(a) The human body is absolutely dependent upon water to cool itself in hot environments. In severe heat it is possible for a person to lose a quart of water each hour. Water lost must be replaced or an individual can become a heat injury. The activity will determine the amount of water necessary to maintain proper body functions, as illustrated below.

ACTIVITY	ILLUSTRATIVE DUTIES	Quarts per man per day for drinking purposes (a guide for planning only) WBGT or WD index* Less than 80°	Greater than 80°
Light	Desk	6	10
Moderate ...	Route march	7	11
Heavy	Forced marches; stevedoring; entrenching; or route marches with heavy loads or in CBR protective clothing.	9	13

*80° wet bulb globe temperature (WBGT) or WD index is approximately equivalent to a dry bulb temperature of 85° in a jungle or 105° in a desert environment.

Water requirements.

(b) The myth that humans can be taught to adjust to decreased water intake has been disproven. When water is in short supply, significant water economy can be accomplished only by limiting physical activity to the coolest part of the day or night.

(2) Salt.

(a) Ordinarily one's normal food intake will contain adequate salt; however, in heat stress situations, unacclimatized persons may require additional intake.

(b) Unless one is sweating continuously or repeatedly, salt tablets will not be required. Extra salt in the cooking, at the table, and in the water is all that is required.

(c) Older people and acclimatized persons tend to have less acute needs for salt replacement.

(d) A convenient way to provide adequate salt is to salt the drinking water 0.1%, in amounts shown below.

Salt Diluting Water

2 ten-grain salt tablets--dissolved in ....1-quart canteen
4 ten-grain salt tablets--dissolved in ....2-quart canteen
1 1/3 level mess kit spoons salt--dissolved in ...5-gallon can
9 level mess kit spoons salt--dissolved in ......lister bag
1 level canteen cup salt--dissolved in ....250-gallon water trailer

Preparation of 0.1 percent salt solution.

(3) Acclimatization. It takes a period of about 2 weeks to become acclimatized, regardless of the physical condition. An acclimatization program should consist of a person being exposed to progressively increasing heat and physical exertion in a new climate condition. Careful and fully developed acclimatization increases resistance, but it does not give complete protection from the ill effects of heat.

(4) Physical conditioning has a significant bearing on the reaction to heat stress.

(a) Debilitating diseases and injuries enhance the likelihood of heat injuries.

(b) Overweight personnel have a <u>much</u> higher incidence of heat injuries.

(5) Environmental factors.

(a) Although heat injuries can occur at temperatures below 0°F., e.g., overexerting and overdressing, most heat injuries occur during periods of high temperature and humidity. As the temperature rises, physical activity should be curtailed, as shown in heat categories below.

GUIDELINES FOR PHYSICAL ACTIVITY

CATEGORY	WBGT INDEX	NONACCLIMATED PERSONNEL	ACCLIMATED PERSONNEL
I	82-84.9°F.	Use discretion in planning intense physical activity. Limit intensity of work and exposure to sun. Provide constant supervision.	Normal duties.
II	85-87.9°F.	Strenuous exercises such as close order drill and physical training will be canceled. Outdoor classes in the sun will be canceled.	Use discretion in planning intense physical activity. Limit intensity of work and exposure to sun. Provide constant supervision.
III	88-89.9°F.	All physical training, strenuous activities, and parades will be canceled.	Strenuous outdoor activities will be minimized for all personnel with less than 12 weeks

			training in hot weather.
IV	90°F. and above	Strenuous activities and nonessential duty be canceled.	Strenuous activities and nonessential duty will be canceled.

Heat categories.

(b) The four basic factors that determine the degree of heat stress exerted by the environment are air temperature, relative humidity, air movement, and heat radiation. These factors can be measured by using a WBGT Index. The WBGT Index is computed as follows:

WBGT = 0.7 x wet bulb temperature

+ 0.2 x black globe temperature

+ 0.1 x dry bulb temperature.

(c) To make a WBGT apparatus, see sketch on following page.

b. Heat cramps. Caused by excessive salt loss from the body.

S. Painful cramps of the voluntary muscles usually in paroxysms lasting from 3-10 minutes with periods of relative comfort between the spasms. Patient may be grimacing and thrashing about with arms and legs drawn up. Skin is usually hot and moist.

O. Blood pressure and temperature will usually be normal. The pulse may be slightly elevated.

A. Heat cramps. Differential diagnosis: Heat exhaustion.

P. Remove to shaded area and give salt in any form to balance loss. IV normal saline 500-1,000 cc. in acute cases, 0.1% salt solution in cool water orally will afford both relief and continued protection. Massaging of cramped muscles will usually help afford immediate relief.

Do not use hot packs on the cramped muscles; that will only make it worse. Do not use saline enemas as that only draws more salt and water from the tissue.

c. Heat exhaustion. Caused by failure of peripheral circulation due to salt loss and dehydration.

S. Profuse sweating (diaphoresis) with cold, wet, and pale skin. Headache, mental confusion, vertigo, incoordination, drowsiness, extreme weakness, anorexia, nausea and vomiting, with visual disturbances. Occasionally, cramps of the extremities or abdominal muscles occur.

O. Temperature taken orally may be subnormal or slightly elevated, rectal temperature is usually elevated (100-101°F.), rapid pulse (140-200) with blood pressure usually lowered.

A. Heat exhaustion. Differential diagnosis: Heat cramps,

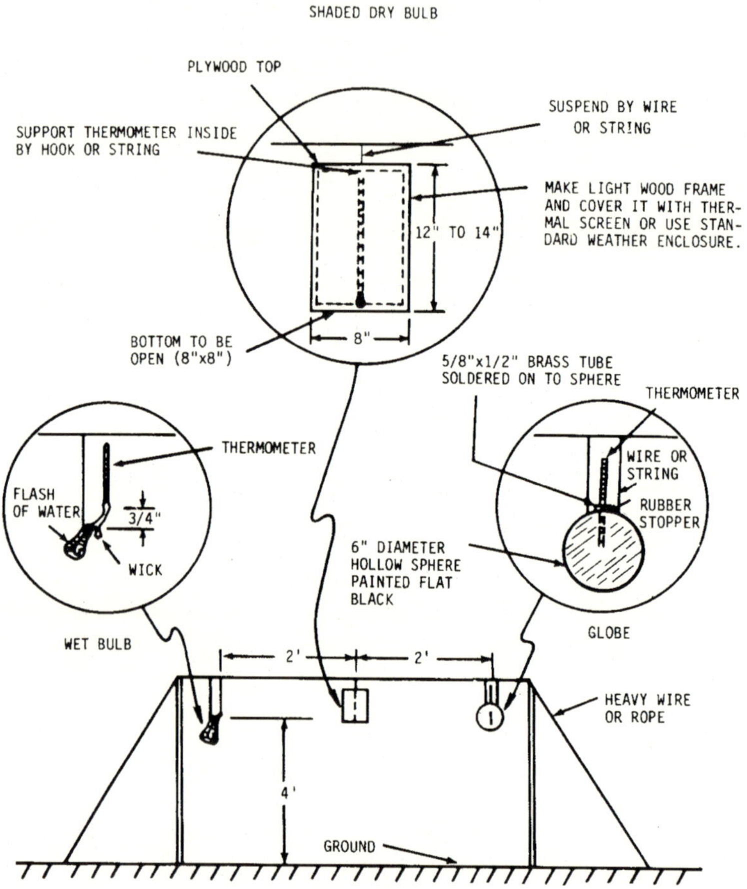

FIGURE 1. WBGT Index of-field apparatus.

heatstroke.

P. Remove patient to a cool, shaded area. Replace fluids and salt by giving patient cool water with 0.1% salt solution; or if he cannot take by mouth, give 1,000 to 1,500 cc. 5% dextrose in normal saline or a normal saline IV (an IV should be started in any case). Stimulation may be required such as tea, coke, coffee (caffeine) or even IM injection of .3 to .5 cc. of 1:1,000 epinephrine. Avoid immediate reexposure to heat.

d. Heatstroke. Caused by a breakdown of the body heat regulating mechanism.

S-O. There may be early symptoms of headache, dizziness, mental confusion, weakness, nausea, involuntary urination, and diminished or absent sweating. There may even be a false sense of exhilaration. Usually, however, the onset is dramatically sudden with collapse and loss of consciousness. Convulsions may occur. The skin is hot, red, and dry. The pulse is full and rapid, with blood pressure normal or elevated. Respirations are rapid and deep. The body temperature is markedly elevated (106-110oF.). As the patient's condition worsens, cyanosis is usually noted. The breathing becomes shallow and irregular. Pulmonary edema, involuntary urination and defecation, vomiting, hemorrhagic tendencies, disturbances of muscle tone, and jaundice and meningitislike symptoms to include tetanuslike body arching. Death may come very rapidly, but if patient survives until the second day, recovery usually occurs. Severe relapses may occur.

A. Heat stroke.

P. Lower the patient's body temperature as rapidly as possible. The longer the body temperature is high the greater the threat of permanent damage or death. Remove the patient's clothes and immerse him in cold water (tub of ice water, if possible). If not available, wet patient down with ice, water, or alcohol and fan him. Rub patient's extremities and trunk briskly to increase circulation to the skin. Temperature must be monitored closely and when temperature drops to 102oF. stop cooling, dry patient off, and wrap him in blankets or place him on heating pads. Usually the temperature will continue to fall, and sometimes will reach as low as 94oF. before it starts to rise again. If the patient's temperature falls below 97oF. be prepared to start the cooling process again when his temperature rises to 97oF. Constantly monitor the patient's body temperature and alternate heating and cooling until his temperature stabilizes. Continue monitoring the temperature every 10 minutes for the next 48 hours.

Care must be used in giving heatstroke patients medication. Sedative drugs disturb the heat regulating center and should be avoided if possible. When sedatives are necessary (as with convulsions), a short acting barbiturate such as sodium Pentothal IV is the drug of choice. If a longer acting drug is needed, phenobarbital should be administered IM. Epinephrine, sodium amytal, and morphine are contraindicated. Atropine or other drugs that may interfere with sweating are also contraindicated. An IV of normal saline or as second choice Ringer's lactate should be started and 1,000-2,000 cc. should be given initially. Subsequent IV infusion is determined by hourly urinary output and serum electrolyte determinations. It is important to recognize that the heat regulating centers may not function correctly for many weeks after an attack. This means the patient must be kept in a fairly controlled environment during this period and monitored at regular intervals. One attack of heatstroke predisposes an individual to further attacks.

11-2. COLD INJURIES.

a. Factors governing cold injuries.

(1) Weather, temperature, humidity, precipitation, and wind modify the rate of body heat loss. Low temperatures and low humidity favor frostbite, whereas higher temperatures together with moisture are usually associated with trench foot. Wind velocity accelerates body heat loss under both wet and cold conditions. (See chart.)

Cooling Power of Wind on Exposed Flesh Expressed as an Equivalent Temperature (under calm conditions)

Estimated wind speed (in mph)	Actual Thermometer Reading (°F.)											
	50	40	30	20	10	0	-10	-20	-30	-40	-50	-60
	EQUIVALENT TEMPERATURE (F.)											
calm	50	40	30	20	10	0	-10	-20	-30	-40	-50	-60
5	48	37	27	16	6	-5	-15	-26	-36	-47	-57	-68
10	40	28	16	4	-9	-21	-33	-46	-58	-70	-83	-95
15	36	22	9	-5	-18	-36	-45	-58	-72	-85	-99	-112
20	32	18	4	-10	-25	-39	-53	-67	-82	-96	-110	-124
25	30	16	0	-15	-29	-44	-59	-74	-88	-104	-118	-133
30	28	13	-2	-18	-33	-48	-63	-79	-94	-109	-125	-140
35	27	11	-4	-20	-35	-49	-67	-82	-98	-113	-129	-145
40	26	10	-6	-21	-37	-53	-69	-85	-100	-116	-132	-148
(wind speeds greater than 40 mph have little additional effect)	LITTLE DANGER (for properly clothed person)				INCREASING DANGER			GREAT DANGER				
					Danger from freezing of exposed flesh							

Trench foot and immersion foot may occur at any point on this chart.

(2) Clothing should be worn loose and in layers. Loose layers of clothing with air space between them worn under an outer wind- and water-resistant garment provide maximum protection. The loose inner layers can and must be removed during periods of strenuous physical exertion to prevent overheating and accumulation of perspiration. Wet clothing loses much of its insulation value.

(3) The very young and very old are more susceptible to cold injuries.

(4) Previous cold injuries definitely increase the risk of subsequent cold injury, not necessarily involving the part previously injured.

(5) Fatigue may cause apathy leading to neglect of acts vital to

survival.

(6) Other injuries resulting in significant blood loss or shock reduce blood flow to extremities and predispose the extremities to cold injury.

(7) Studies show blacks are more vulnerable than whites to cold injuries.

(8) Starvation or semistarvation predisposes to cold injury.

(9) Any drug or medication that affects peripheral circulation or sweating can lead to cold injury.

(10) Alcohol dilates the peripheral blood vessels causing body heat loss, which increases the dangers of hypothermia and frostbite.

(11) Heat injuries, as strange as it sounds, may occur even in extreme cold due to overdressing and overexertion. When this happens, the body temperature regulating mechanism is damaged and the patient can rapidly develop hypothermia leading to death.

b. Clinical manifestations.

(1) Symptoms during exposure.

(a) The lack of warning symptoms emphasizes the insidious nature of cold injury.

(b) There may be tingling, stinging, or at most a dull aching of the affected part followed by numbness.

(c) The skin briefly may appear red and then becomes pale or waxy white. At this stage the part may feel "like a block of wood." If freezing has occurred, the tissue appears "dead white" and is hard or even brittle with complete lack of sensation and movement.

(2) Differentiation. Terms such as chilblain, trench foot (immersion foot), and frostbite are only used to describe how the injury occurred. After rewarming, the tissue injury, which is largely the result of vascular damage, is similar in all forms of cold injury. The major variable is the degree (severity) of injury. Early evaluation of the degree of cold injury is extremely difficult even to the most experienced doctor. Definitive classification of severity into first, second, third, and fourth degree is possible only in retrospect.

(a) First degree. After rewarming, the skin becomes mottled, red, hot, and dry. The skin blanches poorly on pressure and capillary filling is sluggish or absent. There is frequently intense itching or burning and a later deep-seated ache. Swelling begins within 3 hours and may persist for 10 days or more if patient remains on duty, but usually disappears in less than 5 days if patient is kept at bed rest. Peeling of the superficial layers of the skin may begin within 5-10 days after the injury and last for a month.

(b) Second degree. After rewarming, the skin becomes deep red, hot, and dry. Light touch and position sense are frequently absent. Blisters and even huge blebs may appear within 6-12 hours and may extend nearly to the tips of the involved digits. These blebs are a valuable sign identifying the injury as second degree. They dry forming black eschars within 10-24 days; the eschars gradually separate revealing intact skin that is thin, soft, poorly keratinized, and easily traumatized. During rewarming there may be a tingling and burning sensation that increases in intensity to a deep aching and burning sensation. This pain may increase to the point the patient will require medication.

(c) Third degree. Necrosis of skin and cutaneous tissue. Vesicles may be present but they contain blood, are smaller, and do not extend to the tip of the involved digits. Edema of the entire involved area (entire hand or foot) usually appears in an average of 6 days. Most patients have a period of anesthesia lasting from 5-17 days followed by burning, aching, throbbing, or shooting pains lasting for months and recurring during exposure to cold sometimes for the rest of their lives. The skin overlaying the injury forms a black, hard, dry eschar that eventually separates exposing underlying granulation tissue. Healing occurs in an average of 68 days. Trauma and infection due to injury other than cold may result in extensive tissue loss, systemic infection, and even wet gangrene requiring emergency amputation of the affected part.

(d) Fourth degree. Complete necrosis of the entire thickness of the part including bone, resulting in loss of the entire injured part. Upon rewarming the skin may turn deep red, purple, or mottled and cyanotic. In some cases edema develops rapidly reaching a maximum within 6-12 hours; the area may show no significant increase in volume, but rapidly progresses to dry gangrene and mummification. In other cases edema develops slowly and is more pronounced, and the eschar formation is not evident until 2-3 weeks after rewarming. The line of demarcation becomes apparent in an average of 36 days but it takes 60-80 days to extend down to the bone. Usually there is no feeling in the injured area for 3-13 days, then ghost pain begins that may become severe.

(3) Early diagnosis and prognostic signs. As previously pointed out, classification of cold injuries as to degree is a retrospective diagnosis. In the early stages (first 48-72 hours) after rewarming, you can only differentiate between superficial (loss of skin or less) or deep (loss of skin and tissue) cold injuries.

(a) Signs of superficial cold injury.

<u>1.</u> Early development of large, clear blebs extending to tips of the digits.

<u>2.</u> Rapid return of sensations.

<u>3.</u> Return of normal (warm) temperature in injured area.

<u>4.</u> Pink or mildly erythematous skin color that blanches rapidly.

(b) Signs of deep cold injury.

<u>1.</u> Hard, white, cold, and insensitive.

<u>2.</u> Absence of edema.

3. Dark hemorrhagic blebs or lack of blebs or blisters.

4. Early mummification.

5. Systemic signs of tissue necrosis (fever, tachycardia, prostration).

6. Superimposed trauma.

7. Cyanotic or dark red skin color that does not blanch on pressure.

c. Treatment. Because of the progressive nature of cold injuries, the earlier they are detected and treatment started the better.

(1) Individual. A fairly reliable symptom of incipient frostbite of fingers, toes, and exposed skin is the sudden and complete cessation of the sensation of cold or discomfort in the part, often followed by a pleasant feeling of warmth. Prompt and immediate care will usually prevent the development of a more serious cold injury. The part must be rewarmed immediately. To rewarm an ear, nose, or cheek, remove your glove and hold (do not rub) your warm hand against the part until it is rewarmed, then protect the area with a scarf or ear flaps, etc. Fingers can be warmed by placing them under the clothes against the skin of the abdomen or the armpit. Toes can be rewarmed by holding them against a companion's chest or abdomen under his outer clothing.

(2) Initial or emergency treatment. The patient should be restricted from his usual duties or activities until the severity of the injury can be evaluated. All constricting items of clothing (boots, socks, gloves) should be removed from the injury site, and the area must be protected from further cold injury by blankets or available loose clothing. Smoking, drinking of alcohol, and use of medications (salves, ointments) on affected area are prohibited. Do not drain blisters; cover them with loose dry dressing. Give plenty of hot liquids to the patient (soup, coffee, tea, etc.). If a lower extremity is involved, treat the patient as a litter patient with the affected limb level or slightly elevated. If travel by foot is the <u>only</u> means of evacuation, do not thaw frostbitten feet until the patient reaches an aid station and medical help. Once the patient has reached an area of shelter (aid station, hospital) if freezing has occurred and the affected tissue is still frozen, it should be thawed as rapidly as possible in water 104-109°F. (40-42°C.). Thawing is determined by return of sensations (usually), return of color (frequently dark red or purple), and the observation that the tissue is soft. Under no circumstances should snow, ice water, grease, massage, walking, or dry heat be used. Warming above 98°F. (37°C.) is not recommended for nonfreezing cold injuries. Cold injury is no contraindication for narcotics or other pain medications, but accompanying injuries may govern the choice of medications. Tetanus toxoid booster should be given. Prophylatic antibiotics should not be used, but if an infection develops, suitable antibiotics should be started.

(3) Definitive treatment. Absolute bed rest is mandatory for any cold injury involving the feet. Debridement should be postponed until the eschar is completely formed, which in fourth degree cold injuries can take 60-80 days to extend to the bone. Patience, understanding, and constant encouragement are essential to good results.

d. Hypothermia--lowering of the body temperature below normal.

(1) Usually caused by exposure (atmospheric or immersion) to prolonged or extreme cold. Immersion in water 48oF. for 1 hour will usually lower body temperature enough to cause death, but hypothermia in cold environments can be caused by unconsiousness due to wounds, disease, alcohol, etc., in individuals who are inadequately protected.

(2) When the internal body temperature is about 95oF., there is a breakdown of the temperature control centers and the body cannot produce enough heat to maintain temperature balance. Further decline of body temperature is quite rapid. Death usually occurs by the time the internal body temperature has reached 80oF.

(3) Symptoms.

(a) As the body temperature drops, the patient may become delirious, drowsy, or comatose; the skin is pale and cold. Respirations may be markedly reduced in frequency and so shallow that casual observation may fail to note any respiratory movement. The pulse and blood pressure become difficult to take or even unobtainable. Pupils become unreactive to light but usually not dilated, and the patient becomes unresponsive to painful stimuli. The tissue becomes semirigid and passive movements are difficult. Death usually follows due to cardiac arrest or ventricular fibrillation.

(4) Treatment. The primary intent is to raise the body temperature.

(a) First aid. If patient is wet, strip and dry him. Heat him by a fire or by stripping and bundling in blankets or sleeping bag to share body heat. If patient is conscious, give plenty of hot fluids (tea, coffee, soup).

(b) Definitive treatment. Patients with moderate or severe hypothermia (core temperature of less than 32oC. (89.6oF.)) often require aggressive rewarming with individualized supportive care. Either heated blankets or warm baths may be used. Bath should be 40-42oC. (104-107.6oF.) with a rate of rewarming of 1-2oC. per hour. The patient must be closely monitored as active external warming may cause marked peripheral dilatation that predisposes to ventricular fibrillation and hypovolemic shock. CPR may be required. An IV should be initiated as soon as possible and urinary output closely monitored. Metabolic acidosis, pneumonia, renal failure, and ventricular fibrillation may occur even several days after an apparently successful resuscitation and restoration of body temperature. Because of this the patient's vital signs should be closely monitored for several days after rewarming. With proper early care 50-70 percent of moderate to severe hypothermia cases can be saved.

e. Snowblindness.

(1) Cause/definition. The eye is sensitive to ultraviolet radiation just as the skin is. In areas of unbroken ice or snow, approximately 75 percent of the incident ultraviolet radiation is reflected so that the eyes are exposed to reflected as well as direct rays from the sun. The eyes can be exposed to excessive ultraviolet radiation even on grey, overcast days or in forested areas. Such excessive exposure can result in sunburn of the tissues comprising the surface of the eye, as well

as the retina, producing snowblindness.

(2) Signs/symptoms.

(a) Symptoms may not be apparent until as much as 8 to 12 hours after exposure.

(b) Initially, the eyes feel irritated and dry, but as time passes, the eyes feel as though they are full of sand. Blinking and moving the eyes becomes extremely painful, and even exposure to light may cause discomfort. Redness of eyes and excessive tearing may occur. The eyelids are usually red, swollen, and difficult to open.

(3) Complications. A mild case of snowblindness may completely disable an individual for several days; however, in the more severe cases, the damage to the eye may be permanent.

(4) Treatment.

(a) A mild case of snowblindness will heal spontaneously in a few days; however, the pain may be quite severe if the injury is not treated.

(b) Cold compresses and a lightproof bandage should be applied in order to relieve pain.

(c) If available, an opthalmic ointment should be applied hourly, not only to provide relief from pain but also to lessen the inflammatory reaction and course of the injury.

(d) The individual SHOULD NOT rub his eyes.

(e) Local anesthetic agents SHOULD NOT be used. These agents rapidly lose their effectiveness when applied to the eyes, and they may further damage the eye surface.

(5) Prevention.

(a) Snowblindness can be prevented by the consistent use of proper goggles or sunglasses when in areas of unbroken ice or snow. These glasses should be large and curved or have side covers to block reflected light coming from below and from the sides.

(b) If sunglasses or goggles are broken or lost, an emergency pair should be made from a thin piece of leather, cardboard, or other material that is cut the width of the face and provided with horizontal slits over the eyes. The improvised eye protectors can be held in place with string attached to the sides and tied at the back of the head. (See sketch below.)

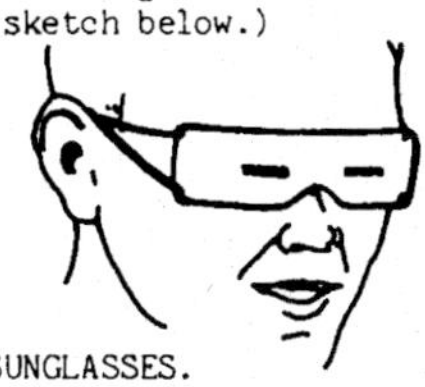

IMPROVISED SUNGLASSES.

CHAPTER 12

BITES (SNAKE, INSECT, AND ANIMAL)

12-1. SNAKE BITES.

a. Classification of poisonous snakes.

(1) Crotalidae (viperine). Frequently called pit vipers (rattlesnake, moccasins, copperhead, bushmaster, fer-de-lance, habu, Russel's viper, etc.).

(2) Elapidae. This family is composed of coral snakes, kraits, cobras, mambas, asps, and others.

(3) Hydrophidae (sea snakes). All are extremely poisonous and many have more toxic venom than cobras.

(4) Colubridae. This family is represented by the backfanged boomslang.

b. Classification of snake venom. Snake venom is broken into two categories: hemotoxic and neurotoxic. Unfortunately snakes are not just hemotoxic or neurotoxic. They are primarily one or the other, but contain elements of both.

(1) Hemotoxic. Members of the Crotalidae family are primarily hemotoxic with the following substances in the venom:

(a) Thrombase. Action mainly at the site of the bite, causing local thrombosis, gangrene, and intravascular clotting.

(b) Hemorrhagin. This is the predominant substance in the venom, causing lysis of the capillary cells with resultant leakage into the tissue. This starts locally and then becomes generalized. Convulsions due to small hemorrhages in the brain sometimes occur.

(c) Anticoagulin. Causes a breaking down of proteins in the fibrin network of the clot.

(2) Neurotoxic. Members of the Elapidae, Colubridae, and Hydrophidae families are primarily neurotoxic with the following substances in the venom:

(a) Neurotoxin. Has paralytic effect on the respiratory center and the 9th, 10th, 11th, and 12th pairs of cranial nerves.

(b) Hemolysin. Found in some varieties; causes lysis of blood cells.

(c) Cardiotoxin. Causes toxic cardiac arrest.

c. Diagnosis of snakebite.

(1) Crotalidae. Symptoms are very marked and onset is rapid.

(a) Tissue swelling at site of bite, gradually spreading to surrounding area. Swelling begins within 3 minutes and may continue for an hour with enough severity to burst the skin.

(b) Excruciating pain at site of bite.

(c) Often presence of fang marks.

(d) Bleeding from major organs that may show up as blood in the urine.

(e) Destruction of blood cells and other tissue cells.

(f) Severe headache and thirst.

(g) A marked fall of B.P. with a corresponding rise in pulse.

(h) Bleeding into surrounding tissue.

NOTE: Death may occur within 24-48 hours if bite is serious and untreated. Even with proper treatment, there is grave danger of loss of a portion of the extremities.

(2) Elapidae and Colubridae. Symptoms not as marked and onset is usually slower than Crotalidae.

(a) Impairment of circulation with irregular heartbeat, drop in B.P., weakness, and exhaustion terminating in shock.

(b) Severe headache, dizziness, blurred vision, hearing difficulty, confusion, and unconsciousness.

(c) Muscular incoordination and muscular twitching.

(d) Respiratory difficulty leading to respiratory paralysis.

(e) Irregularities of skin sensations such as tingling, parasthesia, excessive perspiration, and numbness of the lips and the soles of the feet.

(f) Chills and often rapid onset of a fever.

(g) Nausea, vomiting, and diarrhea.

(3) Hydrophidae. Neurotoxic, bite is usually painless, does not swell, and often there is no clue that treatment should be started. Poisoning should be suspected in those who have been in coastal waters frequented by sea snakes within 1-2 hours before complaining of:

(a) Muscular aches, pains, and stiffness of movement.

(b) Pain on passive movement of arm, thigh, neck, or trunk muscles.

(c) Urine becomes reddish brown within 3 hours.

(d) There is a consistent appearance of neurotoxic symptoms as outlined in Elapidae diagnosis.

NOTE: Without treatment death usually occurs within 12-24 hours.

d. Treatment of snakebite.

(1) General treatment for all snakebites.

(a) Kill the snake if possible, but do not spend more than a few minutes and avoid overexertion in the attempt. Try not to crush the head as this is the primary source of exact species identification.

(b) Have patient lie down. Immediately immobilize injured part. Keep patient warm and quiet.

(c) Tetanus booster and antibiotics are indicated.

(d) Symptomatic treatment as necessary.

(2) Treatment for Crotalidae (viperine).

(a) General treatment for all snakebites (see para d (1) above).

(b) If bitten on a large area of the body (i.e., thigh, calf, forearm, etc.), make an incision 1/8 to 1/4 inch deep along or in the direction of muscle (not across the tissue) through the puncture sites. (Do not make an X cut. Do not cut into joints, tendons, etc.) Then suction using a mechanical device; use mouth only as a last resort and then only if you have no cavities, cuts, or sores in the mouth.

NOTE: Incision and suction should not be used if antivenom can be given within 1 hour or if 1 hour or more has elapsed since the bite.

(c) Do not use a tourniquet, constricting bands, or cold packs.

(d) Do not allow the patient to eat any food or to drink alcohol.

(e) Have patient drink small amounts of water at frequent intervals.

(f) Initiate IV D5W, normal saline, or Ringer's to help prevent hemolytic shock.

(g) Administer specific antivenom, if available and species is known, or polyvalent antivenom as soon as possible.

1. Inject 0.1 cc. subcutaneously and observe patient for 15 minutes for symptoms of allergy such as itching, swelling, and redness at injection site.

2. If patient is not allergic, inject the antivenom in one dose IM at a site other than the bite area.

3. If patient is allergic to the antivenom, but there is no doubt that he has an effective bite by a very dangerous species and will surely die without the antivenom, inject divided doses of 1.0 cc. IM very slowly. Be prepared to treat anaphylactic reactions should they

occur.

(h) Use morphine or other suitable pain relievers as necessary.

(3) Treatment for Elapidae and Colubridae (boomslang).

(a) Apply a tourniquet around the affected limb, over a single bone (above the knee or elbow) proximal to the bite, tight enough to stop arterial flow. This tourniquet should be released for 30 seconds every 20 minutes to allow fresh blood into the affected area.

(b) Administer antivenom using the same rules and precautions as for viperine bites.

(c) General treatment for all snakebites (see para d (1) above).

(d) Do not use morphine or any drugs that cause respiratory depression.

(4) Treatment for Hydrophidae (sea snakes).

(a) Antivenom is the only treatment other than symptomatic care.

(b) Incision and suction are of no value.

12-2. INSECT AND SPIDER BITES.

a. Insect bites. Of all deaths per year due to bites, 40% are caused by insect bites compared to 33% for snake bites, 18% for spider bites, and 9% for animal bites.

(1) Bees, wasp, hornets, yellow jackets, and ants. Most of this group sting their victims and often leave the stingers and venom sac embedded in the skin. The stinger should be removed immediately to prevent more venom from entering the victim. Toxins from this group are similar to the venom of viperine snakes in having a hemolysin factor, but their primary effect seems to be the strong histamine they contain.

(a) Symptoms. Stinging, burning sensation with swelling. This swelling, when caused by stings around the head and neck, may be severe enough to impair the airway.

(b) Treatment.

1. Apply a paste of baking soda (sodium bicarbonate) or apply strong household ammonia to reduce discomfort. Infiltration of lidocaine into sting area often helps.

2. In severe cases give Benadryl 4 mg. per kg. IV stat. with 10 cc. of 10% calcium gluconate. Inject 2 to 4 cc. fairly fast until patient has a burning sensation in the tongue, palm, or soles of his feet. Then slow the injection of the remainder to avoid flushing.

3. If patient is allergic to the venom, treat the anaphylactic reaction.

(2) Centipedes, millipedes, and caterpillars.

(a) Centipedes are venomous with hollow fangs like snakes. If bitten, the patient will have immediate severe pain followed by redness and swelling. Sometimes necrosis with ulcer formation may occur.

(b) Millipedes secrete a toxin by glands in the body. When the fluid touches the skin, it produces burning and itching.

(c) Many caterpillars have hollow venom-containing hairs on their bodies. If these hairs contact the skin, they cause severe burning pain, redness, swelling, and necrosis of tissue. Scotch tape on the sting is effective in removing the broken off hairs from the skin.

(d) Treatment. Very similar to that of bee, wasp, and hornet stings. Antihistamines, ice, and pain medication are helpful. Treat anaphylactic reactions.

b. Spider and scorpion bites.

(1) Black widow spider. Only the female bites and has a neurotoxic venom. Identified by red hourglass on abdomen.

(a) Symptoms. Initial pain is not severe, but severe local pain rapidly develops. The pain gradually spreads over the entire body and settles in the abdomen and legs. Abdominal cramps and progressive abdominal rigidity may occur. Weakness, tremors, sweating, salivation, nausea, vomiting, and/or a rash may occur. Anaphylactic reactions can occur. Symptoms usually begin to regress after several hours and are usually gone in a few days.

(b) Treatment.

1. Calcium gluconate 10 cc. of 10% solution IM or injected slowly IV.

2. Robaxin 10 cc. given slowly IV over a 5-10 min period followed by 10 cc. in 250 cc. of D5W in IV drip over 4 hours.

3. Patients under 14 and over 50 should receive the specific antivenom if they are not allergic to horse serum.

4. Supportive care as necessary, tetanus booster, antibiotics, etc.

(2) Brown house spider (recluse). Identified by dark brown violin on the back of a small light brown spider.

(a) Symptoms. There is no pain or so little pain that most of the time the patient is not aware he is bitten. A few hours later a painful, red area with a mottled cyanotic center appears. A macular rash sometimes occurs. Necrosis does not occur in all bites, but usually after 2-3 days there is an area of discoloration that does not blanch with finger pressure. The area turns dark and mummified in a week or two. The margins separate and the eschar falls off leaving an open ulcer. Secondary infection and regional lymphadenopathy usually become evident at this stage. Many times the patient is unaware of any cause for the ulcer. The outstanding feature of brown recluse bites is the ulcer does not heal, but persists for weeks or months. Physical exam reveals a hard indurated area of skin and superficial fascia with undermined edges.

In many cases there is a systemic reaction, in addition to the ulcer, that is serious and may lead to death. The systemic reactions occur chiefly in children and are marked by fever, chills, joint pain, splenomegaly, vomiting, and a generalized rash. These systemic reactions may occur at any time as long as the ulcer is present.

(b) Treatment. There is no antivenom for brown recluse bites. It is necessary to excise all the indurated skin and fascia before healing will start. If the ulcer is not excised, it may continue to grow until it is several inches in diameter.

Tetanus prophylaxis and antibiotics are necessary to control secondary infection. Cortisone will arrest the systemic reaction but will not affect the ulcer. Anaphylactic reactions may also occur and must be managed.

(3) .Scorpions. All are poisonous to a greater or lesser degree. Fortunately none of the very poisonous varieties are found in the US, but deaths have been reported due to scorpion stings in the US.

(a) Symptoms. There are two different reactions depending on the species.

1. Severe local reaction only, with pain and swelling around area of sting. Possible prickly sensation around the mouth and a thick feeling tongue.

2. Severe systemic reaction with little or no visible local reaction. Local pain and hyperesthesia may be present. Systemic reaction includes respiratory difficulties, thick feeling tongue, tetanuslike body spasm, drooling, gastric distention, double vision, blindness, involuntary rapid movement of the eyeball, involuntary urination and defecation, hypertension, and heart failure. Death is rare, occurring mainly in children or adults with hypertension.

(b) Treatment.

1. DO NOT give morphine or morphine derivatives, including Demerol, because it has a synergistic effect with scorpion venom. Effective pain relief can be obtained by specific nerve blocks using lidocaine.

2. Ice packs or cold water helps slow spread of toxin and relieve pain.

3. Tetanus prophylaxis and antibiotics are indicated.

4. Specific antivenoms are available for the more toxic varieties.

5. Symptomatic care.

12-3. ANIMAL BITES.

a. Animal bites themselves are not usually serious. The main problem is the diseases that can be transmitted by the bites. Number one among these is rabies.

b. Protective measures for bites.

(1) Capture and isolate animal for 8-10 days.

(a) An animal that is rabid should show unmistakable signs of rabies within 8 days.

(b) If the animal dies, cut off the head, freeze it, and ship it frozen to the nearest laboratory having facilities for rabies determination.

(2) Bites from animals that can't be captured and isolated should be considered as rabid, and patient should receive antirabies vaccine.

c. Treatment.

(1) All bites must be promptly and thoroughly cleaned with soap, Betadine or hexachlorophene and water. Then apply either 40-70% alcohol, tincture of iodine, or 1:10,000 benzalkonium chloride directly into the bite. This mechanical cleansing and disinfecting has been credited with blocking many cases of rabies as well as lessening the chances of other types of infection.

(2) Antitetanus prophylaxis is indicated.

(3) Avoid suturing or cauterizing the wound; use delayed secondary closure if at all possible.

(4) If suturing is absolutely necessary, infiltrate 50% of the first dose of rabies vaccine into wound area.

(5) Immediate judgment as to the advisability of administering antirabies serum is required. Take into account the circumstances of the bite and prevalance of rabies in the area.

(6) Symptomatic treatment as required.

CHAPTER 13

OVERDOSE AND POISONING

13-1. GENERAL PRINCIPLES.

a. ABCs in severe OD.

b. Gradation of coma.

Stage 0: Asleep but arousable.
Stage I: Comatose - withdraws from painful stimuli.
Stage II: Reflexes present - does not withdraw from painful stimuli.
Stage III: Reflexes absent - no respiratory or circulatory depression.
Stage IV: Reflexes absent - respiratory depression and/or circulatory collapse.

c. Removal of toxic drug.

(1) Emesis.

(a) More effective than lavage in awake patient.

(b) Ipecac: 15-30-45 cc. of syrup (not tincture) followed by 1 liter of warm water. Activity helps stimulate vomiting. Never leave ipecac in (cardio toxic).

(c) Apomorphine: 0.1 mg./kg. IV or SQ. Vigorous vomiting difficult to control. May act as respiratory depressant: counteracted by Narcan. (Rarely indicated.)

(2) Lavage.

(a) Use normal saline - 200-300 cc. per pass, or 10 cc./kg. per pass.

(b) Y tube set up with 28-32 Fr. Ewald Tube, larger for undissolved tabs.

(c) If no gag use endotrachial tube to protect airway.

(3) Contraindications to emesis and/or lavage.

(a) Caustics.

(b) Hydrocarbon ingestions that are not potentially lethal.

(4) Activated charcoal.

(a) Dose = 30-50 grams.

(b) Will deactivate ipecac. (Wait until patient stops vomiting.)

(c) Can be given prior to and after lavage.

(5) Purgatives.

(a) Castor oil or mineral oil: contraindicated in pesticide poisoning and hydrocarbon ingestion. Helpful in glutethimide.

(b) Mag citrate: 10 oz. Contraindicated in renal failure.

(c) Sodium sulfate: 250 mg./kg. diluted 1:2 or 1:4.

(6) Forced diuresis with alkalinization of urine.

(a) Especially useful in barbiturate and ASA OD.

(b) Protocol.

500 cc. D_5W x 2
500 cc. NS + 20 KCl at 200-500 cc./hr.
1 Amp $HaHCO_3$/2-3 liters.
Lasix 40 mg. IV q. 4-6 h.
Foley for urethral drainage.

(7) Forced diuresis with acidification of urine.

(a) Especially useful in amphetamine and PCP ODs.

(b) Protocol.

1. Ascorbic acid: 1-2 gm in 500 cc. NS IV q.i.d.

and/or

2. Ammonium chloride: 2.75 mEq./kg./dose in 60 cc. saline P.O q.6h. until urine pH less than 5.

(8) Peritoneal and hemodialysis.

13-2. HYPNOTICS.

a. Barbiturates signs and symptoms.

(1) C.N.S. depression and/or agitation (coma is major toxicity).

(2) Temperature usually decreased.

(3) Pulse usually normal, may be increased.

(4) B.P. normal or decreased.

(5) Respirations normal or decreased (if increased, consider aspiration).

(6) "Barb burns" - skin necrosis at high dosage.

(7) Reflexes normal or decreased.

(8) Myocardial toxicity at high dosages.

(9) Ataxia, nystagmus, and vertigo in early OD.

b. Treatment for barbiturates.

(1) General OD protocol.

(2) Hemodialysis.

c. Nonbarbiturate hypnotics.

Glutethimide (Doriden)
Methyprylon (Noludar)
Quaalude (methaqualone)

(1) Signs and symptoms.

(a) Lethargy.

(b) Mydriasis.

(c) Decreased B.P.

(d) Flaccidity (except Quaalude).*
* Quaalude, Placidyl, or phencyclidine can cause hyperreflexia in the presence of coma.

(e) Respiratory depression.

(2) Treatment as for general OD: Glutethimide especially lethal because of enterohepatic circ and varying levels of coma. Use duodenal NG and cholestyramine.

13-3. C.N.S. STIMULANTS.

Amphetamines and cocaine.

a. Signs and symptoms.

(1) Agitation.

(2) Euphoria.

(3) Tachycardia.

(4) Hypertension.

(5) Hyperpyrexia.

(6) Cramps.

(7) Hallucinations (auditory and visual).

(8) Convulsions and coma.

(9) Perforated nasal septum suggests cocaine.

(10) Toxicity begins at 20-25 mg./kg. for amphetamines.

b. Treatment.

(1) Support and calming, avoid stimulation.

(2) Dialysis for amphetamines, but not for cocaine.

(3) Thorazine 25 mg. or valium 5 mg. as calmative.

(4) Acidify urine for amphetamines.

13-4. ANTICHOLINERGICS.

a. Examples.

(1) Atropine.

(2) Scopolamine.

(3) Belladonnna alkaloids.

(4) Tricyclic antidepressants.

(5) Phenothiazines.

(6) Antihistaminics.

(7) Antispasmodics (Pro-Banthine).

(8) Antiparkinsonian agent.

(9) Toxic plants.

(a) Jimsonweed.

(b) Morning glory seed.

(c) Deadly nightshade.

(d) Certain mushrooms.

(e) Potato leaves and sprouts.

b. Signs and symptoms.

(1) Tachycardia.

(2) Dry flushed skin.

(3) Mydriasis.

(4) Dry mouth.

(5) Nausea and vomiting.

(6) Urinary retention.

(7) Increased intraocular pressure.

(8) Confusion.

(9) Disorientation.

(10) Bizarre behavior.

(11) Paranoia.

(12) Hallucinations.

(13) Hyperpyrexia.

(14) Hypotension.

(15) Convulsions.

c. Treatment.

(1) Cooling.

(2) Support.

(3) Sedation.

(4) Physostigmine in severe OD.

13-5. MAJOR AND MINOR TRANQUILIZERS.

Major - Phenothiazines.
Minor - Librium, valium, Placidyl, meprobamate, etc...

a. Signs and symptoms.

(1) Hypotension.

(2) Lethargy.

(3) Respiratory depression.

(4) Coma.

(5) Seizures.

(6) Extrapyramidal ------ Phenothiazines.

(7) Loss of temperature control.

b. Treatment.

(1) Support and general OD measures.

(2) Gastric lavage or emesis.

(3) Control shock as necessary.

(4) Use barbiturates <u>cautiously</u> for control of convulsions.

13-6. USE OF PHYSOSTIGMINE.

Anticholinesterase - i.e., cholinergic drug counteracts

anticholinergic drugs.

a. Actions.

(1) Pupillary constriction.

(2) Contracts bronchioles, gut, and bladder.

(3) Stimulates salivation and sweating.

(4) Slows heart.

(5) Increases muscle contraction.

(6) C.N.S. stimulant.

b. Definite antidotes for:

(1) Atropine and belladonna alkaloids (jimsonweed).

(2) Tricyclic antidepressants.

c. Contraindications.

(1) Mechanical G.I. obstruction - absolute.

(2) Mechanical GU obstruction - absolute.

(3) Asthma - relative.

(4) COPD - relative.

(5) ASCVD - relative.

(6) Should be used to counteract life-threatening central and peripheral anticholinergic signs, or to reverse coma in the presence of those signs.

d. Central anticholinergic signs.

(1) Short-term memory loss.

(2) Disorientation.

(3) Hallucinations (visual and auditory).

(4) Anxiety and agitation.

(5) Psychosis.

(6) Coma.

(7) Twitchy and jerky movements.

(8) Pyramidal signs (Hyperreflexia, hypertonus, clonus).

e. Peripheral anticholinergic signs.

(1) Tachycardia.

(2) Mydriasis with decreased light reflex.

(3) Dry mucous membranes.

(4) Flushed dry skin.

(5) Decreased bowel sounds.

(6) Urinary retention.

(7) Hyperpyrexia.

f. Physostigmine dosage.

(1) 2 mg. in 10 cc. IV over 2 minutes repeated x 2 at 5-10 minutes.

(2) 2 mg. undiluted IM q. 20 minutes.

(3) 0.5 mg. in children.

g. Dangers of Physostigmine.

(1) Precipitate cholinergic crisis and seizures.

(2) Central (medullary) and peripheral respiratory collapse.

(3) Excess salivary and tracheobronchial secretions.

(4) Bronchospasm and laryngospasm.

(5) Muscle twitching, fasciculations, and paralysis.

(6) Reversible - treat with atropine 1/2 physo dose IM.

h. Indications.

(1) Known OD on belladonna alkaloids or tricyclics who are in marked distress.

(2) Anticholinergic findings and hypertension, hallucinations, coma, convulsions, and dysrhythmias.

13-7. HYDROCARBONS.

a. 1 cc./kg. of hydrocarbon, or less if chlorinated or metal containing solvent. Leads to C.N.S. or respiratory depression.

b. If depression has occurred - intubate with cuffed tube gastric lavage and use general OD procedures.

c. Potentially lethal dose but no depression, use ipecac.

d. If less than 1/2 cc./kg., cathartic only - no emesis or lavage.

e. Activated charcoal is useless.

f. Don't use oil-based cathartics. May lead to lipoid pneumonias.

g. X ray initially and at 6-12 hours if evidence of aspiration (patient coughing).

h. Epinephrine contraindicated (dysrhythmias).

i. Steroids are questionably useful.

j. No antibiotics unless infection documented.

13-8. SALICYLATES: ASA AND METHYL SALICYLATE (OIL OF WINTERGREEN).

a. Symptoms at 100 mg./kg. (2 grains/lb toxic - 3-4 gr/lb fatal).

b. Is severe to fatal at 250-400 mg./kg.

c. Adult ingestion of 10 grams should be considered serious.

d. Symptoms.

(1) Early: Headache, dizziness, tinnitus, blurred vision, confusion, lethargy, diaphoresis, thirst, nausea and vomiting, diarrhea, abdominal pain, hyperpnea.

(2) Severe: Restlessness, incoherence, vertigo, tremor, diplopia, delirium, convulsions, coma, fever to 106°F. in children, respiratory alkalosis in adults and children, occasionally hypoglycemia.

e. Treatment.

(1) Basic principles, especially activated charcoal.

(2) Correct acid-base and electrolyte disturbances.

(3) Alkalinization of urine.

13-9. ACETAMINOPHEN OVERDOSAGE (PARACETAMOL).

a. In adult dosages over 5 grams, should be admitted for observations.

b. 10 grams ingestion is associated with severe hepatotoxicity and death.

c. Peak plasma levels usually occur in 40-120 minutes, may be prolonged in OD.

d. Metabolized in liver and conjugated with glucuronide, sulfate, cysteine, and mercapturic acid.

e. Effects are potentiated by drugs utilizing the same conjugating systems, i.e. ETOH and barbiturates.

f. Plasma levels 4 hours after ingestion.

(1) Greater than 300 mg./ml. leads to liver damage.

(2) Less than 120 mg./ml. does not lead to liver damage.

g. Manifestations.

(1) Pallor.

(2) Nausea, vomiting, and diarrhea.

(3) Hepatotoxicity.

(a) May not appear clinically for 2-6 days.

(b) Right upper quadrant pain.

(c) Increased liver enzymes.

(d) Jaundice.

(e) Encephalopathy.

h. Treatment.

(1) Emesis early.

(2) Charcoal early questionably useful.

(3) N-acetylcysteamine (Mucomist) - not yet approved.

(a) 140 mg./kg. P.O. loading dose.

(b) 70 mg./kg. P.O. q.4h. x 17 doses.

13-10. CAUSTICS.

a. Examples.

(1) Draino, Liquid Plummer, etc...

(2) Liquid and dry bleach.

(3) Acetest tablets.

(4) Lye.

(5) Any strong acid or base.

b. Treatment.

(1) No emesis.

(2) No lavage.

(3) Dilute with cool water.

(4) Do not neutralize with weak acid or base (generates heat and gas).

(5) All caustic ingestions should be scoped and followed by G.I.

or ENT.

c. N.B. - Absence of intra or perioral burns does not preclude ingestion.

13-11. ORGANOPHOSPHATES.

a. Examples. (insecticides replacing DDT).

(1) Organophosphate insecticides - chlorathion, Di-Captan, ethion, disyston, malathion, methyl parathion, parathion, phosphamidon, etc...

(2) Carbamate insecticides - cabofuran, dimeton, mexecarbate, etc...

b. Signs and symptoms consist of increased cholinergic stimulation.

(1) Bronchoconstriction with increased bronchial secretion and pulmonary edema.

(2) Nausea and vomiting.

(3) Abdominal cramps and diarrhea.

(4) Increased sweating.

(5) Increased salivation and lacrimation.

(6) Bradycardia and hypotension.

(7) Miosis (may be unilateral) and blurred vision.

(8) Urinary incontinence.

(9) Muscle cramps, weakness, fasciculations, and arreflexia.

(10) Headache.

(11) Restlessness.

(12) Convulsions.

(13) Coma.

c. Treatment.

(1) Mild intoxication requires removal from further exposure.

(2) Severe poisoning.

(a) Support (including removal of secretions).

(b) Decontamination.

(c) Administration of anticholinergic agent.

1. Atropine - 2-4 mg. IV slow q. 15 minutes.

2. PAM pralidoxime - only useful if administered within 24 hours (1 gram over several minutes, children 10-12 mg./kg.)

13-12. CYANIDE.

a. Sources of cyanide (amygdalin).

(1) Nitroprusside therapy.

(2) Laetrile.

(3) Various fruit pits such as peach, apricot, chokecherry, plum, lima beans, apple seeds, various grasses.

(4) Synthetic rubber.

(5) Some fumigant gasses.

(6) Photographic chemicals.

(7) Salts for electroplating, gold and silver extraction, metal cleaning, dehairing hides.

(8) Cyanamide (for fertilizing).

b. Signs and symptoms of cyanide poisoning.

(1) Smell of bitter almonds.

(2) Headache.

(3) Vertigo and faintness. C.N.S.

(4) Excitability.

(5) Opisthotonus and trismus.

(6) Convulsions and coma.

(7) Burning tongue.

(8) Salivation. Oral ingestion

(9) Nausea.

(10) Hypertension with bradycardia and blocks early.

(11) Hypotension, tachycardia, and cardiovascular collapse - late.

c. Treatment.

(1) 100% O_2 by bag and mask.

(2) Cyanide antidote kit:

(a) Amy nitrite by inhalation followed by,

(b) Sodium nitrite IV 10 ml. over 4 minutes (0.2 ml./kg. IV for peds), and

(c) 50 ml. of 25% sodium thiosulfate IV (1 ml./kg. IV for peds).

13-13. ARSENIC.

a. Sources.

(1) Herbicides.

(2) Insecticides.

(3) Rodenticides.

(4) Fungicides.

(5) Paints.

(6) Tanning agents.

(7) Some veterinary medicines.

b. Signs and symptoms (levels in urine, hair, and nails).

(1) Smell of garlic.

(2) Mees' lines in nails after 2-3 weeks.

(3) Hyperpyrexia.

(4) Tremor and convulsions.

(5) Coma.

(6) Nausea, vomiting, and diarrhea.

(7) Liver and kidney damage.

(8) Polyneuropathy.

(9) G.I. complaints may preceed neuropathy, and by 2-3 weeks in acute cases.

c. Treatment.

(1) If acute, lavage or emesis.

(2) General support.

(3) Dimercaprol (BAL). (See chapter 14.)

(4) Follow urine arsenic levels.

13-14. METHEMOGLOBINEMIA.

a. Hemoglobin with Fe in the ferric state.

b. Incapable of reversible transport.

c. Causative agents (oxydizers).

(1) Inorganic agents:
Copper chlorates, chromates, nitrates, nitrites.

(2) Drugs:
Acetanilid, phenacetin, PAS, sulfonamide, lidocaine, benzocaine, nitroglycerin, chloroquine, menthol, primaquine, etc...

(3) Miscellaneous:
Alloxan, naphtalene, quinones anilines nitrosobenzene.

d. Symptoms.

(1) Cyanosis with level 727 (slate gray).

(2) Normal pO_2.

(3) Dyspnea.

(4) Tachycardia.

(5) Stupor and coma.

(6) Nonspecific symptoms.

(7) Blood looks like Hershey's Chocolate.

e. Treatment.

(1) Support.

(2) O_2.

(3) Time.

(4) Methylene blue - 1-2 mg./kg. IV slowly or 3-5 mg./kg. orally.

13-15. CARBON MONOXIDE.

a. Sources.

(1) Car exhausts.

(2) Poorly ventilated furnaces and fireplaces.

(3) Smoke inhalation.

b. Symptoms.

(1) Depends on level - become toxic over 20%, 10% if found in smoking.

(2) Cherry red lips and mucous membranes.

(3) Headache.

(4) Muscle weakness.

(5) Palpitations.

(6) Dizziness.

(7) Confusion.

(8) Coma and death.

c. Treatment.

100% O_2 under hyperbaric conditions for at least 1 hour; maintain body warmth and blood pressure. Give 50 ml. 50% glucose p.r.n. for brain edema.

13-16. LEAD POISONING (PLUMBISM).

a. Sources.

(1) Lead based paint.

(2) Cooking utensils - ceramic or earthenware with lead glaze.

(3) Plumbing.

(4) Stills.

(5) Industrial exposure:

(a) Smelters.

(b) Battery workers.

(c) Painters (auto).

(d) Demolition experts.

b. Signs and symptoms.

(1) Chronic.

(a) Vague aches and pains (may mimic other neuropathies).

(b) Wrist and ankle drop.

(c) Chronic nephritis.

(d) Anemia Hg 10 with basophilic stippling.

(e) Increased urinary aminolevulinic acid (ALA).

(f) Abdominal lead and leadlines on X ray.

(2) Acute.

(a) Metallic taste.

(b) Anorexia.

(c) Constipation and vomiting.

(d) Abdominal pain.

(e) Personality changes.

(f) Lethargy.

(g) Clumsiness.

(h) Ataxia.

(i) Convulsions.

(j) Coma.

(k) Anemia with basophilic stippling.

(l) Increased urinary ALA and coproporphyrins.

(m) Abdominal lead and lead lines on X ray.

(n) Blackstools (leadsulfide).

c. Treatment.

(1) Isolation from further contaminations.

(2) General OD principles.

(3) General support.

(4) Chelation.

(a) BAL 4 mg./kg. IM over 4 h.

(b) EDTA 50-75 mg./kg./day 1 m. 5-7 day courses.

(c) D-penicillamine 20-40 mg./kg./day as outpatient.

13-17. IRON INTOXICATION.

a. Source is usually prescription or over the counter Fe containing preparations.

b. Toxic to lethal dose of 150-300 mg./kg.

c. Signs and symptoms.

(1) Stage I.

(a) 30-120 minutes.

(b) Vomiting and diarrhea (may be bloody).

(2) Stage II.

(a) 6-12 hours.

(b) Latent or improvement.

(3) Stage III.

(a) 18-72 hours.

(b) Cardiovascular collapse.

(c) Coma.

(d) Convulsions.

(e) Coagulation defects.

(f) Hyperpyrexia.

(g) Metabolic acidosis.

(h) Liver failure.

(4) Stage IV.

(a) 4-6 weeks.

(b) Pyloric stenosis and G.I. scarring.

d. Treatment.

(1) Lavage with 5% sodium bicarbonate or emesis if pills still visible on abdominal X rays.

(2) Baseline blood work to include serum Fe.

(3) Chelation only in inpatients (Desferal).

(a) Used in all definitely lethal doses, 300 mg./kg.

(b) Serum Fe TIBC.

(c) Coma, convulsions, and shock.

(d) 40 mg./kg. Desferal 1., to be repeated at expanding time intervals. Do not exceed 1 gm IM initially followed by 500 mg. q.4h. x 2. Never exceed 6 gm in 27 hours.

(e) Urine will turn brown.

(f) Supportive treatment.

CHAPTER 14

NUCLEAR, BIOLOGICAL, CHEMICAL (NBC)

14-1. NUCLEAR. The major problems resulting from nuclear detonation are mass casualties and the destruction of medical care facilities.

a. Of the injured survivors, about one-third of the injuries will be caused by blast effects, one-third by thermal effects (burns), and one-third by both blast and thermal effects. Some in each of these groups will receive radiation from initial radiation and/or radioactive fallout.

(1) Initial treatment for these casualties will be first aid or self aid until they can get to or be brought to a functioning medical care facility.

(2) Once the casualties reach a treatment facility, they must be classified as to the type and urgency of treatment required so appropriate priorities can be established for treatment, evacuation, and hospitalization. This classification is known as triage. Triage is divided into four categories:

(a) Minimal (priority I). Requires only minor treatment, usually on an ambulatory or outpatient basis. This group includes small lacerations and contusions, closed fractures of small bones, second degree burns of less than 20% of the body that are not life threatening, and moderate psychological disorders.

(b) Immediate (priority II). Individuals with life-threatening conditions or moderate injuries that are treatable with a minimum expenditure of time, personnel, and supplies, and who have a good chance of recovery. Conditions include hemorrhage from an accessible site, rapidly correctable mechanical defects (sucking chest wound, respiratory obstruction or distress), severe crushing wounds and incomplete amputations, and open fractures of major bones.

(c) Delayed (priority III). After emergency care, these individuals may have definitive treatment delayed without significant jeopardy to recovery. These include moderate lacerations without bleeding, closed fractures of major bones, noncritical central nervous system (C.N.S.) injuries, and second degree burns between 20 and 40% of the body surface.

(d) Expectant (priority IV). Individuals requiring extensive therapy beyond our means and to the detriment of others. They receive emergency, comfort, and conservative care to the maximum extent possible. Included are critical respiratory and C.N.S. injuries, penetrating abdominal wounds, multiple severe injuries, and severe burns of over 40% of the body surface.

b. Burn and blast injuries are covered in chapter 10.

c. Radiation injuries (acute radiation syndrome) are directly related to the dose (amount) of radiation received. The dose is accumulative.

(1) 50-200 rad. Approximately 6 hours after exposure the individual may have no symptoms to transient mild headaches. There may be

a slight decrease in the ability to conduct normal duties. Less than 5% of individuals in the upper part of the exposure range will require hospitalization. Average hospital stay will be 45-60 days with no deaths.

(2) 200-500 rad. Approximately 4-6 hours after exposure, individuals will experience headaches, malaise, nausea, and vomiting. Symptoms are not relieved by antiemetics in the upper exposure range. Individual can perform routine tasks but any activity requiring moderate to heavy exertion will be hampered for 6-20 hours. After this period, individuals will appear to recover and enter a latent period of 17-21 days. If individual has received 300 rads or more, large quantities of hair will be lost between 12-18 days after exposure. Following the latent stage, symptoms will return, requiring 90% of the personnel to be hospitalized for 60-90 days. Probably less than 5% of those at the lower dose range will die, the percentage increasing toward the upper end of the dose range.

(3) 500-1000 rad. Approximately 1-4 hours after exposure, severe and prolonged nausea and vomiting develop that are difficult to control. Diarrhea and fever develop early in individuals in the upper part of the exposure range. Simple routine tasks can be performed by individuals in the lower dose range. Significant incapacitation is seen in the upper ranges. Initial symptoms last for more than 24 hours, then go into a latent period lasting 7-10 days. Following the latent stage the symptoms return requiring 100% of the individuals to be hospitalized. Of those in the lower range 50% will die, the percentage increasing toward the upper range. All deaths occur within 45 days. The survivors require 90-120 days hospitalization before recovery.

(4) 1000 rad or more. Less than 1 hour after exposure individuals develop severe vomiting, diarrhea, and prostration. There is no latent period. All require hospitalization and die within 30 days.

d. Treatment for radiation exposure includes washing individual thoroughly to remove any radioactive contamination, symptomatic treatment, and prevention of secondary infections.

14-2. BIOLOGICAL WARFARE (BW).

a. Biological agents are divided into two main classes:

(1) Living organisms such as bacteria, viruses, rickettsiae, and fungi.

(2) Poisonous products or toxins produced by living organisms.

b. The most practical method of initiating infection in BW is through the dispersal of agents as minute, airborne particles (aerosols) over a target where they may be inhaled. An aerosol may be effective for some time after delivery, as it will be deposited on clothing, equipment, and soil. When the clothing is used later, or dust is stirred up, personnel may be subject to a "secondary" aerosol.

c. Agents may be able to use portals of entry into the body other than the respiratory tract. Individuals may be infected by ingestion of contaminated food and water or even by direct contact with the skin or mucous membranes through abraided or broken skin.

d. Early warning, immediate detection, and rapid identification of the agent used in a BW attack are of primary importance.

(1) Early warning can sometimes be supplied by intelligence sources, but early warning is not always available.

(2) Immediate detection can be by seeing a plane spraying or by bombs, shells, or mines producing dense clouds near your area. Immediate detection may not occur; for example, in the case of sabotage or an attack launched a considerable distance upwind from you, the first indication may be the appearance of casualties.

(3) Rapid identification of the biological agent. Due to the concentration and/or portal of entry (respiratory tract), there may be a more rapid onset and wide variances to normal symptoms of even common diseases. This can make diagnosis and treatment extremely difficult. Clinical samples should be collected from the first casualties and sent to the nearest laboratory, if possible.

e. Individual protection prior to and during a BW attack.

(1) Maintain body in the best possible physical condition.

(2) If a BW attack is detected,

(a) Use mask.

(b) Button clothing and tie clothing with string or extra shoelaces at the wrists and ankles. If special protective clothing is available, put it on.

(c) Put on gloves, if available.

(d) While in the contaminated area, practice the procedures outlined above.

(e) Upon leaving the area, decontaminate to the extent the situation permits. If bathing facilities and fresh clothing are available, carefully remove contaminated clothing and thoroughly wash the body and protective mask in soap and water prior to removing the mask. Then don fresh clothing. Give special attention to decontamination and treatment of skin lesions.

f. Group protection. The best protection is a pressurized shelter using filtered, forced air. A building or shelter without this feature provides only limited protection from aerosols. Eventually, microorganisms will penetrate through cracks and constitute a respiratory hazard unless the protective mask is worn. As in the case of individual protective measures, utilization of shelters depends upon early warning.

(1) Protection of food and water depends entirely on following good preventive medicine and veterinary procedures (see chapters 20 and 21). Some biological agents cannot be destroyed by normal water purification techniques. When biological agents are known to have been used, all drinking water must be boiled in addition to normal water treatment measures.

(2) Proper hygiene and sanitation procedures must be used (see chapter 20).

(3) Immunizations must be kept current.

g. Pending identification of the agent, measures should be taken to prevent epidemics as soon as possible after initial exposure. These measures include isolation, quarantine, and restriction of personnel movement. After identification of the agent and if it is not capable of producing an epidemic, these restrictive measures can be relaxed.

14-3. CHEMICAL WARFARE. This section deals mainly with the diagnosis and treatment of specific chemical agents.

a. General considerations.

(1) Chemical casualties who have not been decontaminated may endanger unprotected personnel. Handlers of these patients should wear protective masks, impermeable protective gloves, and chemical protective clothing. If conditions permit, an aid station should be established upwind from the contaminated area. The casualties should be undressed and washed thoroughly, downwind of the aid station, before being brought into the aid station.

(2) Most chemical agents can poison food and water. Suspect food and water must be examined by chemical test procedures, if available. If testing equipment is not available, avoid using the water or food, or get an animal to eat or drink a portion and watch it for at least an hour for adverse reactions. Canned foodstuff is completely protected, but the container might be contaminated and should be washed thoroughly with copious amounts of uncontaminated water. Avoid foodstuff that is not well sealed from vapor and liquid agents.

b. Nerve agents.

(1) Nerve agents are among the deadliest chemical agents. They include (GA) tabun, (GB) sarin, (GO) soman, and VX. They are colorless to light brown liquids, some of which are volatile. They are usually odorless, except for GA which has a faint, sweet fruity odor. Toxic liquids are tasteless. They range from nonpersistent to persistent. Nerve agents may be absorbed through the skin, respiratory tract, gastrointestinal tract, and the eyes. However, significant absorption through the skin takes a period of minutes and prompt decontamination is imperative.

(2) Effects of nerve agents.

Site of Action	Signs and Symptoms
	Following Local Exposure
Pupils	Constricted (miosis), marked, usually maximal (pinpoint), sometimes unequal.
Ciliary body	Frontal headache, eye pain on focusing, slight dimness of vision, occasional nausea and vomiting.
Conjunctivae	Hyperemia.
Nasal mucous membranes	Rhinorrhea, hyperemia.

Bronchial tree	Tightness in chest, sometimes with prolonged wheezing expiration suggestive of bronchoconstriction or increased secretion, cough.
	<u>Following Systemic Absorption</u>
Bronchial tree	Tightness in chest, with prolonged wheezing expiration suggestive of bronchoconstriction or increased secretion, dyspnea, slight pain in chest, increased bronchial secretion, cough, pulmonary edema, cyanosis.
Gastrointestinal	Anorexia, nausea, vomiting, abdominal cramps, epigastric and substernal tightness (cardiospasm) with "heartburn" and eructation, diarrhea, tenesmus, involuntary defecation.
Sweat glands	Increased sweating.
Salivary glands	Increased salivation.
Lacrimal glands	Increased lacrimation.
Heart	Slight bradycardia.
Pupils	Slight miosis, occasionally unequal, later maximal miosis (pinpoint).
Ciliary body	Blurring of vision.
Bladder	Frequency, involuntary micturition.
Striated muscle	Easy fatigue, mild weakness, muscular twitching, fasciculations, cramps, generalized weakness, including muscles of respiration, with dyspnea and cyanosis.
Sympathetic ganglia	Pallor, occasional elevation of blood pressure.
Central Nervous System	Giddiness, tension, anxiety, jitteriness, restlessness, emotional lability, excessive dreaming, insomnia, nightmares, headaches, tremor, withdrawal and depression, drowsiness, difficulty concentrating, slowness on recall, confusion, slurred speech, ataxia, generalized weakness, coma, with absence of reflexes, Cheyne-Stokes respirations, convulsions, depression of respiratory and circulatory centers, with dyspnea cyanosis, and fall in blood pressure.

(a) Nerve agents are cumulative in their effect. Daily exposure to concentrations of a nerve agent insufficient to cause symptoms following a single exposure may result in symptoms following several days of exposure.

(b) Suspect nerve agent poisoning if any of the following occurs:

1. A feeling of tightness or constriction in the chest.

2. Unexplained runny nose.

3. Difficulty in breathing, either on inhaling or exhaling.

4. Small, pinpoint-size pupils seen in a mirror or in the eyes of individuals in the vicinity. (On exposure to vapor or aerosol, the pupils become pinpointed immediately. If the nerve agent is absorbed through the skin only or by ingestion of contaminated food or water, the pinpointing will be delayed or even absent.)

5. A drawing, slightly painful sensation in the eyes or unexplained dimness of vision occurring with pinpoint pupils.

(3) Treatment of nerve agent poisoning.

(a) Immediately don the protective mask and hood at the first indication of any chemical attack.

(b) Immediately remove any liquid contamination. (If a drop or a splash of liquid nerve agent gets in the eyes, immediately irrigate the eyes with copious amounts of water).

(c) Administer 2 mg. of atropine as soon as any local or systemic nerve agent symptoms are noted. (Do not give for preventive purposes before exposure to nerve agent.) If the patient has mild symptoms due to nerve agents, the IM injection of 2 mg. atropine should be repeated at 20-minute intervals, 10-minute intervals if moderate to severe symptoms are present, or until signs of atropinization (dry mouth, blurry near vision) are achieved. A mild degree of atropinization should be maintained for at least 24 hours by IM or oral administration of 1-2 mg. of atropine every 1/2 to 4 hours.

1. Atropine can be given IM, IV, or orally. Atropine given IM requires about 8 minutes before effects are noticed. Given IV, effects begin within 1 minute and reach maximum effect within 6 minutes. Atropine tablets require 20 minutes before effects are felt and 50 minutes before maximum effect takes place.

2. Atropine effects include dryness of the mouth and throat, with slight difficulty in swallowing. Patient may have a feeling of warmth, slight flushing, rapid pulse, some hesitancy of urination, and an occasional desire to belch. Pupils may be dilated slightly but react to light and near vision is blurred. Some individuals may experience mild drowsiness, slowness of memory, and the feeling his body movements are slow. Further doses of 2 mg. of atropine intensify the symptoms and prolong the effects. Effects of one to two 2 mg. injections last 3-5

hours, and the effects of four injections given at close intervals last 6-12 hours.

3. Patients with moderately severe nerve agent symptoms have increased tolerance for atropine, so fairly large doses may be administered before signs of atropinization appear.

(d) Severe nerve agent exposure may rapidly cause unconsciousness, muscular paralysis, and cessation of breathing. If this occurs, artificial respiration is required along with the atropine injections. If the patient is in severe respiratory distress or is convulsing, 4-6 mg. of atropine should be injected IV. If relief does not occur and bronchial secretions and salivation does not decrease, give 2 mg. of atropine q. 3-8 minutes until relief occurs and secretions diminish. In severe nerve agent poisoning the effect of each injection of atropine may be transient, lasting only 3-10 minutes. This requires the patient to be monitored closely and atropine repeated as needed. A mild atropinization should be maintained for at least 48 hours.

(e) Pralidoximine chloride (2-Pam Cl or Protopam Cl) can be used to increase the effectiveness of therapy in nerve agent poisoning. 2-Pam Cl reduces the time during which artificial respiration is required. Dosage: 2-Pam Cl, 1 gm in 100 ml. of sterile water, normal saline, or 5% dextrose and water; IV slowly over 15-30 minutes.

c. Blister agents (vesicants).

(1) Vesicants act on the eyes, lungs, and skin causing burns and blisters. They damage the respiratory tract when inhaled and cause vomiting and diarrhea when absorbed. Most vesicants are insidious in action causing little or no pain at the time of exposure. Lewisite and phosgene oxime cause immediate pain on contact. Vesicants poison food and water and make other supplies dangerous to handle. The severity of a chemical burn is directly related to the concentration of the agent and the duration of contact with the skin.

(2) Mustard (HD). An oily liquid ranging from colorless when pure to dark brown. Mustard is heavier than water, but small droplets float on water surfaces. It is only slightly soluble in water, but freely soluble in fats, oils, gasoline, kerosene, acetone, and alcohol. These solvents do not destroy mustard. Mustard is a persistent agent. It smells like garlic or horseradish. Even very small repeated exposures to mustard are cumulative in effect.

(a) Symptoms.

1. Eye effects. In a single exposure the eye is the most vulnerable. In mild exposure there is a latent period of 4-12 hours followed by tearing and a gritty feeling in the eyes. The conjunctiva and lids become red and edematous. Heavy exposure has a latent period of 1-3 hours followed by severe irritation and lesions. Ischemic necrosis of the conjunctivae, edema, photophobia, and blepharospasm may obstruct vision. Dense corneal opacification with deep ulceration and vascularization may occur.

2. Effects on the skin. Latent period depends on weather conditions. In hot, humid weather latency may be as short as 1 hour; in cool weather after mild vapor exposure, latency may be several

days. Normal latency is 6-12 hours. Initial symptom is erythema, resembling sunburn, followed by multiple pinpoint lesions that enlarge and form the typical blisters. The blisters are usually large, domed, thin walled, superficial, translucent, yellowish, and surrounded by erythema. The blister fluid is clear, thin, and straw colored at first; later it is yellowish and tending to coagulate. Liquid contaminaton of the skin usually results in a ring of vesicles around a gray-white area that does not blister.

3. Respiratory effects. Develop slowly taking several days to reach maximal severity. Symptoms begin with hoarseness (may progress to loss of voice). A cough, which is worse at night, appears early and later becomes productive. Fever, dyspnea, and moist rales may develop into bronchopneumonia.

4. Systemic and gastrointestinal effects. Ingestion of contaminated food or water produces nausea, vomiting, abdominal pain, diarrhea, and prostration. Skin exposure may cause malaise, vomiting, and fever appearing about the same time as the erythema. With severe exposure, symptoms may be so marked as to result in prostration. Severe systemic mustard poisoning may present C.N.S. symptoms such as cerebral depression, bradycardia, and cardiac irregularities.

(b) Treatment of mustard agent.

1. Immediately don protective mask and hood.

2. Immediately remove any liquid contamination. (Speed in decontamination of the eye is absolutely essential. Rinse the eye with copious amounts of water.)

3. After rinsing the eyes, apply a steroid antibiotic eye ointment. Patients with severe photophobia and blepharospasm should have 1 drop of 1% atropic sulfate instilled in the eye t.i.d. The eyes must not be bandaged or the lids allowed to stick together.

4. All blisters should be opened and the fluid drained with care, as the fluid itself may be irritating and cause secondary erythema and blisters. Area should be cleansed with tap water or saline and burn cream applied (10% Sulfamylon burn cream).

5. Respiratory tract injuries are treated symptomatically with steam inhalation.

6. The biggest part of the treatment is symptomatic and preventing or treating secondary infections.

(3) Nitrogen mustard (HN). Oily, colorless, pale yellow liquids; some have a faint fishy odor, while others are odorless.

(a) Effects of HN on the eye. Slight to moderate exposure produces symptoms within 20 minutes that wax and wane until they become persistent about 2 1/2 hours later and reach their maximum in 8-10 hours. Severe exposure causes immediate symptoms that progress for 24 hours. In general the symptoms are the same as mustard, but more severe and requiring intensive and early treatment.

(b) The most specific effect is in the blood and lymph

tissue. Within 5-10 days after exposure, anemia may develop and W.B.C. can fall to less than 500.

(c) Treatment of HN is generally the same as for mustard, but frequent checks of the hematocrit and W.B.C. are necessary.

(4) Arsenical vesicants. Colorless to brown liquids, soluble in most organic solvents but poorly soluble in water. They are generally more volatile than mustard and have fruity to geraniumlike odors. Vapors are unlikely to cause significant injuries. Liquids will cause severe burns of the skin and eyes and can gradually penetrate rubber and most impermeable fabrics.

(a) Liquid agent symptoms:

1. Effects on the eye include immediate pain and blepharospasm on contact. Edema follows rapidly, causing the eye to close within an hour. Severe exposure can cause permanent injury or blindness.

2. Effects on the skin are more severe than those from liquid mustard. Stinging pain is usually felt 10 to 20 seconds after contact. The pain increases in severity with penetration and in a few minutes becomes a deep aching pain. About 5 minutes after contact a gray area of dead skin appears resembling that seen in corrosive burns. Erythema resembles that caused by mustard, but is accompanied by more pain. Itching and irritation persist for about 24 hours whether or not a blister develops. Blisters are often well developed in 12 hours and are painful at first (mustard blisters are relatively painless). The pain lessens in 48-72 hours.

3. Respiratory effects are similar to those produced by mustard agent. Systemic absorption of arsenicals causes a change in the capillary permeability. This can permit sufficient fluid loss from the blood stream to cause hemoconcentration, shock, and death. Acute systemic poisoning from large skin burns causes pulmonary edema, diarrhea, restlessness, weakness, subnormal temperature, and low blood pressure.

(b) Treatment. Mask and immediately decontaminate any liquid agent (flush contaminated eyes with copious amounts of water). Treatment for the eyes is mainly symptomatic; atropine sulfate opthalmic ointment or atropine drops should be used in conjunction with an opthalmic antibiotic ointment. BAL ointment should be applied to areas of skin contamination BEFORE any blistering appears and remain on the area for at least 5 minutes. (BAL ointment occasionally causes stinging, itching, or urticarial wheals. Frequent application on the same area of skin causes mild dermatitis.) Treatment of blisters is the same as for mustard agents.

(c) Indication for systemic treatment.

1. Cough with dyspnea and frothy sputum, which may be blood tinged, and other signs of pulmonary edema.

2. Skin contamination the size of the palm of the hand or larger in which there is gray or dead-white blanching of the skin or in which erythema develops over the area within 30 minutes.

(d) Two types of treatment may be used.

1. Local neutralization by liberal application of BAL ointment that must remain on the affected area. Remove any other protective ointment before applying BAL ointment.

2. IM injection of dimercaprol (BAL) 10% solution in oil. For mild to moderate poisoning give 2.5 mg./kg. (1.5 ml./60 kg.) q.4h. x 2 days, then one injection q.12h. the third day, fourth to the tenth day give one injection once or twice a day. For severe poisoning give 3 mg./kg. (1.8 ml./60 kg.) q.4h. x 2 days, third day give one injection q.6h., fourth through fourteenth day one injection twice a day. Up to 5 mg./kg. can be given in severe cases.

Symptoms caused by BAL include dryness of the mouth and throat, mild tearing, slight reddening of the eyes, feeling of constriction in the throat, burning sensation of the lips, generalized muscular aching, abdominal pain, mild restlessness and sweating of the hands, apprehension, mild nausea and vomiting on eating, and a transient rise in blood pressure. Symptoms start 15-30 minutes after injection and last about 30 minutes. Unless they are severe or prolonged, they are not a contraindication for continuing therapy.

(5) Phosgene oxime (CX). A powerful irritant that is especially effective as a liquid. It has a disagreeable penetrating odor and is readily soluble in water.

(a) Phosgene oxime is violently irritating to mucous membranes of the eyes and nose. Even low concentrations can cause tearing. Any exposure to liquid or vapor that produces pain will also produce skin necrosis at the site of contact. The area becomes blanched and is surrounded by an erythematous ring within 30 seconds. This is followed by a wheal within 30 minutes. Within 24 hours the original blanched area acquires a brown pigmentation. An eschar forms at about 1 week and sloughs at about 3 weeks. Itching may be present throughout the entire course of healing. Healing may take 2 months or more.

(b) Decontamination is not effective after pain starts, but the contaminated area should be flushed with copious amounts of water to remove any agent that has not yet reacted with the tissue. Treat as any other ulcerated necrotic skin lesion, plus supportive care, as needed.

(6) Mixtures of blister agents. Arsenical vesicants are often mixed with mustard to confuse and make diagnosis difficult. These mixtures do not produce more severe lesions than either agent alone.

d. Choking agents (lung irritants). Best known of these agents is phosgene, a colorless gas with an odor of new mown hay, grass, or green corn. Phosgene is a nonpersistent agent that is broken down rapidly by water (fog, rain, heavy vegetation).

(1) During and immediately after exposure there is likely to be coughing, choking, a feeling of tightness in the chest, nausea, occasionally vomiting, headache, and tearing. There may be an initial slowing of the pulse followed by an increase. These symptoms may not appear, but if they do, a latent period follows that commonly lasts 2-24 hours but may be shorter. Following the latent period, signs and symptoms of pulmonary edema develop. They start with rapid shallow breathing, painful cough, and cyanosis. Nausea and vomiting may appear. As edema progresses, discomfort, apprehension, and dyspnea increase and frothy

sputum is raised. Rales and rhonchi are heard throughout the chest, and breath sounds are diminished. Patient may develop a shocklike state, with clammy skin, low blood pressure, and feeble rapid heart action.

(2) Protective mask offers adequate protection. Treatment is rest, oxygen therapy, cautious use of IV therapy, codeine for cough control, and antibiotic therapy to prevent secondary infections. Do not use expectorants or atropine. Patients who survive the first 48 hours usually recover.

e. Blood agents (cyanides). Hydrocyanic acid (AC) and cyanogen chloride (CK) are the important agents in this group. AC is a colorless, highly volatile liquid that is highly soluble and stable in water. It has a faint odor like peach kernels or bitter almonds. It is nonpersistent. CK is a colorless, highly volatile liquid that is slightly soluble in water but dissolves readily in organic solvents. It has a pungent, biting odor and is nonpersistent.

(1) Symptoms produced by AC depend upon the concentration of the agent and duration of exposure. Typically, either death occurs rapidly or recovery takes place within a few minutes after removal from the toxic area. Moderate exposure causes vertigo, nausea, and headaches followed by convulsions and coma. Severe exposure causes an increase in the depth of respiration within a few seconds, cessation of regular respiration within 1 minute, occasional shallow gasps, and finally cessation of heart action within a few minutes.

(2) Symptoms of CK are immediate intense irritation of the nose, throat, and eyes, with coughing, tightness in the chest, and tearing. The patient may become dizzy and increasingly dyspneic. Unconsciousness is followed by failing respiration and death within a few minutes. Convulsions, retching, and involuntary urination and defecation may occur. If effects are not fatal, signs and symptoms of pulmonary edema may develop: persistent cough with frothy sputum, rales in the chest, severe dyspnea, and marked cyanosis.

(3) Mask immediately. Crush 2 ampules of amyl nitrite and insert into the region of the eyelenses of the mask. Repeat every 4-5 minutes until a total of 8 ampules have been used or normal respiration has resumed. Give artificial respiration if patient is not breathing. Second step in emergency treatment is IV administration of 10 ml. of 3% sodium nitrite over a 1-minute period plus 50 ml. of a 25% solution of sodium thiosulfate given slowly IV. Further treatment is symptomatic. Recovery from AC or CK may disclose residual C.N.S. damage with irrationality, altered reflexes, and unsteady gait that may last for weeks, months, or be permanent.

f. Incapacitating agents. Agents producing a temporary disabling condition that persists for hours to days after exposure to the agent has ceased.

(1) Signs and symptoms produced by incapacitating agents.

Signs and symptoms	Possible etiology
Restlessness, dizziness, or giddiness; failure to obey orders, confusion, erratic behavior, stumbling or staggering, vomiting.	Anticholinergics, indoles, cannabinols. Anxiety reaction. Other intoxications (e.g., alcohol, bromides, barbiturates, lead).
Dryness of mouth, tachycardia at rest, elevated temperature, flushing of face; blurred vision, pupillary dilation; slurred or nonsensical speech, hallucinatory behavior, disrobing, mumbling and picking behavior, stupor and coma.	Anticholinergics (e.g., BZ).
Inappropriate smiling or laughing, irrational fear, distractability, difficulty expressing self, perceptual distortions; labile increase in pupil size, heart rate, B.P.; stomach cramps and vomiting may occur.	Indoles (e.g., LSD). (Schizophrenic psychosis may mimic in some respects.)
Euphoric, relaxed, unconcerned daydreaming attitude, easy laughter; hypotension and dizziness on sudden standing.	Cannabinols (e.g., marihuana).
Tremor, clinging or pleading, crying; clear answers, decrease in disturbance with reassurance; history of nervousness or immaturity, phobias.	Anxiety reaction.

(2) General treatment consists of close observation, restraint and confinement as required, supportive care with fluids, and appropriate clothing. Underlying medical problems should be treated as needed. If the specific agent can be identified, treat appropriately.

g. Vomiting agents. Produce a strong pepperlike irritation in the upper respiratory tract with irritation and tearing of the eyes. Principal agents of this group are DA, DM, and DC that are usually dispersed by heat as fine particulate smoke. When concentrated, DM smoke is canary yellow,

DA and DC smokes are white. All are colorless when diluted with air.

(1) Vomiting agents produce a feeling of pain and fullness in the nose and sinuses accompanied by severe headache, intense burning in the throat, tightness and pain in the chest, irritation and tearing of the eyes, uncontrollable coughing, violent and persistent sneezing, runny nose, and ropy saliva flow from the mouth. Nausea and vomiting are prominent and mental depression may occur. Onset of symptoms may be delayed several minutes after exposure. Mild exposure symptoms resemble those of a severe cold.

(2) Most individuals recover promptly after removal from the contaminated area. The few that don't can receive symptomatic relief by inhaling chloroform vapors either directly from a bottle or by pouring a few drops into the cupped palms and breathing. Chloroform is inhaled until the symptoms or irritation subside and is repeated when the symptoms become severe again. Do not use to the point of anesthesia. Aspirin may be given to relieve the headache and general discomfort.

h. Irritant agents (CS, CN, CA). CS has a pungent pepperlike odor. It is faster acting, about 10 times more potent, and less toxic than CN. CN has an apple blossom odor, and CA has a sour fruit odor.

(1) With CS there is marked burning pain and tearing of the eyes, runny nose, coughing, and dyspnea. Following heavy exposure there may be nausea and vomiting. Warm moist skin, especially on the face, neck, ears, and body folds, is susceptible to irritation by CS. CS causes a stinging burning sensation even at moderately low concentration. Higher concentrations may cause an irritant dermatitis with edema and (rarely) blisters. An increase in the stinging is usually noted upon leaving the contaminated area, but usually subsides in 5-10 minutes. CN and CA cause basically the same reaction as CS, but require a higher concentration and are more toxic.

(2) When it is safe to do so, remove mask and blot eyes. Do not rub the eyes. Flush the eyes with copious amounts of water. To prevent skin reaction, rinse the body with water or 5 or 10% sodium bicarbonate in water. Delayed erythema (irritant dermatitis) may be treated with a bland shake lotion. Most persons affected by irritant agents require no medical treatment. Severe reactions of the eyes or skin may take days or weeks to heal depending on their severity.

CHAPTER 15

SHOCK

15-1. SHOCK. A breakdown of effective circulation at the cellular level and/or failure of the peripheral circulatory system. Failure causes tissue perfusion to become inadaquate to feed the body cells.

15-2. CAUSES. Different types of shock result from different kinds of failure in the circulatory system.

a. Hypovolemic shock (peripheral resistance). Caused by hemorrhage, burns (loss of plasma), and/or decreased body water and electrolytes (vomiting and bowel obstruction or diarrhea).

b. Cardiogenic shock (resistance to heart muscle, pump failure). Caused by myocardial infarction, cardiac arrhythmias, and congestive heart failure. Pump failure of the heart causes a reduction in blood flow and then blood backs up behind the heart, causing an increase in venous pressure.

c. Neurogenic shock. Caused by spinal injuries, spinal anesthesia, trauma, manipulation of fractures, and some head wounds. There is a failure of arterial resistance with a pooling of blood in dilated capillary vessels. Cardiac activity increases in an attempt to increase the blood volume to preserve capillary pressure.

d. Septic shock. Caused by wound infection, peritonitis, meningitis, etc. Septic shock is usually caused by gram-negative bacteria causing a septicemia (invasion of the blood by pathogenic bacteria or their toxins). Hypovolemia develops as a result of pooling of blood in the capillaries and a loss of fluid from the vascular space as a result of a generalized increase in capillary permeability. There is also a possibility of a direct toxic effect on the heart with depressed cardiac function. Peripheral resistance is usually decreased but can increase as shock worsens.

e. Anaphylactic shock. Acute, often explosive, systemic reaction characterized by urticaria, respiratory distress, vascular collapse, and occasionally vomiting, cramps, diarrhea.

(1) Signs and symptoms. Usually occurs in 1-15 minutes; patient becomes agitated, uneasy, and flushed. Palpitations, paresthesia, pruritus, throbbing in the ears, coughing, sneezing and difficulty in breathing, followed by dizziness, disorientation, collapse, coma, and death.

(2) Treatment.

(a) Epinephrine solution, 1:1,000, 0.4-1 ml., IV stat. Repeat every 5-10 min p.r.n.

(b) Recumbent position, elevate legs, establish airway (tracheostomy if necessary).

(c) Diphenhydramine HCl, 5-20 mg. IV p.r.n.

(d) Aminophylline solution, 250-500 mg. IV slowly for severe asthma without shock.

(e) IV fluids to correct hypovolemia if present.

(f) Hydrocortisone sodium succinate, 100-250 mg. IV over 30 seconds for hypotension control if needed.

(g) +for injected antigen (e.g., vaccination) a constricting band (rarely a tourniquet) should be applied proximal to the injection site. An additional 0.1-0.2 ml. epinephrine (1:1,000) may be injected into the site to reduce systemic absorption.

(h) +oxygen should be utilized if available at 4-6 liters/minute.

(i) Definitive care p.r.n. and continue observation for 24 hours.

15-3. SIGNS AND SYMPTOMS OF SHOCK.

a. Shock chart.

Degree of Shock	Blood Volume Loss	B.P. (approx)	Pulse	Temp	Color	Circulation	Thirst	Mental State
Mild	Up to 20%	Up to 20% Increase	Normal	Cool	Pale	Slowing	Normal	Clear Distinct
Moderate	20-40%	Decrease 20-40%	Increased	Cool	Pale	Slowing	Definite	Clear With Apathy
Severe	40% or More	Decreased Below 40%	Weak to Absent	Cold	Ashen to Cyanotic	Very Sluggish	Severe	Apathetic to Comatose

b. The patient appears anxious and looks tired. Later he appears apathetic or exhausted. If bleeding continues, the patient will go into a coma and die.

c. The skin usually feels cool, is pale and mottled, and nail beds blanch easily.

d. The pulse and blood pressure are not totally accurate.

(1) Decreased blood pressure is always significant.

(2) In a healthy adult, blood pressure may remain normal until large volumes of blood are lost.

(3) Respirations, heart beat, and pulse are usually increased, but this increase may not occur in the prone position. If the patient is in shock and you sit him up, the systolic blood pressure will show a decrease of up to 15 mm. and you will observe an increase of 15 beats or more in the pulse.

15-4. TREATMENT.

a. Hemorrhagic shock - low peripheral vein pressure. You can expect early collapse of the usual IV routes; venous cutdown may be indicated.

b. Primary therapy for hypovolemic and hemorrhagic shock.

(1) Standard IV fluids listed in order of effectiveness.

(a) Whole blood - administer with crystalloid solutions.

(b) Plasma - administer with crystalloid solutions.

(c) Serum albumin - administer with crystalloid solutions.

(d) Dextran - should administer with crystalloid solutions.

(e) Lactated Ringer's solution (crystalloid).

(f) Normal saline (crystalloid).

(g) D5W - use alone only if nothing else is available (crystalloid).

(2) To insure adequate IV fluids you should monitor the urinary output.

(3) Keep patient warm and dry and place in the shock position unless contraindicated, e.g., head wounds, chest wounds.

(4) Analgesics such as morphine should be given for pain as necessary.

(5) Broad spectrum antibiotic treatment should be started as soon as possible as a prophylaxis for large wounds or burns.

CHAPTER 16

EMERGENCY WAR SURGERY

16-1. PRIORITIES OF TREATMENT.

a. The following priorities for surgical intervention are recommended. Injuries are dealt with on an individual basis.

b. Follow the rule of ABC.

A - Airway. Insure it is clear.

B - Breathing. Insure patient is able to breath, e.g., no sucking chest wounds, etc.

C - Circulation. Insure heart is beating and there is adequate circulating blood volume.

c. First priority.

(1) Asphyxia, respiratory obstruction from mechanical causes, sucking chest wounds, tension pneumothorax, and maxillofacial wounds in which asphyxia exists or is likely to develop.

(2) Shock caused by major external hemorrhage, major internal hemorrhage, visceral injuries, massive muscle damage, major fractures, multiple wounds, and severe burns over 20% of the body.

d. Second priority.

(1) Visceral injuries, including perforations of the gastrointestinal tract, wounds of the biliary and pancreatic systems, wounds of the genitourinary tract, and thoracic wounds without asphyxia.

(2) Vascular injuries requiring repair. All injuries in which the use of a tourniquet is necessary fall into this group.

(3) Closed cerebral injuries with increasing loss of conciousness.

(4) Burns of 20% of certain locations; hands, feet, genitalia, and perineum

e. Third priority.

(1) Brain and spinal injuries in which decompression is required.

(2) Soft-tissue wounds in which debridement is necessary but in which muscle damage is less than major.

(3) Lesser fractures and dislocations.

(4) Injuries of the eye.

(5) Maxillofacial injuries without asphyxia.

(6) Burns of other locations under 20%.

16-2. SOFT TISSUE INJURIES.

a. In the following surgical procedures we will assume that the medic knows how to prepare a patient for surgery and set up for sterile procedures.

b. The primary objective in the treatment of soft tissue injuries is localization or isolation of the deleterious effects of the injury. To best accomplish this objective, remove all foreign substances and devitalized tissue and maintain an adequate blood supply to the injured part. This can be achieved by a two-step procedure.

(1) Step one is a thorough debridement of the injured area, accomplished as early as possible after the injury (when delay is unavoidable, systemic antibiotics should be started). The wound is left open, with few exceptions, to granulate.

(2) Step two is a delayed primary closure (DPC) within 4-10 days after injury. The wound must be kept clean during this time and antibiotics are usualy indicated. The indication for a DPC is the clean appearance of the wound during this time.

c. Antibiotic wound therapy. Should be started prior to debridement.

(1) Penicillin (aqueous) - 10 million units IV q.8h. x 3 days then reevaluate.

(2) Kanamycin - 500 mg. IM q.12h. x 3 days then reevaluate.

(3) Tetanus toxoid - 0.5 cc. IM or SQ once (test for allergy only if not previously immunized).

d. Wound debridement.

(1) An incision is made in the skin and fascia long enough to give good exposure. Good exposure is required for accurate evaluation. Incisions are made over both the entry and exit wound along the longitudinal axis of extremities (S-shaped crossing joint creases). Avoid making an incision over superficial bones. When excising skin only, cut 2-3 cm. from the wound edge.

(2) Skin, fascia, and muscle should be separated to give adequate exposure. Muscles should be separated into their groups and each muscle group debrided separately.

(3) Distinguishing tissue viability. Use the four Cs: color, consistency, contractility, and circulation; color being the least desirable.

	Viable	Dead or Dying
Color	Bright reddish brown	Dark, cyanotic
Consistency	Springy	Mushy

Contractility	Contracts when pinched or cut	Does not contract when pinched or cut
Circulation	Bleeds when cut	Does not bleed when cut

(4) Steps of debridement. All devitalized muscle must be removed; if not, the chance of infection is greater. It is better to take good muscle tissue and have some deformity than to leave devitalized muscle and have infection. The preferred method of debridement is to cut along one side of a muscle group in strips or in blocks and not piecemeal or in small bunches.

(a) Remove all blood clots, foreign material, and debris from the wound during exploration of the wound with a gloved finger.

(b) Vital structures like major nerves and blood vessels must be protected from damage.

(c) All procedures must be carried out gently with precision and skill.

(d) Major blood vessels must be repaired promptly.

(e) All foreign bodies must be removed, including small detached bone fragments, but time should not be wasted looking for elusive metallic fragments that would require more extensive dissection.

(f) Tendons usually do not require extensive debridement. Trim loose frayed edges and ends. Repair should not be performed during initial treatment.

(g) Hemostasis must be precise.

(h) Repeated irrigations of the wound with physiologic salt solution during the operation will keep the wound clean and free of foreign material. <u>This step cannot be overemphasized</u>.

(i) When debridement is complete, all blood vessels, nerves, and tendons should be covered with soft tissue to prevent drying and maceration.

(j) Joint synovium should be closed or at least the joint capsule. The skin and subcutaneous tissue is left open in any case.

(k) Dependent drainage of deep wounds must be employed.

(l) Liberal fasciotomy of an extremity is often an additional precaution that allows for postoperative swelling. Use when the five Ps are present distal to an injury or wound (pain, pallor, pulselessness, puffiness, and paresthesia).

(m) <u>DO NOT</u> dress the wound with an occlusive dressing, but place a few wide strips of fine-mesh gauze between the walls of the wound; place fluffed gauze in the pocket that is formed, then dress the wound to protect but not constrict.

(n) All wounds will be left open with the exception of

wounds of the face, sucking chest wounds, head wounds, wounds of the joint capsule or synovial membrane, and wounds of the peritoneum.

(o) Immobilization and correct positioning of the injured part promotes healing, and these measures should be used even if no fracture is present.

16-3. VASCULAR INJURIES. Although a vascular injury is extremely serious, you must consider the equipment available, other injuries to the patient, and other casualties.

a. Accurate diagnosis of a vascular injury may not be possible until exploration is undertaken, but the following signs and symptoms may be used as evidence of arterial damage:

(1) Extremity may be pale, waxy, mottled, cyanotic, and cold.

(2) Pulse may be absent, but the presence of a pulse does not rule out arterial injury.

(3) Analgesia, loss of voluntary motion of extremity, muscle spasm or contracture may be present.

(4) External hemorrhage, like bright red spurting blood, may or may not be present.

(5) The affected limb may be larger than the intact limb.

b. There is no set time when a vascular injury must be repaired to insure saving the limb, but the longer the time lag, the greater the failure rate. The best results are obtained within 6 to 10 hours of the injury.

c. You probably will not be able to undertake major vascular repairs, but you should have the equipment to handle arterial lacerations caused by low velocity missiles or sharp instruments.

(1) Clamps of a noncrushing type should be applied to the injured artery, the first proximal to the injury and the second distal.

(2) Keep the artery moist with a saline solution.

(3) All debridement accomplished by the standard technique should be completed before arterial repair is begun.

(4) Run a Fogarty balloon catheter distally in the artery to determine the patency. This will also clear any distal thrombus.

(5) Use a continuous suture of 5-0 or 6-0 synthetic suture with a fine curved, noncutting swaged needle.

(6) Release the clamps and observe for leaks.

(7) Dress the wound as a soft tissue injury.

(8) Keep the extremity at heart level.

(9) Begin active muscle exercises while patient is still in bed.

d. When the muscle tissue is of questionable viability after arterial continuity has been restored, the patient is observed for:

(1) A decrease in urinary output.

(2) Increasing pain toxicity, confusion, and fever.

(3) Increase in pulse rate.

(4) Evidence of clostridial myositis.

e. If this evidence is present, excision of necrotic muscle tissue or early amputation may be called for. It is usually safe to hold off on amputation for up to 5 days until a line of demarcation is established.

16-4. BONE AND JOINT INJURIES.

a. For all open bone and joint injuries, the following principles apply:

(1) Initial determination of the extent of the wound and the structures involved.

(2) Generous extensile incision and removal of foreign material, debridement, and removal of small bone chips.

(3) Arthrotomy.

(4) Vascular repair and fasciotomy.

(5) Wound is left open for delayed primary closure.

(6) Bulky nonocclusive dressing and immobilization of fractures, nonfractures, and joint injuries.

(7) Documentation of everything observed.

b. War wound therapy is indicated in all open bone or joint injuries.

16-5. PERIPHERAL NERVE INJURIES.

a. The field medic does not have the equipment or the expertise to perform nerve repair. Nor is it really necessary.

b. Closed nerve injuries are never surgically explored. Open injuries of nerves are handled as any other soft-tissue injury with the nerve left intact and covered with muscle tissue to prevent exposure.

16-6. AMPUTATIONS.

a. Amputations are performed to save life and are done at the lowest level possible. All attempts should be made to save the knee and elbow joints even if this means having a short stump.

b. Indications for amputation are:

(1) Massive gas gangrene (clostridial myositis).

(2) Overwhelming local infection that endangers life despite antibiotic therapy and surgical measures.

(3) Established death of a limb.

(4) Massive injuries in which structures of a limb are obviously nonviable.

(5) Secondary hemorrhage in the presence of severe infection.

(6) Extremities with severe involvement of skin, muscle, and bone with anesthetic terminus and irreparable nerve damage.

c. Under combat conditions the most acceptable type of amputation is the open circular technique.

(1) A circumferential incision is made through the skin and deep fascia at the lowest viable level. This layer is allowed to retract.

(2) The muscle bundles are exposed and then divided circumferentially at the new level of the skin edge. The muscle bundles will retract promptly exposing the bone.

(3) Upward pressure is placed on the proximal muscle stump and the bone is then transected at a still higher level. The surgical wound will have the appearance of an inverted cone.

(4) Blood vessels are isolated, clamped, and ligated as they are encountered. Bone wax is applied to the open end of the bone to prevent oozing.

(5) Major nerves are transected at the highest level possible.

(6) Never close an amputation primarily.

(7) Cold injuries are not indications for emergency amputation. Wait until the edges demarcate.

d. A layer of fine mesh gauze is placed over the wound and the recess is packed loosely with fluffed gauze. A stockinette is then applied over the stump securing the stockinette above the stump using liquid adhesive. The stump is then wrapped with ace wraps using compression decreasing proximally and 5 to 6 pounds of traction is applied. Continued traction will result in secondary skin closure over the stump.

16-7. REGIONAL INJURIES.

a. Craniocerebral injuries. Serious injuries to the head require more extensive surgery than can be done in the field. There are some expedient measures, however, that can be taken to give the patient a chance. These are:

(1) Prophylactic antibiotic therapy.

(2) Grossly devitalized and contaminated soft tissue and bone should be removed, along with any foreign material, visible on inspection, superficial to the dura. The dura should not be attacked.

(3) Gently irrigate the wound with physiologic salt solution and ligate all bleeding vessels. Gelfoam can be used to control oozing.

(4) If possible, the scalp wound should be loosely approximated to provide temporary coverage.

(5) Sterile petroleum-impregnated gauze should be laid over the wound. A thick gauze dressing should be placed over that and held in place by a bandage.

(6) High priority should be given for evacuation.

(7) Mark the medical record prominently and call attention to the incompleteness of treatment.

b. Spinal cord injuries.

(1) The primary aim of early surgical treatment of open spinal cord injuries is the prevention of localized or general infection including meningeal infections.

(2) The patient is placed on a frame made with two stretchers. He is sandwiched face down between the stretchers with holes cut out of the stretchers to expose the injury, the genitals, and the face.

(3) General debridement is then performed, with special care given to isolating the spinal wound from an abdominal wound when present.

(4) If dura is visualized and appears lacerated, place gelfoam over area and close overlying muscles and skin with sutures.

(5) Prophylactic antibiotic therapy should be initiated.

c. Maxillofacial injuries.

(1) The primary concern in facial injuries is the maintenance of a patent airway.

(2) Once an airway is opened, minimal debridement is performed and the wound is closed primarily.

(3) Prophylactic antibiotic therapy should be initiated.

(4) Fractures are handled in the best way possible. The main thing is to immobilize the fracture.

d. Eye injuries.

(1) Conjunctival foreign body.

(a) Pull eyelid away from eye.

(b) Pass a sterile wet cotton applicator across the conjunctival surface. Touching the object with the wet applicator makes it stick to the applicator.

(2) Corneal foreign body.

(a) Place a fluorescein strip in the corner of the eye, then examine the cornea with the aid of a magnifying device and strong illumination.

(b) Remove the foreign body with a sterile wet cotton applicator.

(c) Apply an antibiotic opthalmic ointment.

(d) Reexamine the eye for secondary infections 24 hours later.

(3) Lacerations of eyelid.

(a) Lid laceration not involving the lid margin can be sutured like any other laceration.

(b) If the lid margin is lacerated, the patient should be evacuated for specialized care to prevent permanent notching.

(4) Laceration of conjunctiva.

(a) Superficial lacerations of the conjunctiva do not require sutures.

(b) Apply broad-spectrum antibiotic opthalmic ointment until the laceration heals.

(5) Deep laceration or puncture wounds of the eye, foreign bodies that can't be removed, or vitreous hemorrhage (blood in the vitreous body may obscure a retinal detachment).

(a) Apply anesthetic drops to the eye.

(b) Bandage both eyes lightly and cover injured eye with an eye shield.

(c) Evacuate as soon as possible.

e. Ear injuries.

(1) You are limited to surgical repair of the external ear.

(2) Perform minimal debridement.

(3) Close lacerations in layers, being careful to realign the cartilage.

(4) Initiate prophylactic antibiotic therapy.

f. Neck injuries. Wounds of the neck are very serious and usually complicated.

(1) Establish and maintain a patent airway.

(2) Carefully debride the wound.

(3) Initiate prophylactic antibiotic therapy.

g. Chest injuries.

(1) The treatment of chest wounds is based upon the following special principles of management.

(a) Normal pleural and pericardial pressures must be maintained.

(b) The pleural space must be kept empty.

(c) The bronchial tree must be kept clean.

(d) Ventilation sufficient for adequate oxygenation and removal of carbon dioxide must be assured.

(e) The amount of hemorrhage must be estimated and blood replaced as necessary.

(2) Pneumothorax.

(a) Seal the wound(s) airtight.

(b) Place a chest tube anteriorly in the second interspace.

(c) Hook the chest tube into a closed drainage system with a waterseal.

(3) Hemothorax.

(a) Seal the wound(s) airtight.

(b) Place a chest tube through the chest wall in the midaxillary line for the removal of blood and fluid.

(4) Cardiac tamponade (fluid buildup in the pericardial sack causing muffled heart sounds and added pressure on the heart).

(a) Pericardium must be aspirated.

1. Insert cardiac needle in the angle between the xiphisternum and the costal margin.

2. Pass the needle upward and backward at a 45-degree angle into the pericardium.

3. Remove only enough fluid to improve the patient's blood pressure and pulse.

(b) Continue to monitor the patient's heart sounds, pulse, and blood pressure.

(5) Severe flail chest.

(a) Immediately intubate.

(b) Place a chest tube in the same way as with pneumothorax.

(c) Initiate positive pressure breathing.

(d) For lesser degrees of flail chest, strap the affected side with a firm dressing.

h. Abdominal injuries. The only abdominal wound we will discuss is evisceration.

(1) Stabilize the patient.

(2) Initiate prophylactic antibiotic therapy.

(3) Remove bowels from abdominal cavity and check for nicks and cuts.

(4) Suture or tag any nicks or cuts.

(5) Irrigate the abdominal cavity with sterile saline solution and remove all foreign material.

(6) Replace all good bowel into the abdominal cavity leaving the sutured and/or tagged bowel outside.

(7) Close the abdominal cavity partially and in layers leaving the tagged and sutured bowels outside on a sterile dressing to drain.

(8) Keep the patient NPO.

(9) Evacuate as soon as possible.

CHAPTER 17

ANESTHESIA

17-1. CHOICE OF ANESTHESIA.

a. In a general hospital 70-75 percent of surgery is performed under general anesthesia and the remainder under regional or local anesthesia. Operating outside a hospital these percentages should be turned around.

b. General anesthesia carries a risk with it no matter how simple the surgical procedure. Local anesthesia is often preferable to general anesthesia for the following reasons: The technique is simple and minimal equipment is required; there is less bleeding, nausea, and vomiting and less disturbance to body functions; it can be used when general anesthesia is contraindicated (e.g., recent ingestion of food by the patient); less postoperative observation and patient care are required; and there is a much lower incidence of pulmonary complications.

c. Regional anesthesia (regional block) produces complete sensory block; it prevents nerve impulses from passing by injecting the anesthetic solution around the nerve trunk at a distance from the area to be anesthetized. Regional blocks can be used almost anywhere in the body, but we will confine the blocks to dental and the upper extremities.

17-2. LOCAL ANESTHETICS.

a. Doses of local anesthetics for topical use:

Drug	Concentration	Duration	Maximal Dose
Cocaine	4%	30 min	200 mg.
Lidocaine (Xylocaine)	2-4%	15 min	200 mg.
Tetracaine (Pontocaine)	0.5%	45 min	50 mg.
Benzocaine	2-10%	Several hours	

b. Doses of local anesthetics for infiltration and nerve blocks:

Drug	Concentration	Duration	Maximal Dose
Procaine (Novocain)	2-4%	1/2 hr	1,000 mg.
Lidocaine (Xylocaine)	1-2%	1-2 hr	500 mg.
Mepivacaine (Carbocaine)	1-2%	1-2 hr	500 mg.
Tetracaine (Pontocaine)	0.1 0.25%	2-3 hr	75 mg.
Chloroprocaine (Nesacaine)	1-2%		1,000 mg.
Piperocaine (Metycaine)	1-2%		750 mg.
Hexylcaine (Cyclaine)	1-2%		500 mg.
Prilocaine (Citanest)	1-2%		500 mg.
Bupivacaine (Marcaine)	0.5%	5-7 hr	200 mg.
Etidocaine (Duranest)	0.5-1%	4-6 hr	300 mg.

c. Local anesthetic drugs (except cocaine) dilate the blood vessels, causing an increased rate of absorption and decreased duration of anesthetic action. A vasoconstrictor drug (epinephrine) may be added to injectable local anesthetic solutions to prolong and increase the anesthetic effect. Epinephrine counteracts the depressing action of local anesthetics on the heart and circulation. Epinephrine is used in concentrations of 1:100,000 (1 mg./100 ml.) or 1:200,000 (1 mg./200 ml.).

Stronger solutions should not be used because they may cause tissue damage due to ischemia.

Contraindications to adding epinephrine to local anesthetics are:

(1) Patients with history of hypertension, thyrotoxicosis, diabetes, or heart disease.

(2) Surgery on fingers or toes because severe vasospasm and ischemia of the extremities may occur.

d. Local anesthetics are used either topically or by infiltrating (injecting) the anesthesia directly around the area of surgery.

17-3. REGIONAL NERVE BLOCKS.

a. Nerve blocks are extremely effective, but in order to succeed with a nerve block you must know the anatomy of the area you want to block.

b. Premedication should be given before a nerve block is performed. Often premedication will make a block successful, especially if the patient interprets touch and motion as pain.

(1) 100 mg. (1 1/2 gr.) of phenobarbital by mouth can be given 1 1/2 to 2 hours before the block is performed.

(2) 50 to 100 mg. of phenobarbital can be given IV just before the block is performed.

(3) An alternate would be 1/8 to 1/4 gr. morphine prior to the block.

c. Axillary block of the brachial plexus.

(1) Indications. Surgery or setting fractures of the arm, forearm, and hand.

(2) Contraindications. Local infection or inflammation of the axillary nodes.

(3) Axillary blocks are used because of ease and accuracy of placement of the needle as well as the minimal incidence of complications. Additional advantages are that the axillary block can be repeated if necessary during the course of a lengthy operation and it is easily applied to a child or a somewhat uncooperative patient.

(4) The brachial plexus, axillary artery, and axillary vein are enclosed in a neurovascular compartment in the axilla. Solution injected into this sheath is limited and can spread only up or down, parallel to the neurovascular bundle.

(5) Technique. The axilla should be shaved and the arm abducted 90 degrees with the forearm flexed at a right angle and lying flat on a table. A pneumatic tourniquet (B.P. cuff) is placed just below the axilla to direct the local anesthetic toward the supraclavicular region.

The tourniquet is removed after the injection is completed. Standing at the patient's side, palpate the axillary artery as high as possible and fix it with your index finger against the humerus. Using a 23-gage needle (or smaller; larger needles can cause hematomas if the artery is punctured), raise a skin wheal. Insert the needle at a 45-degree angle in the direction of the artery until pulsations of the axillary artery are transmitted to the needle.

This is most often preceded by a palpable click as the needle penetrates the deep fascia forming the axillary sheath. If there is paresthesia radiating down the arm to the fingers or if you aspirate blood, you are in the right area. If you aspirate blood, withdraw the needle slowly until the aspiration of blood stops. In either case you can then inject 30-40 ml. of 1% lidocaine with 1:200,000 epinephrine.

The intercostobrachial nerve that innervates the skin of the upper half of the medial and posterior side of the arm is sometimes missed but can be anesthetized by a subcutaneous injection of 3 ml. of 1% lidocaine and 1:200,000 epinephrine over the axillary artery.

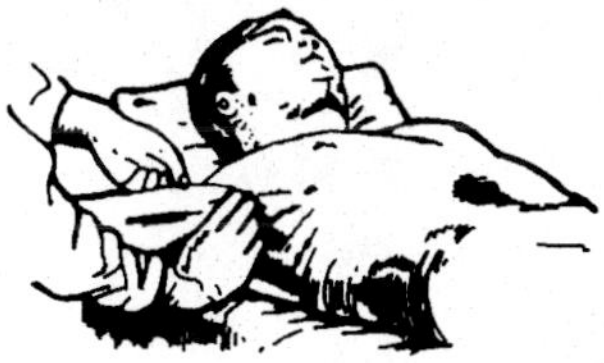

AXILLARY BLOCK OF THE BRACHIAL PLEXUS.

d. Nerve block of the wrist.

(1) Indications. Surgery or setting fractures of the hand or fingers.

(2) There are three major nerves that innervate the hand and fingers: the radial nerve, the median nerve, and the ulnar nerve. To completely block the hand and fingers, all three nerves must be blocked.

(3) For these blocks use the principle "No paresthesia no anesthesia."

(4) No more than 50 mg. of anesthesia should be used for the entire block.

(a) The radial nerve innervates the thumb and the back of the first three fingers. It is anesthetized by subcutaneous infiltration at the dorsolateral aspect of the wrist, using slow careful movement of the needle to insure an even distribution of the anesthetic solution.

1. Technique. Form a skin wheal, using a 22-gage needle (or smaller) at the point shown in the drawing. Working through the skin wheal with the syringe parallel to the nerve, elicit paresthesia (an electric shocklike sensation) in the thumb and the back of the first three fingers. When paresthesia is achieved, aspirate to insure you are not in a blood vessel, then inject 10 ml. of 1% lidocaine in a ring fashion. Begin lateral to the radial artery and extend the ring to the center of the back of the hand using slow, careful movement to insure even distribution. No

more than 20 cc. of 1% lidocaine should be used for the entire procedure.

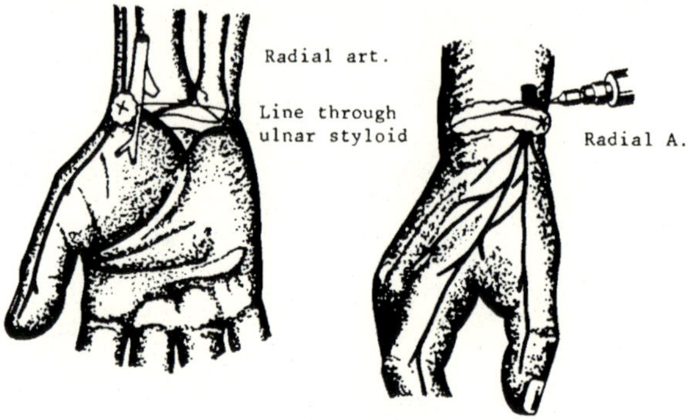

LANDMARKS AND METHODS OF BLOCKING THE RADIAL NERVE AT THE WRIST.

2. Complications. IV injection and/or hematoma of the joint.

(b) Median nerve innervates the palm of the hand, the index finger, the middle finger, and the radial side of the ring finger.

1. Technique. Locate the palmaris longus ligament and form a skin wheal, using a 22-gage needle (or smaller), just to the radial side of the palmaris longus. Working through the skin wheal, attempt to elicit paresthesia in the palm of the hand and fingers. When paresthesia is achieved, aspirate, then inject 5 ml. of 1% lidocaine. Then begin at the wheal and using slow, careful movements to insure even distribution, inject in a line right and left of the median nerve as depicted in the drawing.

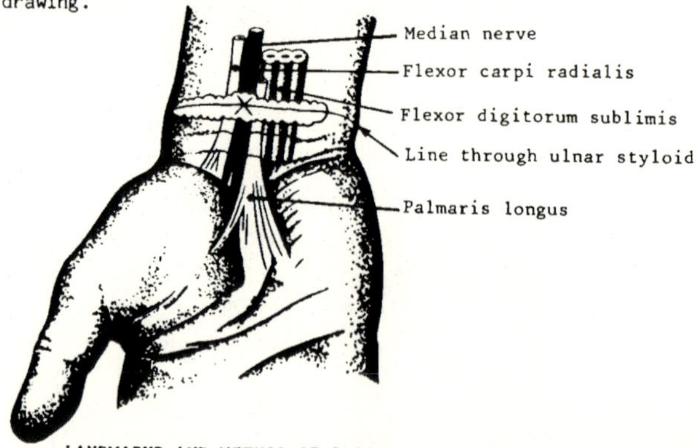

LANDMARKS AND METHOD OF BLOCKING THE MEDIAN NERVE AT THE WRIST.

The injection to the right and left might not be necessary, but occasionally there are collateral nerves that have moved down into the palm, and this will anesthetize them also.

2. Complications. IV injection and/or hematoma.

(c) Ulnar nerve innervates the ulnar side of the ring finger, the little finger, the ulnar side of the palm, and the back of the little and ring fingers.

1. Technique. Locate the flexor carpi ulnaris (see drawing) by palpation on a line through the ulnar styloid. Using a 22-gage needle, raise a skin wheal just lateral to the flexor carpi ulnaris. Working through the skin wheal, introduce the needle in the direction of and parallel to the nerve. After achieving paresthesia and aspiration, inject 5 ml. of 1% lidocaine with 1:200,000 epinephrine.

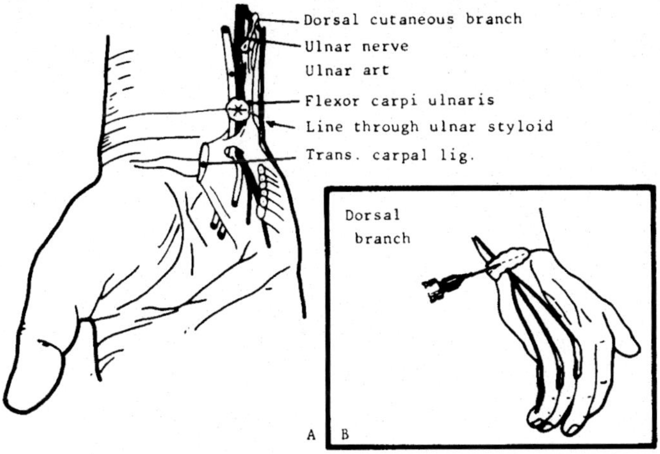

LANDMARKS AND METHODS OF BLOCKING THE ULNAR NERVE AT THE WRIST.

A. Volar Branch B. Dorsal Branch.

Once this is done begin at the skin wheal and extend the anesthesia dorsally in a ring fashion to the center of the back of the hand, using slow careful movement to insure even distribution of the anesthesia in the subcutaneous layer.

2. Complications. IV injection and/or hematoma.

e. Digital block (fingers & toes).

(1) No premedication is necessary.

(2) Do not use vasoconstrictor agents (epinephrine).

(3) Do not exceed 8 cc. of anesthesia per digit.

(a) Technique. Raise a skin wheal on the dorsolateral sides of the digit at the interdigital folds (see drawing).

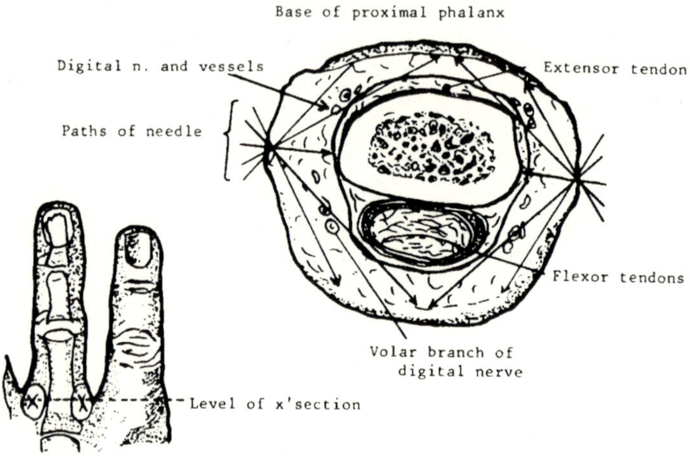

LANDMARKS AND METHOD OF BLOCKING DIGITS.

Working through the wheals in a fan-shaped method, place a ring of local anesthetic around the digit (see drawing). Massage the digit where the anesthesia was deposited to facilitate spread of the solution.

(b) Repeat the block if analgesia is inadequate.

(c) Complications. IV injection and/or hematoma.

17-4. GENERAL ANESTHESIA.

a. Ideally, the patient should have a complete physical and history done at least a day before surgery. Special examinations and laboratory work should be done as needed. The patient should have a good night's sleep and be placed N.P.O. 6-8 hours prior to surgery. The operation should be explained to the patient to help calm his fears. Finally, the patient should receive the proper premedication.

b. Premedication.

(1) Produces psychic sedation (relaxes and calms the patient, making administration of anesthesia easier).

(2) Reduces metabolic rate and decreases reflex irritability.

(3) Reduces quantity of anesthetic drug necessary.

(4) Minimizes or abolishes secretions of saliva and mucus.

(5) There are a wide range of sedatives, narcotic analgesics,

tranquilizers, and belladonna compounds (atropine and scopolamine) that can be used as preanesthesia medication. You must determine which is best for your situation. A good example is:

(a) Adult premedication.

1. Place patient N.P.O. 6-8 hours preoperatively.

2. 100 mg. pentobarbital P.O. at bedtime.

3. 100 mg. pentobarbital IM 2 hours preoperatively.

4. 0.5 mg. atropine SQ 1 hour preoperatively.

(b) Child premedication.

Age	Weight		Pentobarbital or Secobarbital	Morphine	Atropine or Scopolamine
Newborn	7 lb	3.2 kg.	----	----	0.1 mg.
6 months	16 lb	7.3 kg.	----	----	0.1 mg.
1 year	22 lb	10 kg.	35 mg.	1 mg.	0.2 mg.
2 years	26.5 lb	12 kg.	50 mg.	1.2 mg.	0.3 mg.
4 years	33 lb	15 kg.	65 mg.	1.5 mg.	0.3 mg.
6 years	44 lb	20 kg.	75 mg.	2 mg.	0.4 mg.
8 years	55 lb	25 kg.	90 mg.	2.5 mg.	0.4 mg.
10 years	66 lb	30 kg.	100 mg.	3 mg.	0.4 mg.
12 years	88 lb	40 kg.	100 mg.	4 mg.	0.4 mg.

1. N.P.O. 6-8 hours preoperatively.

2. _____ mg. pentobarbital, IM 2 hours preoperatively.

3. _____ mg. atropine, SQ 1 hour preoperatively.

c. Ether anesthesia. Used for all types of surgery, particularly that requiring muscle relaxation. It is probably the safest of the inhalation anesthesias. Induction of ether anesthesia is prolonged because of its irritating effects. To shorten the induction period the patient can be preanesthetized ("knocked down") with a nonirritating rapid-acting drug such as sodium pentothal.

(1) Advantages.

(a) Reliable signs of anesthesia depth.

(b) Stimulation of respiration.

(c) Bronchodilation.

(d) Does not depress circulation.

(e) Good muscle relaxation.

(f) Relatively nontoxic and safe. (Death rate is lower than any other anesthesia.)

(2) Disadvantages.

(a) Prolonged induction and recovery.

(b) Irritating action causes secretions of mucus from upper airway.

(c) Emetic action is dangerous in patients with full stomach. (Aspiration pneumonia.)

d. Sodium pentothal. Used for minor procedures of approximately 30 minutes or less. Can also be used as a "knock down" for ether anesthesia.

(1) Technique. Slowly inject the drug through an existing IV. Do not exceed 2 cc. in the first 15 seconds; then stop and wait (patient will be narcotized in 30-40 seconds). Having the patient count will let you know how it is affecting him. Slowly inject 1/2 to 1 cc. from time to time as required.

(2) Disadvantage.

(a) The anesthesia is noncontrollable.

(b) Laryngeal spasm may develop.

(c) The necessary effective dose is difficult to estimate.

(d) A severe respiratory depression ensues.

(e) Pentothal is a barbiturate that does not possess any analgesic properties.

(f) The muscular relaxation is not satisfactory.

(3) Signs of anesthesia. No reliable signs of anesthesia exist. The anesthetist must attempt to maintain the patient between the zones of decreased reflex activity and respiratory and circulatory failure.

(4) Complications.

(a) Respiratory failure.

(b) Hypotension.

(c) Laryngeal spasm.

(d) Slough of skin. Solutions of the sodium salts of barbiturates are alkaline and cause damage to tissues in event of seepage.

(e) Phlebothrombosis.

(f) Prolonged somnolence.

(g) Operations of undetermined length. Large amounts of the drug may be necessary to complete the operation. This causes a marked depression of respiration and circulation from cumulative effects.

(h) Shock from trauma or hemorrhage. Irreversible

respiratory failure or enhancement of hypotension may occur.

(5) Precautions.

(a) The limit should be approximately 1 gram of the drug for an adult.

(b) Be positive that the drug is completely dissolved and that the solution is clear before performing venipuncture. Undissolved particles act as foreign bodies in the solution and may cause "reactions."

(c) Inject the solution slowly. Do not inject more than 6 cc. of a 2-1/2% solution at any one time at the onset.

e. Open drop method of inhalation anesthesia. The simplest method requiring the least equipment.

(1) Make a wire frame in a cup shape to fit over the nose and mouth. Pad and tape the bottom edges to make a better fit and protect the patient's face. Place one or two unfolded 4 X 4s over the top to completely cover the frame and tape the edges down. Cut two notches in the cork going into the ether container, one for air to enter the container and one for the wick that will drop the anesthesia on the mask.

(2) By regulating the amount of anesthesia dripped on the mask, you can regulate the depth of anesthesia.

(3) Oxygen can be fed into the mask by running a small tube under the edge of the mask; however, the higher the flow of oxygen the lower the concentration of anesthesia.

(4) Condensation of water vapors on the gauze interferes with vaporization of the anesthesia. The colder the gauze the more rapid the condensation of moisture in the expired air. Replace the gauze as required to correct the impaired vaporization.

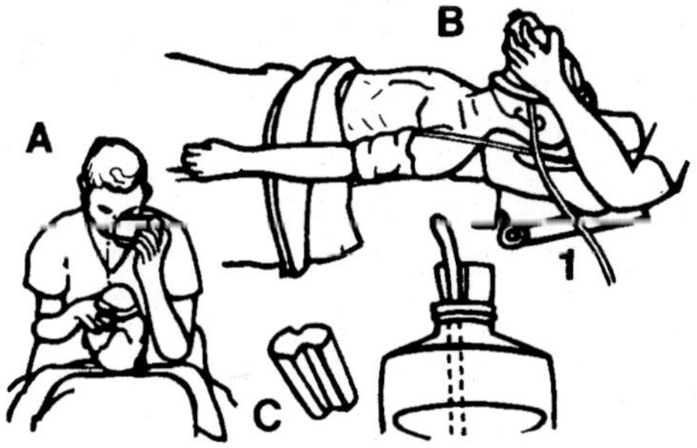

TECHNIQUE OF "OPEN DROP" ANESTHESIA. A - Method of supporting the head with the arms. B - Lateral view showing support of head and insufflation of oxygen (1) beneath the mask. C - Cork cut and wick in place to drip ether.

f. Stages and signs of anesthesia. Anesthesia is divided into four stages, and the third or surgical stage is subdivided into four planes.

STAGE I - ANALGESIA

STAGE II - DELIRIUM

STAGE III - SURGICAL

Plane 1

Plane 2

Plane 3

Plane 4

STAGE IV - RESPIRATORY PARALYSIS

(1) STAGE I. The Stage of Analgesia is that period from the beginning of induction to the loss of consciousness.

(a) Analgesia is the loss of the sense of pain without the loss of consciousness or sense of touch. Pain sense is progressively depressed during this stage. The point of pain abolition is known as total analgesia, and the approach to total analgesia is relative analgesia. The danger and difficulty in achieving and maintaining total analgesia is its proximity to the second stage. It is sometimes attempted, however, in dentistry, obstetrics, and to a small extent in minor surgery.

(b) False anesthesia as a manifestation of hysteria may occur in this stage. The signs may indicate quiet surgical anesthesia, i.e., regular rhythmic respiration with apparent loss of eyelid reflex. Starting the preparation or the operation at this point may precipitate fatal ventricular fibrillation. The only way of differentiating between false anesthesia and true surgical anesthesia is the length of time elapsed since induction. Three or four minutes may be long enough to reach Stage III with cyclopropane and pentothal, but it is not when using ether. When in doubt, wait much longer than you would otherwise wait before starting a procedure.

(c) "Brain anesthesia" is another phenomenon that may be encountered. The brain has a very rich blood supply and high partial pressure of the agent may cause the brain to become saturated with the first few respirations giving the appearance of surgical anesthesia. Subsequently, the agent will diffuse out of the brain almost as rapidly as it diffused in, and the signs will become a more accurate index.

(2) STAGE II. This is the Stage of Delirium or excitement stage and represents the period of the earliest loss of consciousness. The hazards of the second stage are physical injury and ventricular fibrillation.

(a) The higher cerebral or voluntary control centers are abolished, leaving the secondary centers free. Response to stimulation or to dreams the patient may be having is exaggerated and is frequently expressed in violent physical activity. This violence may be initiated by external stimulation such as instruments being knocked together, talking, moving the patient or the operating table, etc. The excitement will be more pronounced in patients who are afraid. (Who isn't afraid when coming to the operating room?)

(b) The stages of anesthesia are the same whether the patient is going to sleep or waking up. Emergence delirium is less frequently violent than that of induction because of several factors. First, external stimulation is seldom as great; and second, postoperative surgical depression limits the amount of activity. Remember that nonshocking procedures done under short-acting drugs leave the patient potentially as active during emergence as during induction.

(c) Ventricular fibrillation occurs most frequently in the group from 5 to 35 years of age, but may occur at any age. This danger also increases in proportion to the degree of fear--probably due to increased adrenalin output accompanying fear.

(d) Management of the second stage consists of:

1. Reducing nervous irritability by use of adequate premedication.

2. Proper restraint of the patient.

3. Avoidance of external stimuli.

4. Rapid, smooth induction.

(3) STAGE III. The Surgical Stage.

(a) Plane 1. Entrance into Plane 1 is marked by the appearance of full, rhythmic, and mechanical respiration. The tidal volume and respiratory rate are increased depending on the efficiency of respiration in the preceding stages. If the first and second stages have been uneventful, the increase in volume is about 25% above normal. If the course has been stormy with consequent carbon dioxide retention, the volume may be twice normal. If hyperpnea has preceded this stage, it is possible that the respiratory volume may be below normal. Within a minute or so, however, the balance between the respiratory threshold and the carbon dioxide tension should be established at a moderate hyperpnea.

1. Inspiration is shorter and slightly quicker than expiration, and there is a pause at the end of expiration.

2. Premedication has a direct bearing on the rate and volume throughout the anesthesia. Other things being equal, the minute volume is decreased in proportion to the threshold elevation by the preanesthetic drug.

3. Response to reflex stimulation is still present and minute volume is also directly proportionate to the amount of stimulation from the operative field.

(b) Plane 2. The tidal volume is usually somewhat decreased while the rate may be either decreased or increased. As the rate increases, the pause at the end of expiration becomes shorter so that both phases are more nearly equal in length. The response to reflex stimulation from the operative site is somewhat less than in Plane 1.

(c) Plane 3. Entrance into this plane is marked by beginning paralysis of the intercostal muscles. The first evidence of this paralysis is a delayed thoracic inspiratory effort. That is, the diaphragm begins its excursion before the intercostals cause thoracic expansion. This phenomenon can be felt before it is visible. The pause between inspiration and expiration becomes progressively longer at the expense of inspiration. Inspiration becomes a quick jerky movement. The progressive intercostal paralysis gradually decreases the tidal volume with progression downward.

The lower border of Plane 3 is marked by the completion of intercostal paralysis. The bony thorax is stationary, and there is decided retraction of the intercostal spaces with each inspiration. It should be remembered that intercostal retraction also occurs with respiratory obstruction.

(d) Plane 4. At this point the diaphragmatic excursion is greater than at any other period of anesthesia. The resistance to its descent, which is normally provided by the expansion of the bony thorax, is absent; therefore, it becomes a quick jerky movement. This movement, long before intercostal paralysis is complete, is annoying to the surgeon working in the abdomen. He may complain that the patient is "pushing" and may attempt, to alleviate the condition by deepening the anesthesia, resulting in aggravation on the part of the surgeon and consternation on the part of the anesthetist when the patient suddenly stops breathing.

Diaphragmatic paralysis begins, and there is a marked decrease in tidal volume, progressing rapidly as diaphragmatic paralysis increases. Inspiration becomes more shallow and gasping, and the rhythm is very irregular.

(4) STAGE IV. Complete diaphragmatic paralysis or cessation of respiration marks the entrance into Stage IV, and death ensues within 1 to 5 minutes unless corrective measures are instituted immediately.

(5) Eye signs. It is the degree of activity of the motor muscles of the eyeball that serves as an anesthetic guide, not the type of activity. Preanesthetic medication may retard eyeball activity, but it does not destroy its value as an anesthetic guide. The protruding eyeball is usually not as active as the normal one.

(a) Stage I. Eyeball activity is normal or under voluntary control.

(b) Stage II. The motor muscles undergo a period of excitation activity. The mechanism is not completely understood, but it is believed that it is the result of the impulses "running riot" in the central nervous system. These "berserk impulses" result in the stimulation of first one nucleus then another. This is manifested in the hyperactivity of the eyeball in Stage II.

(c) Stage III.

1. Plane 1. The hyperactivity is still present upon entrance into Plane 1 and decreases progressively as anesthesia is carried downward. This may be explained on the basis of progressive depression of the central nervous system with consequent diminution of stimulation of the various centers.

2. Plane 2. Complete cessation of activity marks entrance into Plane 2. From this point on down, the eyes should be fixed concentrically because the muscles are paralyzed and flaccid. Eccentric fixation should suggest the possibility of hypoxia.

(d) Reflexes.

1. Conjunctiva palpebral. Present in Stages I and II. Absent in Stage III, Plane 1. The eyelids close when the tip of the finger brushes the margin of the upper lid.

2. Lid. Present in Stages I and II. Absent in Stage III, Plane 1. Tested by gently raising the upper eyelid with the finger. If the reflex is present, the lid will attempt to close either at once or after a few seconds' exposure. If it is absent, no effort to close the lid will occur.

(6) Muscular reflexes.

(a) Vomiting occurs at the extreme lower border of Stage II.

(b) Swallowing occurs at the extreme upper border of Plane 1.

(c) Jaw sign is tested by pushing the jaw forward and up from the angle. In light anesthesia there will be a marked change in respiration in response. The response will not be marked in mid Plane 2, and in lower Plane 2 there should be no change in respiration.

(d) Pharyngeal reflex is abolished in mid Plane 1.

(e) Laryngeal reflex response to direct stimulation is abolished at the junction of Plane 1 and Plane 2. The response to reflex stimulation is abolished in mid Plane 2.

(f) Reflex response to skin traumatism is usually abolished by anesthesia in the upper half of Plane 1.

(g) Skeletal muscles are relaxed in the following order:

1. Small - Plane 1

2. Large - Plane 2

3. Abdominal - Mid Plane 2

4. Diaphragm - Plane 4

(h) Smooth muscle tone (intestinal tract and blood vessels) is lost in lower Plane 3.

GRAPH I STAGES AND SIGNS FOR ETHER, VINAMAR, VINETHENE ANESTHESIA

STAGES	PLANES	BREATHING	EYEBALL	LID REFLEX
I		Regular, inspiration slightly greater than expiration and increased rate	Voluntary movement 0-4+ and moist	Present
II		Irregular in rate and amplitude	Involuntary movement 0-4+ and moist	Present
III	1.	Rhythmical and exaggerated respiration	Slight movement then centrally fixed and moist	Absent
III	2.	Inspiration and expiration equal with decreasing amplitude	Fixed; Lusterless	Absent
III	3.	Beginning intercostal paralysis with lessening amplitude; inspiration less than expiration	Fixed; Lusterless	Absent
III	4.	Intercostal paralysis complete; shallow, jerky with tracheal tug and prolonged expiration	Fixed; Lusterless	Absent
IV MEDULLARY PARALYSIS		Apnea	Fixed; Lusterless	Absent

GRAPH I STAGES & SIGNS FOR ETHER, VINAMAR, OR VINETHENE ANESTHESIA (CONT'D)

PUPILS	LARYNGEAL REFLEXES	BLOOD PRESSURE	PULSE	MUSCLE RELAXATION
Normal or slight dilatation and reaction to light.	Present	Slightly increased	Slightly accelerated	None
Dilated but react to light (sympathetic response)	Possible retching, gagging, or vomiting present up to lower part of Plane I			
Constricted		Normal	Normal	Jaw slightly relaxed
Slightly dilated	Absent			Beginning abdominal relaxation
Moderately dilated				Complete abdominal relaxation
Widely dilated		Slight hypotension	Accelerated	Complete muscle relaxation
Fully dilated (paralytic dilatation)		Marked hypotension	Weak and irregular	Flaccid paralysis

GRAPH II STAGES + SIGNS FOR SODIUM PENTOTHAL

STAGES	PLANES	BREATHING	EYEBALL		LID REFLEX
I		Decreased rate and amplitude immediately upon induction	Voluntary movements 0-2+		Present but sluggish
II		← No delirium			
III	LIGHT	Slow and shallow, progressive decrease in amplitude (Progressive decrease in tidal volume)	Fixed	Moist	Absent
III	DEEP	Minimal amplitude & rate, assisted respirations indicated (Progressive decrease in tidal volume)	Fixed	Lusterless	Absent
IV MEDULLARY PARALYSIS		Apnea (Progressive decrease in tidal volume)	Fixed	Lusterless	Absent

GRAPH II STAGES + SIGNS FOR SODIUM PENTOTHAL

PUPILS	LARYNGEAL REFLEXES	BLOOD PRESSURE	PULSE	MUSCLE RELAXATION
Normal to slight dilatation	Present	Unchanged	Unchanged	None
Normal, sluggish reaction to light	Present, pharyngeal tube or mucus may initiate laryngospasm			Slight, but none at pharynx, larynx, or abdomer; reaction to afferent stimuli
Normal, no reaction to light; dilatation is a toxic sign	Absent	Moderate hypotension	Rapid & weak	Relaxation of larynx, pharynx, and peripheral muscles; no reaction to afferent stimuli
No light reaction, may show hippus or wide paralytic dilatation		Marked hypotension	Slow, weak & irregular	Flaccid

GRAPH III STAGES & SIGNS FOR ETHYLENE, NITROUS OXIDE, OR TRICHLORETHYLE....ANESTHESIA

STAGES	PLANES		BREATHING	EYEBALL	
I			Regular, inspiration slightly greater than expiration	Voluntary movements 0-4+	
II			Rapid and irregular in rate and amplitude	Involuntary movements 4+ & moist	
III	LIGHT		Exaggerated and machinelike, prolonged inspiration, possible phonation	Slight activity then centrally fixed and moist	
	MEDIUM	Oxygen starvation characteristics	Deep, regular & accelerated, inspiration & expiration equal. may sob	Fixed and downward rotation	Lusterless
	DEEP		Irregular, slow & shallow with prolonged expiration, may be spasmatic, sobbing & crowing		
IV MEDULLARY PARALYSIS			Opnea	Eccentric and jerky	

GRAPH III STAGES & SIGNS FOR ETHYLENE, NITROUS OXIDE, OR TRICHLORETHYLE...ANESTHESIA (CONT'D)

LID REFLEX	PUPILS	LARYNCEAL REFLEXES	BLOOD PRESS	PULSE
Reflex present	Constricted or dilated	Present	Normal	Normal
Reflex present, lids - resistant	Dilated (sympathetic response)	Swallowing with tendency to retching gagging, or vomiting	Unchanged	Slightly accelerated
Reflex - faintly present & lids slightly resistant	Small and sluggish to light			
Reflex - absent, lids open	Small to moderate, NO light reaction	Absent	Slight hypertension	
Reflex absent and lids open and stiff	Dilated (danger sign)	Absent reflex with tendercy to gasping, retching and vomiting		Increasing rate
	Maximum dilatation, may become irregular		Marked hypertension	Weak and irregular

GRAPH III STAGES & SIGNS FOR ETHYLENE, NITROUS OXIDE, OR TRICHLORETHYLE....ANESTHESIA (CONT'D)

MUSCLE RELAXATION	CENTRAL NERVOUS DEPRESSION (EEG) cps = cycles per sec. mvs = microvolts
None	Intermediate frequency, 8-13 cycles per sec; low voltage, less than 50 microvolts
Exaggerated reflex and rigidity	Low frequency, 4-6 cps; low voltages, less than 50 microvolts
None	Mixed wave forms 4-6 cps, and 40-70 mvs, superimposed upon slow frequency 2-3 cps, 100-150 microvolts
Slight	
Absent with rigidity & spasm	Continuation of mixed wave patterns with burst suppression, rhythmicity is lost; frequencies are relatively slow 3-5 cps, but the amplitude remains high, over 200 mvs
Spastic	

CHAPTER 18

IV THERAPY (FLUIDS AND ELECTROLYTES, BASICS)

18-1. GENERAL. Assuming you will be deployed and not have the capabilities to determine serum electrolytes, the following information is presented to keep you and your patient out of trouble. First, let's consider the composition of some common IV fluids (see table below).

Solution	Na	K	Cl	HCO_3	Ca	Mg	Calories	CH_2O gm
Ringer's lactate	130	4	109	(28)	3	-	-	-
Normal saline	154	-	154	-	-	-	-	-
D5W	-	-	-	-	-	-	200	50
D5NS	154	-	154	-	-	-	200	50
D5 .2NS	34	-	30	-	-	-	200	50
D5 .45NS	77	-	74	-	-	-	200	50
D10W	-	-	-	-	-	-	400	100
Ringer's solution	147	4	155	-	4	-	-	-

Na = Sodium, K = Potassium, Cl = Chlorine, HCO_3 = Bicarbonate, Ca = Calcium, Mg = Magnesium, CH_2O = Carbohydrates

18-2. COMMON PROBLEMS.

a. Now, what type of solution would you use for daily maintenance of an N.P.O. patient? Considering the daily requirements of Na (70 mEq.), K (40-60 mEq.), CHO (150-200 gm) and water to be 2 liters, the following should be given:

1,000 cc. D10W + 20 mEq. KCl over 12 hours
500 cc. D10W + 10 mEq. KCl over 6 hours
500 cc. D5NS + 10 mEq. KCl over 6 hours

b. Daily fluid requirement for infants and children according to body weight.

0-10 kg. - 100 cc./kg.

11-20 kg. - $\frac{100 \text{ cc./kg.}}{10}$ + 50 cc./kg.

21 kg. and over - $\frac{100 \text{ cc./kg.}}{20}$ + 50 cc./kg. + 25 cc.

c. Next, how would you replace fluid removed by an NG tube - in addition to daily maintenance requirements? Electrolytes common to gastric secretions are Na (40 mEq. per liter), K (10 mEq./L.), and Cl (140 mEq./L.). An appropriate replacement would be daily maintenance plus 1 liter per liter loss replacement of D5 .2NS + 20 mEq. KCl.

d. For the last common problem, consider replacement of fluid lost by diarrhea. Electrolytes common to diarrheal fluid are Na (50 mEq./L.), K (35 mEq./L.), Cl (40 mEq./L.) and HCO_3 (45 mEq./L.). Appropriate fluid for diarrheal losses would be daily maintenance plus liter for liter replacement with 1,000 cc. D5W + 35 mEq. KCl + 45 mEq. $NaHCO_3$.

18-3. ADJUSTMENT FOR INCREASED BODY TEMPERATURE, ENVIRONMENTAL TEMPERATURE, AND HYPERVENTILATION.

Fever	Environmental Temperature	Respiratory Rate	Additional Fluid Allowance
101°F. or less	85°F. or less	35 or less	None
101-103°F.	85-95°F.	Over 35	500 cc. H_2O
Over 103°F.	95°F. or less	-	1,000 cc. H_2O

18-4. BURNS - FLUID THERAPY.

a. Brooke Formula - first 24 hours.

(1) Colloids (plasma, plasmanate, or dextran) .5 ml./kg./% body surface burned.

(2) Electrolyte solution (Lactated Ringer's) 1.5 ml./kg./% body surface burned.

(3) H_2O requirement (D5W) 2,000 cc. for adults - for children correspondingly less.

ROUGH GUIDE FOR H_2O REQUIREMENT IN CHILDREN:

During first 2 yrs - 120 cc./kg.
2d - 5th yr - 100 cc./kg.
5th - 8th yr - 80 cc./kg.
8th - 12th yr - 50 cc./kg.

BURNS COVERING MORE THAN 50% OF THE BODY SURFACE ARE CALCULATED AS 50% OR EXCESS FLUID WILL BE GIVEN!!!

b. In the second 24 hours about one-half the colloid and electrolyte requirement of the first 24 hours is needed.

CHAPTER 19

DENTAL EMERGENCIES AND TREATMENT

19-1. GENERAL.

a. A tooth is divided into two major parts: the crown (portion of the tooth normally visible in the mouth) and the root or roots (portion embedded in the socket and partially covered by soft tissue).

b. The crown has five surfaces: the occlusal or biting surface, the lingual or tongue side surface, the facial or cheek side surface, and the other two surfaces (mesial and distal) that come in contact with adjacent teeth (mesial being the contacting surface nearest the midline and distal the farthest from the midline). All surfaces may be affected by dental decay (caries).

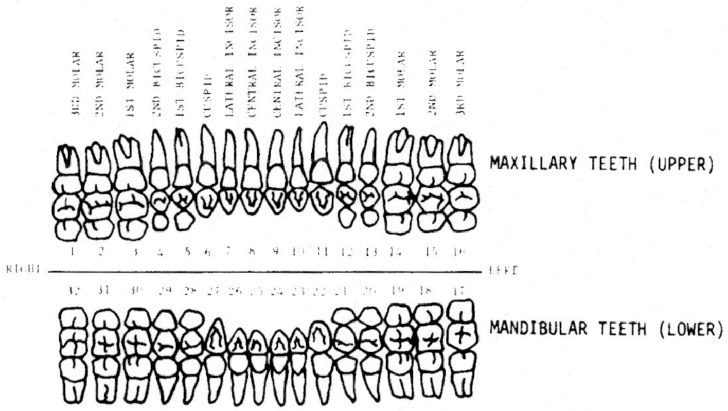

19-2. TOOTHACHES. Toothaches are usually associated with one of the following: caries (decay); tooth, crown, or root fractures; and acute periapical (root end) abscess.

19-3. CARIOUS LESIONS IN VITAL TEETH.

a. Diagnosis. Finding the offending tooth may be difficult. The patient with a toothache resulting from a carious lesion will usually present the following symptoms:

(1) Intermittent or continuous pain that is usually intense.

(2) Pain may be caused by heat, cold, sweet, acid, or salt substances.

(3) The tooth will usually be grossly carious (decayed).

(4) The carious enamel and dentin are discolored.

(5) Tapping the tooth with an instrument will usually elicit pain.

b. Diagnostic test.

(1) Thermal tests can be used; however, if hot and cold are used, a normal tooth must be tested also and used as a basis for comparison. The application of cold to normal teeth elicits pain in most instances, but the response ceases soon after the stimulus is removed. A diseased tooth, compared to a normal tooth, varies in its reaction to the temperature test. For example, a reaction to cold persists after application stops and the tooth responds very little to heat or the reaction to heat persists after application and the tooth appears to respond very little or not at all to cold.

(2) Thermal test procedure.

(a) Isolate the teeth to be tested from the saliva with gauze packs.

(b) Cold test. Spray a cotton-tipped applicator with ethyl chloride and place the cold surface on the tooth crown. Note the response and its duration. (Ice may also be used). A vital tooth will give a painful response to cold.

(c) Heat test. Heat an instrument (e.g., a mouth mirror handle) and touch against the tooth. Note the response and duration.

(d) Test an unsuspected tooth for comparison.

(e) Check vitality by touching sound dentin (pain upon touching dentin indicates vitality).

c. Treatment.

(1) This treatment regimen will only work on teeth that are still vital. Eugenol is an agent that will sooth hyperemic pulp tissue if treated indirectly (if not in direct contact with the pulp). If a mix of zinc oxide and eugenol is applied directly to vital pulp, it will kill the pulp.

(2) After finding the source of pain, local anesthetic will probably be necessary to carry out the following:

(a) Remove as much of the soft decayed material as possible with a spoon-shaped instrument. If the patient is properly anesthetized he should feel no pain.

(b) Irrigate the cavity with warm water until loose debris has been flushed out.

(c) Isolate the tooth with gauze packs and gently dry the cavity with cotton pledgets.

(d) Mix zinc oxide powder with two or three drops of eugenol on a clean dry surface (parchment pad) until a thick puttylike mix is obtained.

(e) Fill the cavity with the zinc oxide-eugenol paste, tamping it gently (use the Woodson Plastic Instrument #2 or #3).

(f) Relieve interference with opposing teeth by having the patient bite several times. Surplus filling material is easily removed by lightly rubbing the tooth with a moist cotton pledget. The pain should disappear in a few minutes and the paste will harden within an hour. Caution the patient not to chew on the treated tooth.

(g) If zinc oxide powder is not available, a cotton pledget impregnated with eugenol may be left in the cavity.

(h) Instruct the patient that the procedure is temporary and definitive care must be given by a dental officer.

19-4. TOOTH CROWN FRACTURES. The anterior (front) teeth are particularly susceptible to injuries that result in fracture of the crown. The classification and emergency treatment for the majority of these injuries are summarized below.

a. Simple fractures of the crown involving little or no dentin. Treatment: Smooth the rough edges of the tooth.

b. Extensive fractures of the crown involving considerable dentin but not the pulp. Treatment:

(1) Wash the tooth with warm saline.

(2) Isolate and dry the tooth.

(3) Cover the exposed dentin with a zinc oxide-eugenol paste (it is difficult to achieve retention in anterior fractures). A copper band or an aluminum crown, trimmed and contoured to avoid lacerating the gingiva, may be filled with this paste and placed over the tooth. An alternative method is to incorporate cotton fibers into a mix of zinc oxide and eugenol (the fibers give additional strength) and place this over the involved tooth, using the adjacent teeth and the spaces between them for retention. Have the patient bite to be sure neither the bands or the "splint" interfere with bringing the teeth together.

(4) Have the patient see a dentist as soon as possible.

c. Extensive fractures involving the dentin and exposed pulp. Treatment:

(1) Anesthetize the tooth.

(2) Isolate and dry the tooth.

(3) Wash gently with warm saline.

(4) Cover the pulp and dentin with a mix of calcium hydroxide and dycal (DO NOT USE ZINC OXIDE AND EUGENOL AS IT CAUSES NECROSIS OF THE PULP), allow to harden (if the mix if moistened with water after placement, the hardening will be more rapid).

(5) The efficiency of this treatment regimen depends on the size of the pulp exposure. If the exposure is larger than 1.5 mm. consider

extraction. If all you have available is zinc oxide eugenol, you must also consider extraction.

19-5. ACUTE PERIAPICAL (ROOT END) ABSCESS.

a. Diagnosis.

(1) Patient gives history of repeated episodes of pain that has gradually become more continuous and intense.

(2) The accumulating pus causes increased pressure and the tooth will feel "long" to the patient. It will seem to be the first tooth to strike when the teeth are brought together.

(3) There is severe pain on percussion. This is a most significant sign. Always begin percussion on a tooth that appears normal and progress to the suspected tooth.

(4) Swelling may be present.

(5) Malaise, anorexia, and elevated temperature are sometimes noted. If severe, antibiotics should be considered, but only if these signs are present.

(6) The gingival tissues around the tooth are often tender and inflamed.

(7) An untreated periapical abscess may burrow through alveolar bone and appear as a bright red elevation of the soft tissues in the area.

b. Treatment. Drainage usually provides immediate relief from pain. Two methods may be used to accomplish adequate drainage:

(1) If the abscess has "pointed," incise the fluctuant area of the soft tissue associated with the acute infection. Local anesthesia is neither necessary nor easy to obtain.

(2) Establish drainage from the tooth; stabilize the tooth firmly with the fingers, remove the soft decay with a spoon-shaped instrument until an opening into the pulp chamber is made. Finger pressure on the gingiva near the root of the tooth should force pus out through the chamber opening. Pain will usually subside immediately.

c. Untreated acute periapical abscess.

(1) The common course of an untreated acute periapical abscess is as follows:

(a) Accumulation of pus and destruction of bone at the root end of the tooth.

(b) Invasion of the marrow spaces and destruction of trabeculae (suppurative osteitis).

(c) Destruction of the cortex and displacement of the periosteum by suppurative material (subperiosteal abscess).

(d) Rupture of the periosteum with resulting gingival

swelling (gum boil or parulis).

(e) Spontaneous drainage by rupture of the parulis.

(2) This chain of events can usually be halted at any of the stages by removal of the cause. Extraction is usually indicated. If treatment is not given, spontaneous drainage, while affording welcome relief to the patient, does not suffice. The acute process is merely converted to a chronic state that may flare up at any time, especially during periods of lowered resistance. The spread of the primary periapical abscess is usually in the direction of least resistance. As a general rule, it may be stated that the cortical bone nearest the abscess site will be the point of breakthrough, but positively identifying the involved tooth by its closeness to the abscess or parulis is an unreliable procedure. Certainly a tooth should not be extracted without further diagnostic evidence. The path of progression and the possibility of serious sequelae resulting from further spread of the infectious process is determined by the anatomy of the region. The following general statements may be made:

(a) Periapical abscess spread is usually toward the lateral aspect of the jaw.

(b) If the primary infection involves the palatal root of an upper tooth, the abscess usually drains in the palate (palatal roots are present in the upper molars and the first bicuspids). Abscesses on all other roots in the maxillary dentin tend to burrow through to the facial side.

(c) Periapical abscesses developing on the lingual surface of the mandible at a level producing drainage into the mouth are rare.

(d) Drainage may be extraoral. A periapical abscess may perforate the cortical bone and produce a pathway for drainage that opens onto a skin surface without involving the oral mucosa. The external application of heat may promote this untoward result.

(e) When the spread of a mandibular periapical abscess is directed lingually, the level of bone perforation dictates its course. If the breakthrough is above the attachments of the muscles of the floor of the mouth, sublingual infection results. If below these attachments, the avenue of spread is through the facial spaces of the neck, and grave, possibly fatal complications (e.g., Ludwig's angina) may result.

(3) Treatment. In more advanced cases, drainage is still essential. Antibiotics should be administered and their administration continued for several days subsequent to the remission of symptoms. In soft tissue abscesses, the application of heat is often helpful in localizing the suppuration. Emergency treatment centers around prevension of serious sequelae by drainage, if indicated, and the maintenance of high blood levels of antibiotics. It is highy probable that the extraction of the offending tooth will be necessary, but it is preferable to wait until the acute symptoms have subsided.

19-6. PERIODONTAL ABSCESS.

a. Diagnosis. A deep, throbbing, well-localized pain and tenderness of the soft tissues surrounding the tooth are characteristic. The patient frequently complains that the involved tooth seems elevated in its socket.

This acute suppurative process occurs in the periodontal tissues alongside the root of a tooth and involves the alveolar bone, periodontal ligament, and gingival tissues. It usually presents the following signs and symptoms:

(1) Redness and swelling of the surrounding gingiva.

(2) Sensitivity of the tooth to percussion.

(3) Mobility of the tooth.

(4) Cervical lymphadenopathy.

(5) General malaise and elevation of temperature.

b. Etiology. This condition results from irritation from a foreign body, subgingival calculus (tartar, hard calcium deposits on the teeth) or local trauma, and subsequent bacterial invasion of the periodontal tissues.

c. Treatment.

(1) Carefully probe the gingival crevice to establish drainage and locate the foreign body.

(2) Spread the tissues gently and irrigate with warm water to remove remaining pus and debris from the abscess area.

(3) Remove any foreign bodies.

(4) Instruct the patient to use a hot saline mouth rinse hourly.

19-7. ACUTE NECROTIZING ULCERATIVE GINGIVITIS (Vincent's infection, trench mouth).

a. Diagnosis. Constant gnawing pain and marked gingival sensitivity are usually the outstanding complaints. These subjective symptoms are accompanied by pronounced gingival hemorrhage, fetid odor, foul metallic taste, general malaise, and anorexia. Necrosis and ulceration are the principal characteristics of this painful inflammatory disease of the gingival tissues. Necrotic lesions commonly appear between the teeth. These are craterlike ulcerations covered by a grayish pseudomembrane. Cervical lymphadenitis and elevation of temperature may develop after the onset of acute oral symptoms. Untreated lesions are destructive with progressive involvement of the gingival tissues and underlaying structures.

b. Etiology. Although it was felt for many years that fusospirochetal organisms were solely responsible, the precise cause has not been proven. It is considered to be an infection arising as a result of the action of ordinarily harmless surface parasites exposed to an altered environment. General health, diet, fatigue, stress, and lack of oral hygiene are the most important precipitating factors. This disease is not considered to be transmissable; however, the fusospirochetal organisms are very virulent.

c. Treatment. The primary problem in therapy is the establishment of good oral hygiene. Simple emergency treatment is outlined as follows:

(1) First day.

(a) Wear surgical or exam gloves when working on this if possible.

(b) Swab the teeth and gingiva thoroughly with a 1:1 aqueous solution of 3% hydrogen perioxide on a cotton-tipped applicator twice.

(c) Instruct the patient to rinse his mouth at hourly intervals with this same solution. Issue the patient one pint of hydrogen peroxide. Caution him not to use this treatment for more than 2 days (due to possibility of precipitating a fungal infection).

(d) Place the patient on an adequate soft diet and advise a copious fluid intake.

(e) Have patient return in 24 hours.

(2) Second day. Patient will be much more comfortable.

(a) Using a soft toothbrush soaked first in hot water, clean the patient's teeth without touching the gingiva.

(b) Maintain the hourly hydrogen peroxide mouthwash regimen.

(c) Have patient brush with a soft toothbrush soaked in hot water every hour.

(d) Have patient return in 24 hours.

(3) Third day. Patient is essentially free of pain.

(a) Clean patient's teeth as before.

(b) Floss between all teeth.

(c) Discontinue hydrogen peroxide mouthwash regimen.

(d) Have patient brush 3-4 times a day.

(e) Tell patient to floss once a day.

(4) The above steps will suffice for the management of the typical acute case. After treatment, the acute form subsides and the chronic phase ensues. Although clinical symptoms are minimal, tissue destruction continues until further corrective measures are completed. Definitive care consists of cleaning and scaling of the teeth, instruction in oral hygiene and, in some cases, recontouring of the tissues involved in the infection. Unless the patient develops systemic involvement, antibiotic therapy should not be instituted. Antibiotic lozenges should never be employed in the management of this disease. As in other oral disorders, the use of silver nitrate or other causitcs is definitely contraindicated.

d. Remarks. Lesions similar to those of acute necrotozing ulcerative gingivitis frequently appear in patients suffering from blood dyscrasias or vitamin deficiencies. Any case of gingivitis that does not respond well within 24 hours requires hematological analysis.

19-8. HERPETIC LESIONS (COLD SORES, FEVER BLISTERS).

a. Diagnosis. Intense pain is the most frequent symptom when the fully developed herpetic ulcer is present. Itching, burning, and a feeling of tissue tautness are characteristics in the early stages. Oral herpetic lesions usually appear as small, localized ulcerations, but extensive involvement is occasionally seen. The vesicular stage (presence of fluid-containing "blisters" characteristic of involvement of the lips) is seldom seen with the mouth. Intraoral vesicles are quickly ruptured and the hepatic lesion then appears as a small eroded area with a bright red, flat or slightly raised border. In later stages, the lesion becomes covered with an all white plaquelike mass of epithelial cell fibrin and debris. Generalized herpetic infections produce large aras of fiery red, swollen, and extremely painful oral mucosa. It is in this type that systemic symptoms are pronounced.

b. Etiology. Lesions are due to the herpes simplex virus. This virus persists throughout the lifetime of the patient in areas near the site of the primary infection. In an otherwise healthy mouth, a degree of lowered resistance must be present in the oral structures for the virus to produce its effects. Predisposing factors include emotional stress, the common cold and other upper respiratory infections, gastrointestinal disorders, nutritional deficiencies, food allergies, and traumatic injuries to the oral mucosa. In females, menstruation and pregnancy often seem to trigger this process.

c. Treatment. Treatment is directed at the symptoms. Antibiotics are ineffective, but in severe cases they may prevent secondary infection. Fluids should be forced to prevent dehydration. Spices, spirits, and smoking should be avoided since they irritate the already painful lesions. Oral hygiene must be maintained.

d. Remarks. Healing usually occurs in about 2 weeks. Scar formation or serious sequelae are exceedingly rare. The primary infection, usually seen during childhood, produces a much more extensive and serious oral involvement than do the later episodes. Lesions are usually larger and more numerous and the pain is consequently greater. Because of the pain, children frequently refuse to eat or drink and dehydration may result.

19-9. PERICORONITIS.

a. Diagnosis. Marked pain in the area of a mandibular third molar is the most constant complaint. Acute inflammation is present in tissue flaps over partially erupted teeth. The clinical picture is that of a markedly red, swollen, suppurative lesion that is very tender and often accompanied by pain radiating to the ear, throat, and the floor of the mouth. The opposing (upper) wisdom tooth may impinge on the swollen flap of tissue thus making chewing virtually impossible. Fever and general malaise are often present. In addition, there may be spasm of the masticatory muscle on the affected side. Involvement of the cervical lymph nodes is common. Principal etiologic factors include trauma from opposing teeth, accumulation of food and debris, and bacteria and their products.

b. Treatment.

(1) Wrap the tip of a blunt instrument with a wisp of cotton. Dip the cotton in 3% hydrogen peroxide and carefully clean the debris from

beneath the tissue flap; pus may be released.

(2) Flush the area using warm saline solution.

(3) Instruct the patient to use a hot saline mouth rinse hourly.

(4) Prescribe an adequate soft diet.

(5) Repeat this treatment at daily intervals until the inflammation subsides.

(6) Stress that oral hygiene must be maintained.

(7) Extraction of the opposing molar must be considered if the inflammation does not subside.

NOTE: Antibiotic therapy should be limited to the treatment of systemic symptoms. Extraction of the offending tooth is usually necessary. Since the inflammatory process tends to recur, definitive dental treatment will be necessary.

19-10. DENTAL ANALGESIA.

a. Maxillary.

(1) Infiltration will provide adequate analgesia of the maxillary teeth. (Analgesia - blocking of pain impulses. Anesthesia - blocking of all nerve impulses.)

(2) Technique. Both facial and palatal injections must be given for maxillary extraction.

(a) Facial injection (see illustrations below).

1. Insert the needle into the mucobuccal fold directly above the tooth.

2. Advance the needle upward about three-eighths of an inch until the needle gently contacts bone (this should approximate the root end).

3. Aspirate to insure that the needle has not entered a blood vessel.

4. Slowly deposit three-fourths of the cartridge's contents.

(b) Palatal injection (see illustrations below).

1. Insert the needle one-half of an inch above the gingival (gum) margin of the tooth.

2. Deposit 3-4 drops of solution - DO NOT BALLOON THE TISSUE.

NOTE: The palatal injection is very painful.

b. Mandibular (Inferior alveolar). Conduction analgesia

supplemented by infiltration is the method of choice in anesthetizing the lower teeth. The inferior alveolar nerve is blocked as it enters the mandibular foramen on the medical aspect of the ramus of the mandible. This foramen is located midway between the anterior and posterior borders of the ramus and approximately one-half of an inch above the biting surface of the lower molars. The width of the ramus at this level can be estimated by placing the thumb on the anterior surface of the ramus (intraorally) and the index finger on the posterior surface extraorally. The inferior alveolar and lingual nerves are anesthetized by a single injection.

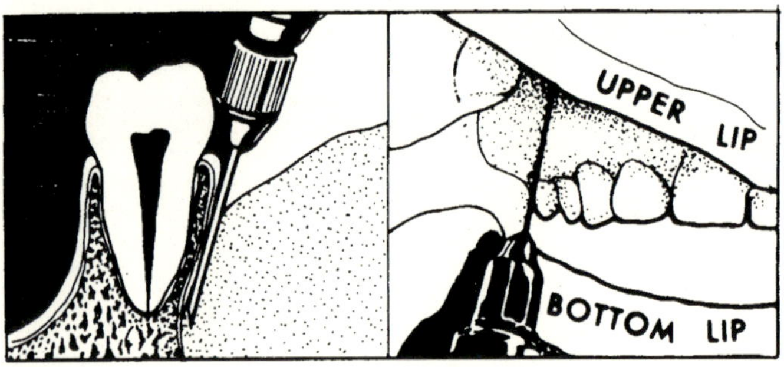

FACIAL INJECTION.

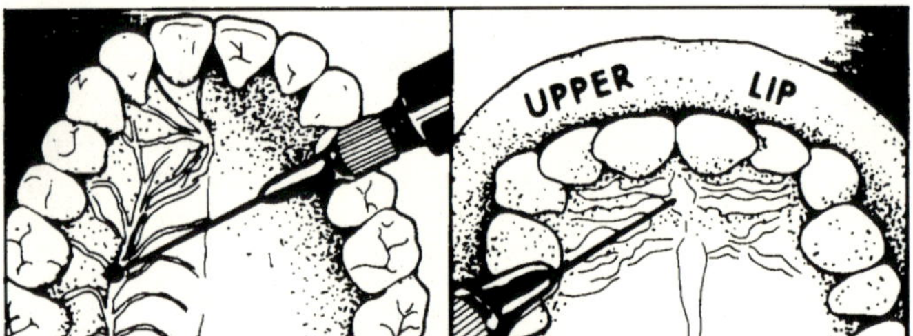

PALATAL INJECTION.

(1) Place the index finger on the biting surface of the lower molars so that the ball of the finger will contact the anterior border of the ramus. The fingernail will then be parallel to the midline.

(2) Place the barrel of the syringe on the lower bicuspids on the side opposite of the side to be anesthetized.

(3) Insert the needle into the tissue of the side to be

anesthetized in the apex of the V-shaped, soft tissue depression about one-half of an inch ahead of the tip of the finger on a line horizontally bisecting the fingernail.

(4) Advance the needle to contact the medical surface of the ramus. A 1-inch soft tissue penetration will usually suffice to position the needle point in the area of the mandibular foramen.

(5) Slowly deposit approximately two-thirds of the cartridge contents.

(6) Swing the barrel of the syringe to the side of the mouth being injected (leaving the needle in the position described in (4) above) and inject the rest of the cartridge contents while withdrawing the needle. This should anesthetize the lingual nerve.

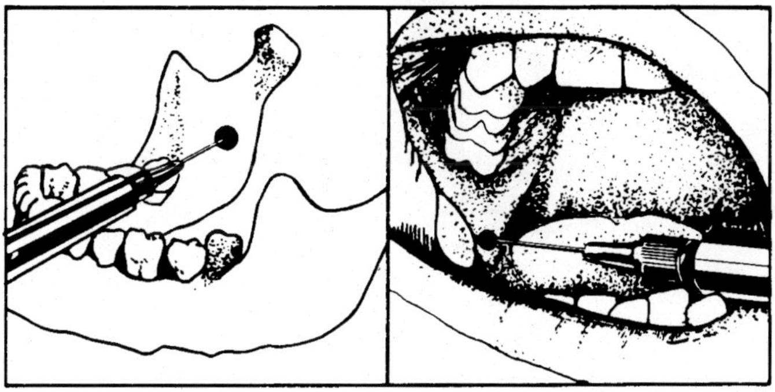

MANDIBULAR INJECTION.

(7) Anesthesia of the area is completed by a long buccal injection (see illustration below). Insert the needle in the mucobuccal fold at a point just anterior to the first molar. Gently pass the needle held parallel to the body of the mandible, with the bevel down, to a point as far back as the third molar, depositing the solution slowly as the needle is being advanced through the tissue.

(8) After a 5-minute interval, the results of the injection are evaluated by checking the following symptoms:

(a) Inferior alveolar nerve (supplies lower teeth, alveolar bone up to the midline).

1. A sensation of swelling and numbness extending to the midline of the lower lip on the injected side.

2. Insensitivity of the facial gingival tissue extending to the midline on the injected side.

(b) Lingual nerve.

1. A swollen numb sensation extending to the midline of the tongue.

2. Insensitivity of the lingual gingival tissue.

(c) DO NOT ATTEMPT EXTRACTION UNTIL THE SIGNS DESCRIBED ABOVE HAVE APPEARED.

19-11. TOOTH EXTRACTION.

a. This section describes only one extraction technique. Although many types of extraction forceps are manufactured, the removal of any erupted tooth can usually be accomplished with one of two instruments: The Maxillary Universal Forceps (150) or the Mandibular Universal Forceps (151).

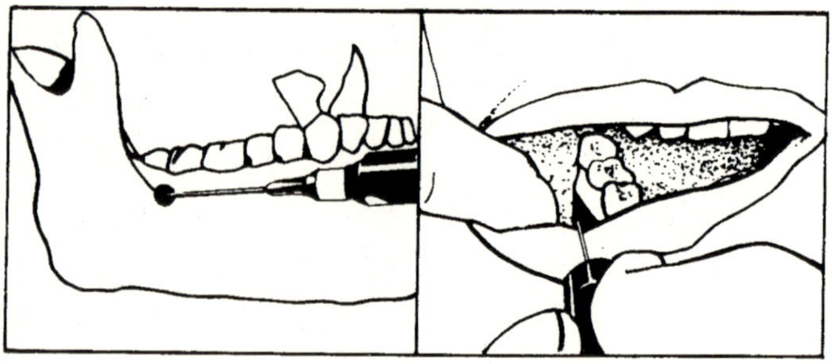

LONG BUCCAL INJECTION.

b. Technique. Break the attachment of the gingival tissue to the tooth by forcing a blunt instrument (Periosteal Elevator, Woodson Plastic Instrument, etc.) into the crevice between the tooth and the gingiva, all the way around the tooth. The tooth-tissue attachment should be broken to the level of the alveolar bone.

Use the free hand to guide the beaks of the forceps under the gingival margin on the facial and lingual aspects of the tooth and to support the alveolar process. Apply pressure toward the root of the tooth to force the tips of the forceps as far down on the root as possible. Slowly rock the tooth with progressively increasing pressure in a facial-lingual direction. This force is used for the loosening of teeth with more than one root (molars and upper first bicuspids). Single-rooted teeth are loosened by combining this rocking motion with a rotary force. When considerable mobility has been established, deliver the tooth by exerting gentle traction. Note the direction in which the tooth tends to move most easily and follow this path for delivery. Inspect the extracted tooth to determine if the roots have been fractured. After the extraction has been completed, compress the sides of the empty socket (this repositions the bone that has been sprung by the extraction force) and place a folded dampened sponge or 2x2 over the wound. Instruct the patient to maintain light biting pressure on this compress for 20 minutes. Repeat if necessary to control hemorrhage. Caution the patient NOT TO RINSE the mouth for at least 12 hours since this may disturb the clot.

19-12. INJURIES OF THE JAWS.

a. General. The immediate treatment of facial trauma consists of the establishment of an airway, the control of hemorrhage, the treatment of shock, and the evaluation of neurologic findings. These basic measures MUST BE CONSIDERED FIRST. Although diagnosis is difficult when edematous distortion and muscular trismus are present, a thorough clinical examination should include inspection and palpation of the oral regions for the following:

(1) Wounds, swelling, and discoloration.

(2) Pain, tenderness, crepitus, and mobility at suspected fracture sites.

(3) Facial asymmetry.

(4) Trismus.

(5) Abnormal mandibular excursions.

(6) Altered biting relationship of the upper and lower teeth.

(7) Segmental alveolar fractures. Exert pressure upon each individual tooth to determine the integrity of the underlying alveolar bone.

b. Dislocations of the mandible.

(1) The usual type of dislocation of the mandible is bilateral and the condyles are displaced anteriorly. The mouth is locked open with the chin protruded. Trismus is present and speech is difficult. In the unilateral type (very rare), the chin is deviated away from the side of the dislocation. Reduction of the dislocated jaw is normally accomplished without anesthesia. Narcotics are effective in relieving pain and apprehension and thereby prompt relaxation of the jaw muscles, but restraint must be exercised in their use. In the more resistant cases, general anesthesia may be indicated. Repositioning of the dislocated mandible is accomplished in the following manner:

(a) Wrap the thumbs with several thicknesses of gauze or towel. This provides protection against snap closure of the mandible.

(b) Place the thumbs lateral to the molar teeth to prevent injury to the thumbs and extend the fingers to grasp the under surface of the mandible. (The thumbs may also be placed on the biting surfaces of the lower molar teeth so that more pressure can be exerted, but when the jaw snaps closed you can get bitten.)

(c) Exert DOWNWARD pressure with the thumbs to bring the condyle of the mandible below the articular eminences. The fourth and fifth fingers may be used to exert an upward pressure on the point of the chin.

(d) Gently but firmly force the mandible FORWARD, then BACK. This will usually return the condyles to normal position.

(e) Caution the patient to avoid excessive opening of the mouth for several weeks.

(f) Prescribe a soft diet.

(2) Normally the pain following repositioning continues for about 72 hours. Analgesics should adequately control this pain. If marked pain persists or if there is a tendency toward recurrence of dislocation, immobilization is indicated. This may be effected by head bandages.

c. Mandibular fractures.

(1) Mandibular fractures must be differentiated from dislocations of the jaw because of the great difference in treatment. Some of the features of fractures are:

(a) Pain.

(b) Abnormal bite relationship between upper and lower teeth; they come together normally on one side and do not touch on the other when the jaws are closed.

(c) Crepitus.

(d) Gross displacement of segments of the jaws.

(2) Once a mandibular fracture has been diagnosed, the patient should be evacuated in a face-down or side position to prevent aspiration of blood, saliva, vomitus, etc. The use of head bandages to immobilize the jaws is not recommended since the backward force exerted may push the tongue (or other soft tissue) back to obstruct the airway. In addition, head bandages make it difficult for a patient to vomit without aspiration. Reducing the fracture at this time is not suggested since the harm done may exceed any benefits derived. If evacuation is not possible and you have to keep the patient, wait until the patient's condition is stable, then line up the upper and lower teeth using wire sutures (0 silk if wire is not available). Wire the upper and lower teeth together as follows:

(a) Form a small loop in the center of the wire and wrap the wire in a figure 8 around two teeth with small loop centered between the teeth.

(b) Repeat this in at least four positions on the top teeth and the same number on the lower teeth, insuring the loops on top and bottom are opposite each other.

(c) Wire the two loops (in each of the four positions) together. This will hold the jaw in position. (See illustration below.)

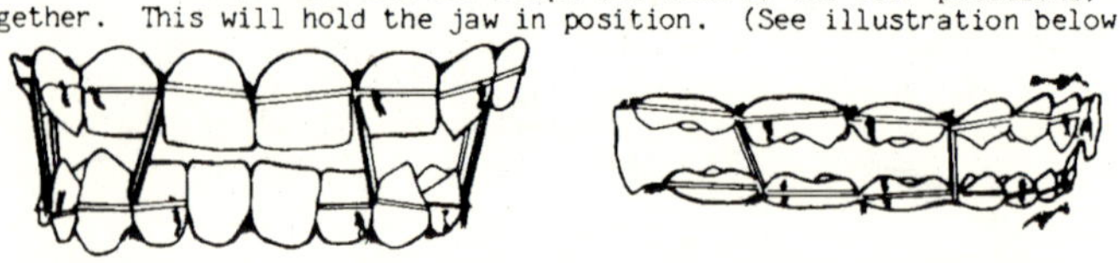

The wires will have to remain in place from 3-6 weeks, and the patient will have to be placed on a liquid diet during this time. After the wires are removed, keep the patient on a soft diet for a couple of weeks; then gradually return him to a normal diet.

CHAPTER 20

PREVENTIVE MEDICINE (PM)

20-1. THE MEDIC'S ROLE IN PREVENTIVE MEDICINE.

a. Plans preventive medicine programs.

b. Advises and recommends preventive medicine measures to the commander.

c. Supervises or performs preventive medicine measures.

d. Insures that preventive medicine programs are implemented properly.

e. Teaches and supervises personnel in preventive medicine measures.

20-2. PERSONAL HYGIENE.

a. Foot care.

(1) Keep feet clean (dry well after bathing).

(2) Massage and powder twice daily if possible.

(3) Change socks daily or when wet.

(4) Keep socks and footgear in good repair.

(5) Keep toenails short with squared off cut.

b. Showering and hand washing.

(1) Shower as often as possible to avoid skin disease.

(2) Wash hands after using latrine and before eating.

(3) If unable to bathe, wash face, underarms, groin, feet, etc.

(4) Desitin, A&D Ointment, or cornstarch in groin and between buttocks helps control rash.

20-3. INDIVIDUAL PROTECTIVE MEASURES.

a. Clothing. The combat uniform worn fully and properly is the best means of initial protection and first line of defense available. It should be worn loosely to permit ventilation and must be worn with the pants bloused into the boots, shirt tail tucked into pants, sleeves down and buttoned to provide protection against insects such as ticks and to lessen exposure to mosquitoes, sandflies, and other disease carriers.

b. Use of M1960-Clothing Repellent (DEET). The full uniform impregnated with M1960 repellent provides additional protection against arthropods. Do not impregnate underclothing and socks. The M1960 repellent kills mites and ticks and repels mosquitoes and other vectors. To mix, use a large container (approximately 15 gallons) and a long stick for stirring; add 1 gallon of DEET to 11 gallons of water. The ratio must remain correct. Soak and saturate the outer clothing only. Wring out excess solution and allow the uniform to dry prior to wearing. This procedure must be repeated each time the uniform is laundered.

c. Individual insect repellent applied to exposed skin areas provides good protection against all insects. Kerosene applied to neck, wrists, and legs at the boot tops will prevent infestation from chiggers, mites, etc.

d. Lindane dust or sulfa powder provides good protection against mites, chiggers, and lice when other repellents are not available.

e. Aerosol insecticides sprayed into containment areas such as living quarters, tents, and bed nets are highly effective against flying insects.

f. If infestation of lice, chiggers, etc., should occur, bathing with a strong soap will rid the individual of the insects. Additionally, clothing must be removed and laundered to prevent reinfestation.

g. Good personal hygiene and protective measures are the basic lines of defense against disease.

20-4. COLLECTIVE PROTECTIVE MEASURES - FIELD SANITATION AND CHEMICAL CONTROL.

a. Pesticides (chemical control) can be valuable aids in the control of arthropods, but these are only to supplement, not replace, good field hygiene and individual measures of protection. Pesticides are poisonous and can be more dangerous than helpful to the environment and the individual if misused. Pesticides can be inhaled or absorbed through the skin if the user is improperly trained to protect himself through the use of respirators, protective masks, gloves, etc.

(1) Classification of pesticides.

(a) Stomach poisons (e.g., lead arsenate) must be ingested by the insect to be effective.

(b) Contact poisons (e.g., DDT, lindane, pyrethrum, and Diazinon) kill by merely coming in contact with the insect. These can be quick kill, short life or residual, long term kill expectancy. NOTE: DDT, lindane, pyrethrum, and Diazinon are either not available in the US or under the scrutiny of US Standards (EPA, FDA, USDA, etc.). However, they may still be accessible for export or available in the OCONUS area of operation. Care must be used in all applications of pesticides. You may find agents such as DDT, if available, very valuable in delousing operations. Do not hesitate to use pesticides in a cautious manner even though they have been banned in the US.

(c) Fumigants kill through the insect's respiratory system and are very dangerous to humans, normally requiring special handling and training; they are not recommended for the use of the medic in any situation.

(2) Toxicity. When you use pesticides, always read the instructions and follow those instructions to prevent harm to yourself and others or to the environment. Never use any pesticide marked "concentrate"; it must be diluted in accordance with its nature and handled only by specially trained personnel. When in doubt, avoid the substance or

contact the group preventive medicine personnel.

b. Equipment available for issue and use in chemical control and in application of pesticides are the hand duster for use with dusts such as DDT and lindane and the hand pressure sprayer for use with liquids.

20-5. FIELD DISINFECTION OF WATER (PURIFICATION).

a. Directions for the use of iodine water purification tablets call for adding one tablet to a quart canteen of clear water, two tablets if cloudy. Recent studies indicate that one tablet may not guarantee complete destruction of Giardia cysts in clear, very cold water. Giardia, an intestinal protozoan parasite, is found worldwide, particularly in cold water. Therefore, two tablets will be used in very cold water, whether cloudy or clear.

b. Canteen (1 quart):

(1) Concept: Any water can be collected in a soldier's canteen and made safe using iodine tablets. (Water Purification Tablets, NSN 6850-00-985-7166.)

(2) Procedures:

(a) CHECK THE WATER. (Use one tablet if clear; use two if cloudy or cold.)

(b) ADD IODINE TABLETS. (Use only steel gray; don't use red or white.)

(c) WAIT 5 MINUTES. (Allow time for the tablets to dissolve.)

(d) SHAKE THE CANTEEN. (Mix the contents well.)

(e) DISINFECT THREADS. (Loosen the cap; turn canteen upside down.)

(f) WAIT 30 MORE MINUTES. (Allow time for the iodine to kill.)

(3) Alternate methods of disinfecting if iodine tablets are not available.

(a) Boil water. Bring to a boil for at least 15 seconds.

(b) Iodine (tincture). Add five or more drops to each canteen.

(c) Bleach (Clorox). Add two or more drops to each canteen.

(d) Chlorine ampules. Break one ampule into a canteen cup; fill cup with water to the bottom rivet and stir; pour half a capful of the slurry into each canteen and wait 30 minutes.

c. Water bag (lister bag - 36 gallons).

(1) Concept: Any water can be poured into a lister bag and made safe using chlorine ampules. (Chlorination Kit, Water Purification, NSN 6850-00-270-6225.)

(2) Procedure:

(a) DISSOLVE THREE AMPULES. (Use a canteen cup as a bowl.)

(b) POUR INTO LISTER BAG. (Stir the bag with a clean stick.)

(c) FLUSH ALL THE TAPS. (Let each run for several seconds.)

(d) WAIT 10 MINUTES. (Allow time for chemical reaction.)

(e) CHECK THE RESIDUAL. (Use the plastic test tube in the kit.)

1. Crush one "OT" tablet in the metal cap.

2. Dump the resulting powder into the plastic test tube.

3. Flush the tap from which you are going to take the sample.

4. Fill test tube with water to bottom of the yellow band.

5. Compare colors: If the water is at least as dark as the yellow band, proceed to step 6; if the water is lighter, more chlorine is needed. Repeat steps 1 through 5 using one or more additional chlorine ampules.

6. WAIT 20 MORE MINUTES. (Allow time for the chlorine residual to kill.) Check residual again before drinking; if chlorine residual is < 5 ppm., repeat steps 1-5.

d. Water cans (5 gallon).

(1) Concept: Water in standard 5-gallon cans can be made safe using chlorine ampules. (Chlorination Kit, Water Purification, NSN 6850-00-270-6225.)

(2) Procedure:

(a) DISSOLVE ONE AMPULE. (Use a canteen cupful of water.)

(b) POUR HALF OF CUP INTO CAN. (Remainder can be poured into a second can.)

(c) DISINFECT THE THREADS. (Loosen cap; turn can upside down and shake; then retighten.)

(d) WAIT 30 MINUTES. (Allow time for chlorine to kill.)

e. Water trailer (400 gallon).

(1) Concept: If the unit's field sanitation team tests the trailer and fails to find a measurable chlorine residue (any degree of yellow is acceptable), the water in the trailer can be made safe using chlorine powder. (Calcium hypochlorite, 6-oz. jar, NSN 6810-00-255-0471) or Chlorination Kit, Water Purification, NSN 6850-00-270-6225.)

(2) Procedure:

(a) DISSOLVE ONE SPOONFUL. (Use a mess kit spoon and a canteen cup.)

(b) POUR INTO TRAILER. (Stir with a clean stick.)

(c) FLUSH TRAILER TAPS. (Let each run for several seconds.)

(d) WAIT 10 MINUTES. (Allow time for chemical reaction.)

(e) CHECK RESIDUAL. (Use the plastic test tube from chlorination kit.)

1. Crush one "OT" tablet in the metal cap.

2. Dump the resulting powder into the plastic test tube.

3. Flush the tap from which you are going to take the sample.

4. Fill test tube with water to bottom of the yellow band.

5. Compare colors: If the water is at least as dark as the yellow band, proceed to step 6; if the water is lighter, more chlorine is needed. Repeat steps 1 through 5 using half a spoonful of powder.

6. WAIT 20 MORE MINUTES. (Allow time for the chlorine residual to kill.) Check residual again before drinking; if chlorine residual is < ppm., repeat steps 1-5.

f. Remarks.

(1) The concept that <u>any</u> water can be made "safe" by chlorination is a misconception. Chlorinating potentially contaminated water does not necessarily make it safe due to amoebic cysts. Filtration is a practical means of removing cysts from the water; however, this may be impractical. Boiling water to a hard roll for at least 15 seconds is another means of making the water safe from amoebic cysts as this action will kill the cysts.

(2) Chlorination, when performed properly, will make water "safe" in regards to killing disease-causing bacteria, such as E. coli; however, only filtration or boiling can kill or remove the amoebic cysts from the water source. All water from unknown sources must be considered dangerous and contaminated. All precautions for the treatment of the water must be utilized.

(3) POL containers or water containers that have been contaminated with POL must not be used for consumable water.

(4) Always check the water for chlorine residual, regardless of the source. When the residual is adequate, no disinfection is necessary. However, if the residual is low, disinfect the water using the procedures described for each container. A minimum of 5 ppm. chlorine residual is required for field water supplies.

20-6. WATER SOURCES.

a. Surface water (lakes, ponds, streams, rivers). Although this source is the least desirable, it is most plentiful and easily accessible. Knowing the best sites to choose to avoid excessive polution and the proper methods of water treatment is the best prevention of waterborne disease. Sometimes water may be unpalatable due to odors or unpleasant taste, but it can be made potable and it may prevent death through dehydration if it is properly treated.

b. Ground water. Wells are usually the most desirable source; however, care must be taken to insure no pollution has been introduced by dumping animal carcasses, garbage, feces, etc. All water of unknown origin must be considered polluted and must be treated.

c. Precipitation. Even with rain and snow (often least common and least dangerous when fresh), precautions must be taken to avoid introducing disease pathogens to the individual; therefore, rain and snow require treatment to the recommended level.

20-7. WASTE DISPOSAL.

a. The term "wastes" includes all types of refuse resulting from the living activities of humans or animals: human wastes (feces and urine); liquid wastes (wash, bath, and liquid kitchen wastes); garbage; and rubbish.

b. The methods that should be used to dispose of wastes depend upon the situation and the location. Burial and burning are the methods most commonly used in the field.

c. Large quantities of all types of wastes, liquid and solid, are generated each day under field conditions. These materials must be removed promptly and thoroughly; otherwise, the camp or bivouac will quickly become an ideal breeding area for flies, rats, and other vermin. Filth-borne diseases such as dysentery (amebic and bacillary), typhoid, paratyphoid, cholera, and plague could become prevalent.

d. Disposal of human wastes:

(1) The devices for disposing of human wastes in the field vary with the situations.

(a) When on the march, each person uses a "cat-hole" latrine during short halts. It is dug approximately 1-foot deep and is completely covered and packed down after use.

(b) In temporary camp of 1 to 3 days the straddle trench is most likely to be used unless more permanent facilities are provided for the unit.

(c) In temporary camps deep pit latrines and urine soakage pits are usually constructed. Until such time as the construction of deep pit latrines can be completed, straddle trench latrines are used. Where the construction of deep pit latrines is not practicable, other types of latrines are used.

(2) Rules common to the construction, maintenance, and closing of latrines.

(a) In determining the type of latrines to be constructed, consider the length of stay, the water level, and the soil conditions. To protect water from contamination, do not extend the depth of a latrine pit or trench below the underground water level.

(b) In determining the location within the camp area for construction of latrines, consider first the protection of food and water from contamination and, secondly, the accessibility to the users.

1. To protect food and water from contamination, select a location that is at least 100 yards from the unit mess and 100 feet from the nearest water source and that drains away from all water sources.

2. Choose a location that is accessible to the users and reasonably near the edge of the camp.

(c) Sufficient latrines should be constructed to serve at least 8 percent of the personnel at one time.

(d) After the latrines have been completed, construct the necessary protective and hygienic devices.

1. Place canvas or brush screens around the latrines or tents over them. In a cold climate the shelters should be heated, if possible.

2. To prevent surface water from flowing into the shelters, dig drainage ditches around them.

3. In each latrine shelter, provide toilet paper on suitable holders with tin cans for covering the toilet paper to keep it from getting wet during bad weather.

4. Install a simple, easily operated handwashing device just outside each latrine shelter. These devices should be kept filled with water at all times so that each individual can wash his hands after he uses the latrine.

5. At night extend cords from trees or stakes to the latrines to serve as guides.

(e) Police the latrines properly and maintain a good fly-control program in the entire camp area to prevent fly breeding and to reduce odors.

1. Keep the lids to the latrine seats closed and all

cracks sealed.

2. Scrub the latrine seats and boxes with soap and water daily.

3. Spray the inside of the shelters with a residual insecticide twice weekly. If a fly problem exists, also spray the pit contents and the interior of the boxes twice weekly with a residual insecticide. Using lime in the pits or burning out the pit contents, except in burn-out latrines, is not effective for fly or odor control; these methods, therefore, are not recommended.

(f) When a latrine pit becomes filled with wastes to 1 foot from the surface or when it is to be abandoned, remove the latrine box and close the pit as follows:

1. Using an approved residual insecticide, spray the pit contents, the side walls, and the ground surface extending 2 feet from the side walls.

2. Fill the pit to the ground level with successive 3-inch layers of earth, packing each layer down before adding the next one; then mound the pit over with at least 1 foot of dirt and spray it again with insecticide. This prevents any fly pupa, which may hatch in the closed latrine, from getting out.

(3) Cat hole latrine. Primarily used when a unit is "on the march or for short-term duration" (1 day). It is 6-12" deep and is covered after use.

(4) Straddle trench latrine. Used for 1 to 3 day bivouac, in nonrocky or nonfrozen soil. Construct 1' wide, 2 1/2' deep, and 4' long. Accommodates two men. Parallel trenches at least 2' apart. Excavated earth is used promptly to cover excreta.

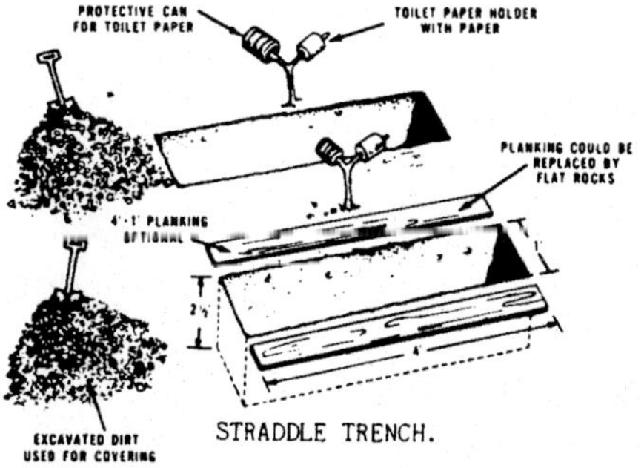

STRADDLE TRENCH.

(5) Deep pit latrine (illustrated on next page). Used in temporary camps; not used in rocky or frozen soil or where the water table is high. Construct 2' wide, 7 1/2' long, and 1' of depth for each week of use. Add 1' of depth for dirt. Maximum depth 6'. Cover with latrine box. Accommodates four men. Wash latrines with soap and water daily.

(6) Mound latrine. Used when the water table is high or in

rocky soil. Build mound 6' wide and 12' long to accommodate a latrine box. Pit is built in mound. Pits have same dimensions as a deep pit latrine. Reinforce walls (if necessary) to avoid cave-ins.

(7) Burn-out latrine (illustrated below). Used in rocky/frozen soil or when the water table is high. Construct with 55-gallon drum; bury half or cut it in half. Cover with flyproof wooden seat. For feces only (not for urinating), burn out daily or when half full. (Use 1 qt. gas to 5 qt. diesel or kerosene.) Use two latrines (one in use, while other is burned).

Burn until only ash remains, and bury ash.

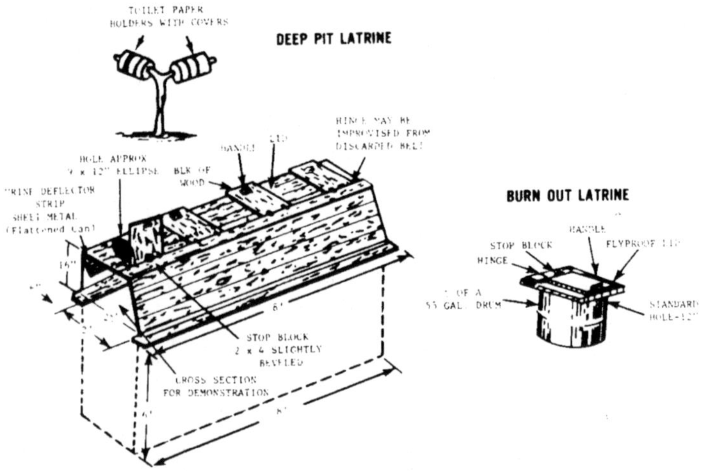

(8) Urinals.

(a) Construct one urinal per latrine facility or enough to serve 5% of the personnel at one time.

(b) Urine soakage pit. Construct 4 cubic feet in length. Fill with rocks, bricks, broken glass, or similar items. Place 1" pipes, 36" long, at each corner 8" deep into pit. Place funnels at the top of the pipes.

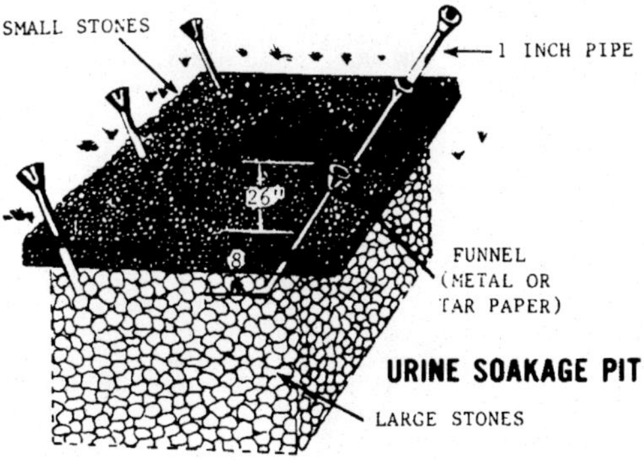

(c) Urine trough. Used when wood is more available than pipe. Allow 10' of trough/100 men. Construct V- or U-shaped trough with metal or tar paper lined wood. Place splash board down the center of trough. Drain into soakage pit or deep pit latrine.

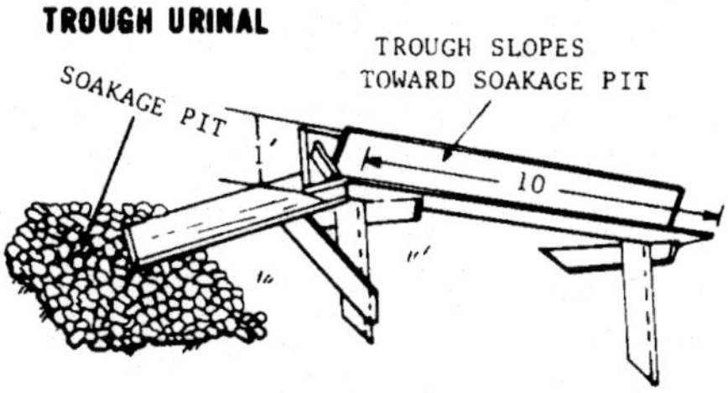

e. Wash, bath, and liquid kitchen wastes:

(1) In the field, wash, bath, and liquid kitchen wastes are disposed of in the soil usually by means of either soakage pits or soakage trenches. In order for the soil to absorb these liquids, the grease and soap as well as any solid particles must first be removed; therefore, each soakage pit or trench used for disposing of wash and liquid kitchen wastes must have a grease trap. In places where heavy clay soil prevents the use of soakage pits or trenches, evaporation beds may be used if the climate is hot and dry.

(2) Soakage pits. In a temporary camp, a soakage pit 4 feet square and 4 feet deep normally will be adequate to dispose of liquid kitchen waste for 200 persons. If the troops are to remain in the camp for 2 weeks, two pits should be constructed for disposal of liquid kitchen waste; each pit should be used on alternate days, thus lessening the possiblity of clogging. Each device provided for washing and bathing must also have a soakage pit under it. These soakage pits are constructed in the same way as a urinal soakage pit except that the urinal pipes are

omitted. A grease trap is provided for each pit, except those under showers. The area under field showers, as well as under drinking devices, should be excavated a few inches and then filled with small, smooth stones to keep the water from standing. If a soakage pit becomes, clogged, it is closed, and a new one is constructed. A soakage pit is closed by covering it with 1 foot of compacted earth.

(3) Soakage trenches. If the ground water level or a rock formation is close to the surface, soakage trenches instead of pits should be used. A soakage trench consists of a pit, 2 feet square and 1 foot deep, with a trench extending outward 6 or more feet from each of its sides. The trenches are 1 foot wide and vary in depth from a foot at the central pit to 1 1/2 feet at the outer ends. The pit and trenches are filled with the same material used in a soakage pit. Two such units should be built to dispose of liquid kitchen waste for every 200 persons, and each unit should be used on alternate days. One unit should be built for each washing device provided. A grease trap is provided for each soakage trench. A soakage trench is closed by covering it with 1 foot of compacted earth. Construction of a soakage pit is the same as for a urine soakage pit minus the pipes.

(4) Grease traps.

(a) Baffle grease trap.

1. A baffle grease trap may be made from a drum or from a watertight box. The drum or box is divided vertically into an entrance chamber and an exit chamber by attaching a wooden baffle. The baffle should be placed so that the entrance chamber will be approximately twice the size of the exit chamber. The baffle should hang to a point within 1 inch of the bottom. A strainer that may be made from a small perforated box filled with straw, hay, or burlap is inserted into the lid above the entrance chamber. A pipe is inserted into the exit chamber about 3 to 6 inches below the top as an outlet to the soakage pit. This baffle grease trap is usually placed on the ground at the side of the soakage pit with the outlet pipe extending 1 foot beneath the surface at the center of the pit. If a grease trap is not watertight, it must be placed partially under the ground.

2. Before the grease trap is used, the chambers are filled with cool water. The waste liquid is poured through the strainer that retains any solids. As the warm liquid strikes the cool water, the grease rises to the surface of the entrance chamber; and the liquid runs under the baffle, filling the exit chamber. When the liquid reaches the outlet pipe near the top of the exit chamber, it runs through this pipe into the soakage pit. Unless the grease trap is of sufficient capacity, the warm greasy liquid poured into the trap will heat the cool water in the trap, thus allowing the grease to remain uncongealed and to pass through the trap. The efficiency of this grease trap can be increased by constructing it with multiple baffles. Also, a series of traps may be used.

3. The baffle grease trap must be properly maintained to prevent clogging of the soakage pit. The grease retained in the trap should be skimmed from the surface of the water daily or as often as required and either buried of burned. The entire trap should be emptied and thoroughly scrubbed with hot, soapy water as often as necessary.

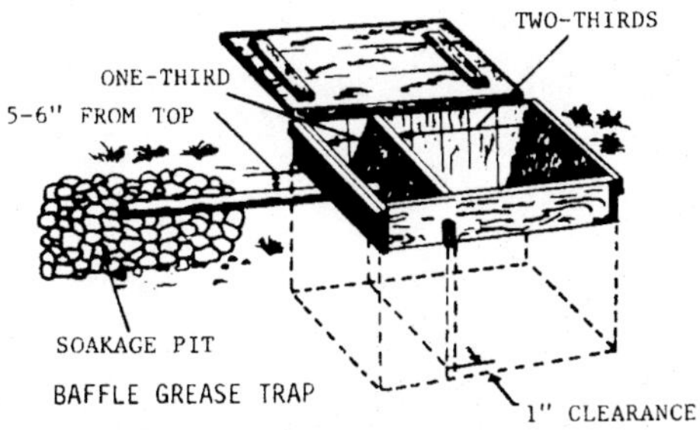

BAFFLE GREASE TRAP

(b) Barrel filter grease trap.

1. The barrel filter grease trap may be made from a 30- to 50-gallon barrel or drum that has the top removed and a number of large holes bored into the bottom. Eight inches of gravel or small stones are placed in the bottom and covered with 12 to 18 inches of ashes or sand. A piece of burlap is fastened to the top of the barrel to serve as a coarse filter. The trap may be placed directly on the soakage pit, or it may be placed on a platform with a trough leading to the pit.

2. Every 2 days the grease trap should be emptied, washed, and refilled as described in 1 above. The material removed should be buried. The burlap filter should be either washed or replaced every day.

FILTER GREASE TRAP

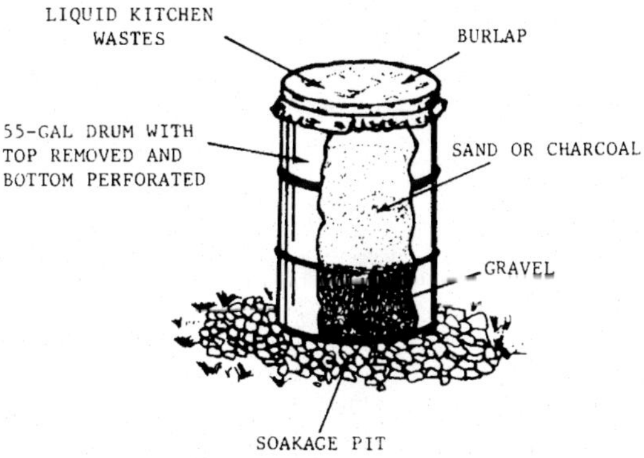

f. Garbage disposal. Garbage is the solid or semisolid waste resulting from the preparation, cooking, and serving of food. It does not include rubbish. Garbage is disposed of by burial or incineration.

(1) Burial. When troops are on the march, in bivouac, or in camps for less than a 1-week duration, garbage is disposed of by burial in pits or trenches. These pits or trenches should not be over 30 yards from

the mess area. Garbage must not, however, be buried closer than 100 feet from any source of water used for cooking or drinking.

(a) Pits are preferred for burying garbage during overnight halts. A pit 4 feet square and 4 feet deep is suitable for 1 day for a unit of 100 men. At the end of the day or such time as the pit is filled to 1 foot below the ground surface, it should be sprayed with insecticide; then it must be filled with earth and mounded over with an additional foot of compacted earth.

(b) The continuous trench is more adaptable to stays of 2 days or more. The trench is first dug about 2 feet wide, 3 to 4 feet deep, and long enough to accommodate the garbage for the first day. As in the pit method, the trench is filled to not more than 1 foot from the top. The trench is extended as required, and the excavated dirt is used to cover and mound the garbage already deposited. This procedure is repeated daily or as often as garbage is dumped. It is a very efficient field expedient for disposing of garbage.

(2) Incineration.

(a) In temporary camps of over 1 week, the garbage is often burned in open incinerators. Excellent types of open incinerators may be constructed from materials that are readily available in any camp area. Since incinerators will not handle wet garbage, it is necessary to separate the liquid from the solid portion. This is done by straining the garbage with a coarse strainer such as an old bucket, salvaged can, or 55-gallon drum in which holes have been punched in the bottom. The solids remaining in the strainer are incinerated, and the liquids are poured through a grease trap into a soakage pit or trench. Field incinerators should be located at least 50 yards downwind from the camp to prevent their being an odor nuisance.

(b) The inclined plane incinerator's effectiveness in combustion and the fact that it is somewhat protected from rain or wind make it an excellent improvised device. Time and skill, however, are required in building it. A sheet metal plane is inserted through telescoped 55-gallon drums from which the ends have been removed. The metal plane should extend approximately 2 feet beyond the upper end of the telescoped drums to serve as a loading or stoking platform. The telescoped drums are positioned on an inclined surface. A grate is placed at the lower end of the telescoped drums, and a wood or fuel oil fire is provided under the grate. After the incinerator becomes hot, drained garbage is placed on the stoking platform. As the garbage becomes dry, it is pushed through the telescoped drums in small amounts to burn. Final burning takes place on the grate. If time does not permit the construction of the inclined plane incinerator, it may be simplified as follows: Dig a fire pit at the bottom of an incline, line it with rocks, and place a grate over it. Place three telescoped drums in a shallow trench up the incline, letting the lower end of the telescoped drums extend somewhat over the fire pit so the flame will be drawn up the drums. The sheet metal plane, if available, should be used, as it permits more thorough drying of the garbage.

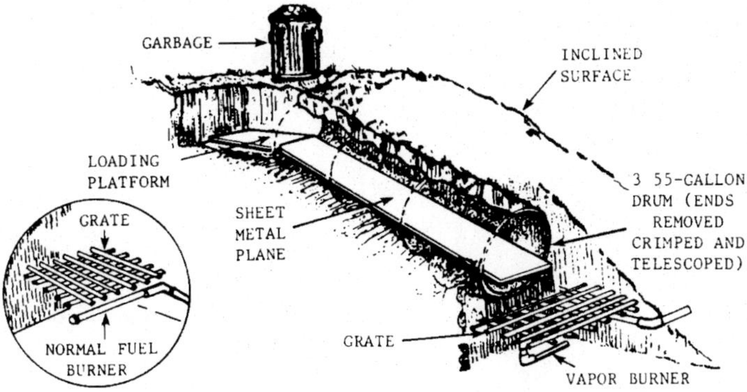

·INCLINED PLANE INCINERATOR.

(c) A barrel incinerator (illustrated below) is made from a 55-gallon drum by cutting out both ends, punching many holes near the bottom, and inserting grates inside the barrel several inches above the holes. The barrel is supported several inches above the ground on stones, bricks, or dirt filled cans, thus allowing space to build a fire under the barrel. The rubbish is put into the barrel on the top grate.

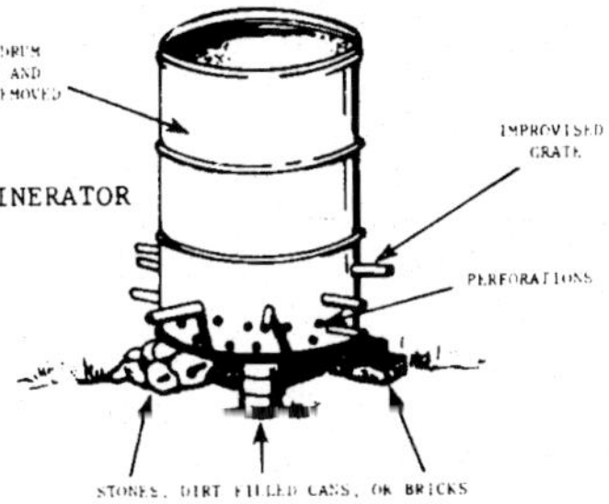

BARREL INCINERATOR

20-8. WASHING DEVICES.

a. Hand washing devices (locate at latrine enclosures and unit messes).

(1) Suspended 5-gallon water can. From a frame over a soakage pit suspend one can of clear water and one can of soapy water so they can be tilted.

(2) Mounted #10 can. Make four holes in the bottom of can and mount it on a stand built over a soakage pit. Have on hand a 5-gallon can of water with a dipper and a bar of soap.

b. Shower devices. (Use soakage pits; a grease trap should be included if soap is used.)

(1) Solar heated shower. Build a drum support to hold 500-600 lbs; color drum a dark, nonreflective shade. Invert a 55-gallon drum on stand. Attach a water control device to bung (top removed). Below valve, attach a tin can with perforated bottom.

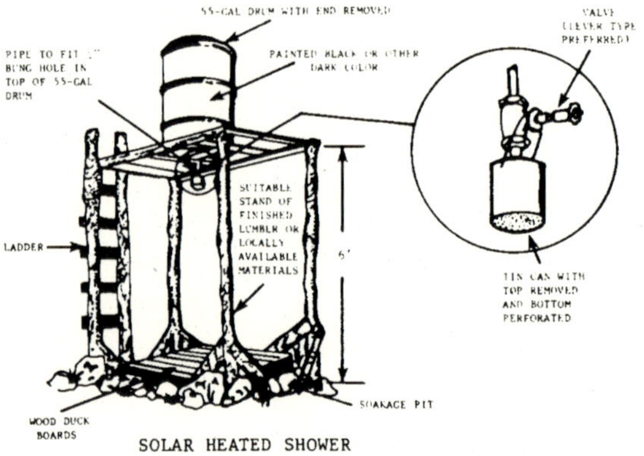

SOLAR HEATED SHOWER

(2) Tilted drum shower. Mount drum so it will tilt. Attach rope to one end of drum and attach safety strap onto the frame at the opposite end. Punch holes in side opposite top. Place rod halfway thru drum and in notches.

(3) Shower utilizing oil-water flash burner. (See diagram on next page.) Mount two 55-gallon drums on an overhead platform. Use pipe fittings to control water and flow. Connect heating drum (15 gallon) to overhead drum by rubber hoses. Place 15-gallon drum on an oil-flash burner.

20-16

SHOWER UTILIZING OIL-WATER FLASH BURNER

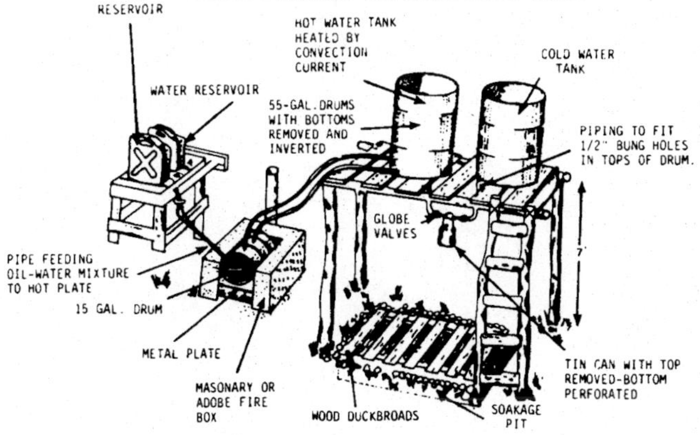

20-9. FOOD SANITATION.

a. Importance of food sanitation. Even the most appetizing food can cause illness if it becomes contaminated with pathogenic organisms through improper handling. Outbreaks of food poisoning, dysentery, infectious hepatitis, and typhoid fever may result from unsanitary practices in kitchens and dining areas. Therefore, persons who handle food must always maintain the highest standards of personal hygiene and sanitation.

b. Food handlers.

(1) All food handlers must be given a thorough physical examination. Those who have communicable diseases or who are known carriers of such diseases are not assigned as food handlers. Even more important than this initial screening is the supervisor's daily on-the-job check of food-handling personnel for signs of illness or infection. This inspection should be thorough enough to make certain that food handlers have no obvious signs of illness or infection; their hands, fingernails, and clothing must be clean, and they must have no boils, rashes, or other skin and wound infections. Food handlers should be instructed to report sore throats, colds, coughs, diarrhea, vomiting, and other symptoms of infection and disease. Questionable cases will be relieved from duties without delay. Food handlers should be provided adequate sanitary facilities, including showers, hand-washing devices, and latrines.

c. Transportation. Vehicles used for transporting food must be clean and completely enclosed.

d. Storage. Perishable food products are stocked at a realistic operating level. They should be refrigerated at 45°F. or below. Vegetables such as potatoes and onions are stored in a dry place on dunnage so air can circulate around them. Acid foods such as citrus fruit drinks must never be stored or served in galvanized iron cans.

e. Cleaning of cooking, serving, and eating utensils. The two procedures that may be used by kitchen personnel in cleaning the cooking, serving, and eating utensils are outlined below:

(1) Procedure to be used when hot water is available. Scrape utensils free of food particles. Wash utensils in warm water containing soap or detergent. Rinse utensils in hot clear water. Disinfect utensils by immersing them in clear water of 180°F. for 30 seconds. If a thermometer is not available to determine the temperature of the water, heat the water to the boiling point. Allow the utensils to air-dry in a place where they are protected against dust, splash, and other sources of contamination.

(2) Procedure to be used when hot water is not available. Scrape utensils free of food particles. Wash utensils in water containing soap or detergent. Rinse utensils with potable water. Disinfect utensils by immersing them in a chlorine-water solution for not less than 30 seconds. This solution is prepared by using Disinfectant, Food Service, as specified on its container. If this disinfectant is not available, an emergency solution can be prepared by mixing at least one level messkit spoonful of calcium hypochlorite (water disinfecting powder) to each 10 gallons of water. If liquid chlorine bleach is available, it may be used. About one-third canteen cup of 5 percent chlorine bleach to each 10 gallons of water will provide the same disinfecting strength. Fresh chlorine-water solutions must be made for rinsing and disinfecting utensils for each 100 persons. Allow the utensils to air-dry in a place where they are protected against dust, splash, and other sources of contamination.

(3) Method of heating water.

(a) Oil-water flash burner.

1. The oil-water flash burner uses diesel or motor oil as fuel. In cold climates it may be necessary to thin these oils with gasoline or kerosene to obtain a good flow. If waste motor oil is to be used as fuel, it must first be strained through a screen or a cloth to remove sludge and lumps.

2. One oil-water flash burner is required for each large can of water to be heated. This burner consists of containers for the oil and the water, a feed pipe, a metal burner plate, shields, and a grate. The containers are equipped with valves, taps, plugs, or siphons for controlling the rate of fuel and water flow. The shields, which prevent strong drafts or rain from cooling the plate, may be made from sheet metal or oil drums.

3. Serious explosion may result from an improperly constructed or operated burner. If the flame of a burner goes out and the fuel is not burned off, turned off, or relighted immediately, a dangerous concentration of gas may build up. If this gas is ignited, an explosion may result. This danger is not as great with the oil-water flash burner as it is with the vapor burner. The automatic relighting device will lessen the possibility of such an explosion. Also the possibility of an explosion in a fuel tank can be considerably decreased by not allowing the fuel to fall below the half-full mark. A visible float-level indicator should be used.

(b) Vapor burner.

1. The vapor burner uses liquids such as diesel oil,

kerosene, or gasoline, or a combination of these. As with the oil-water flash burner, it may be necessary in cold climates to thin the oil with gasoline before use. The construction of this burner requires several sections of pipe, a valve, pipe fittings, and a fuel reservoir. The operation of the vapor burner depends upon vaporization of the fuel by preheating before burning.

2. The pipe is assembled in such a manner that it is doubled under itself. The best size pipe to use is either one-half or three-quarters of an inch in diameter. Very small holes (1/16-inch or less) are drilled in the top of the lower pipe at points where the water containers will be placed. The end of the pipe is capped so that fuel can escape only from the drilled holes. Burning fuel that escapes from the holes in the lower pipe heats the fuel in the upper pipe, causing the fuel to vaporize into gas. The gas produces pressure in the lower pipe and forces the fuel out through the small holes as spray, thus making a better flame. For best operation, the pipes should be placed in a fire trench. The trench should be about 1 foot wide and 15 inches deep. Iron wire should be coiled around lower pipe just above the holes to serve as an automatic relighting device. These wires become red hot after the burner has been in operation for a few minutes. Should one flame go out, the heat from the wires would relight the fuel, thus preventing an accumulation of gas in the trench and a possible explosion.

3. Before lighting the burner, the valve that controls the flow of fuel is opened to allow a small amount of fuel to run out through the holes in the lower pipe. This fuel is then ignited, thus heating the upper pipe and starting the fuel-heat-gas pressure cycle described above. A properly operated burner will produce a blue flame. A yellow flame, which indicates incomplete burning, is caused by too much fuel escaping from the holes. This may be corrected by closing the valve slightly, thus reducing the amount of fuel going to the burner, or by decreasing the size of the holes in the pipe. If the flame is blue, but tends to blow itself out, not enough fuel is getting through the holes. The condition may be corrected by opening the valve slightly, thus allowing more fuel to go to the burner, or by enlarging the holes in the pipe.

(6) Fire trench.

1. When solid fuels are available, a fire trench is one method used for heating. The trench should be about 1 foot wide and 1 foot deep. Its length will depend on the number of water cans to be heated. An 8-foot trench is usually sufficient for three cans. The cans, supported by steel rods or pipes, are placed over the trench; and the fire is built in the trench. Oil drums cut into halves and with the ends removed may be placed around the water containers to increase heating efficiency.

2. Except as a temporary measure, the fire trench is not considered a practical method for heating water. It requires a large amount of solid fuel, such as coal or wood, that ordinarily is not plentiful in the field. Unless windshields are used around the corrugated cans, heating water to the boiling point becomes very difficult. Furthermore, the external heat from the open flame quickly burns out the cans. It also makes standing close enough to wash mess kits uncomfortable and possibly hazardous.

(4) Drums. When corrugated cans are not available, messkit

washing containers may be made from metal drums and used with any of the heating devices. The drums may be used with or without modification in size. In the modification of drums, they should be cut into two-thirds and one-third portions. The two-thirds portions are used as washing containers; the one-third portions are used as needed for supports or shields. Although drums are ordinarily cut crosswise, they may be cut lengthwise. The two-thirds portions of drums cut lengthwise are placed directly on a trench.

(5) Drainage device.

(a) As an aid in draining washing containers, a pipe coupling can be welded into the bottom of each of the three containers; then all three containers can be connected with pipes to one central outlet pipe. This central outlet pipe should be positioned so that the water will pass through a grease trap into a soakage pit.

(b) Plugs or pipes may be screwed into the pipe couplings inside the washing containers to secure the water until drainage is desired. If a pipe is used, it must be cut long enough to extend above the water level.

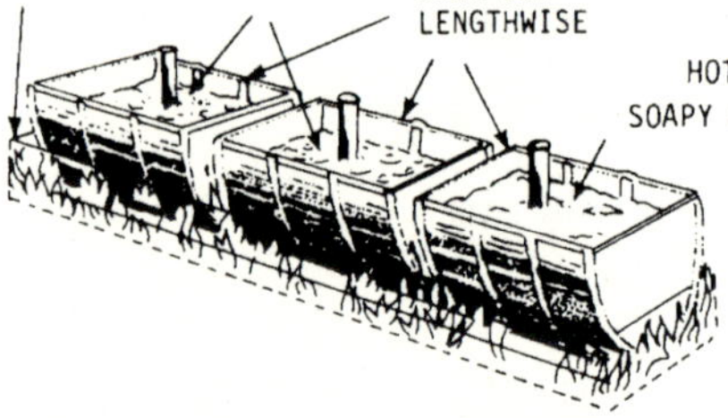

FIRE TRENCH AND DRUMS FOR MESSKIT WASHING SETUP

20-10. ARTHROPOD AND RODENT CONTROL.

a. Rodent control. The key to rodent control is good area police. There are many sophisticated programs that can be instituted; but if insects and rodents are denied a place to live and breed through a good clean-up campaign, a good start has been made in eliminating the problem. Ditches and depressions should be kept free of standing water. Do not allow garbage to remain unburied since it will attract flies and rats. Rats should be live-trapped and burned to kill fleas and mites they may have in their fur.

b. Arthropod control. An effective program for the prevention of arthropod-borne diseases should consist primarily of sanitation measures, but includes the use of personal protective measures and the application of pesticides. Fundamental to the operation of an effective program are a basic understanding of the life cycles of medically important arthropods and a knowledge of where they can be found. The following chart will serve as a reference.

MEDICALLY IMPORTANT ARTHROPODS	APPROXIMATE DURATION OF LIFE CYCLES AT 75oF.	WHERE FOUND
Flies (Example: housefly)	Egg---------10 hours larva------- 5 days pupa-------- 5 days adult-------30 days	Animals or human waste, garbage, grass, decomposing animals, and mud contaminated with organic material.
Mosquitoes (Example: yellow fever mosquito)	Egg--------- 4 days larva-------10 days pupa-------- 2 days adult-------14 days	Standing water found in ponds, tin cans, old tires, and tree holes. (A large variety of places and conditions of breeding have been noted.)
Fleas (Example: oriental rat flea)	Egg--------- 7 days larva-------15 days pupa-------- 8 days adult------365 days	Nests or beds of animals.
Lice (Example: human body louse)	Egg--------- 7 days nymph-------16 days adult-------30 days	Head hair and clothing of humans. Lice cannot exist on a clean human.
Cockroaches (Example: German cockroach)	Egg---------30 days nymph-------60 days adult------200 days	Cracks and crevices that provide warmth, moisture, and food such as around water, garbage, and food facilities.
Ticks and mites	Life cycle completed 6 weeks to 2 years	Tall grass, underbrush, animal watering places, and shady rest areas of animals.

20-11. IMMUNIZATION REQUIREMENTS (MILITARY ALERT FORCES).

IMMUNIZATION	NO. OF SHOTS	BASIC SERIES DOSAGE	INTERVAL	REIMMUNIZATION INTERVAL	REIMMUNIZATION DOSAGE
Smallpox (*1)	2/4 punctures	1 gtt .		3 yr	
Dipt/Tetanus	3	1st) 0.5 cc. 2d) 0.5 cc. 3d) 0.1 cc.	 4-8 wk 12 mo	10 yr (*2)	0.1 cc.
Typhoid	2	1st) 0.5 cc. 2d) 0.5 cc.	 4 wk	3 yr	0.5 cc.
Cholera	2	1st) 0.5 cc. 2d) 1.0 cc.	 1 wk	(*3)	
Plague	2	1st) 1.0 cc. 2d) 0.2 cc.	 3 mos	(*4)	
Yellow Fever	1	0.5 cc. Dilute 1:10	NA	10 yr	0.5 cc.
Polio	3	1st) 2 gtt. (*5) 2d) 2 gtt. (*5) 3d) 2 gtt. (*5)	 6-8 wk 12 mos	S/C	NA
Influenza	1	0.5 cc. (*6)	NA	1 yr	

General: All inoculations may be given either IM or SQ, with the exception of plague that must be given IM and smallpox that is given by the technique described below.

*1 Smallpox — Reaction should be read 6-8 days after administration. Primary vaccination: Typical vesicle formation. Revaccination: Major - vesicular or pustular lesion or an area of induration or congestion surrounding a central crusted or ulcerous lesion. Minor - any other reaction. If minor, check procedures and revaccinate one time only. Punctures are given intradermally, 4 times with single needle or 2 times bifurcated needle initially and 30 times single needle or 15 times bifurcated needle for the revaccination.

NOTE: Do not clean the skin unless grossly dirty, then only with acetone. Never use alcohol to clean skin and allow the skin to dry before giving the vaccination.

*2 Dipth/Tetanus: If the basic series has been completed within the last 5 years, no booster is required for minor injuries. If there is doubt, or the injury is severe or a burn, a booster should be given and the dosage increased from 0.1 cc. to 0.5 cc. When in doubt whether tetanus diphtheria should be given, administer only tetanus toxoid.

*3	Cholera:	Reimmunization is required only upon deployment to Area II as outlined in AR 40-562 and while residing in Area II or as recommended by the World Health Organization (WHO). Revaccination is required every 6 months at 0.5 cc. dosage, SQ or IM.
*4	Plague:	Reimmunization is required only upon deployment to Area IIP as outlined in AR 40-562 and while residing in Area IIP or as recommended by the World Health Organization (WHO). Revaccination is required every 6 months at 0.2 cc. dosage, IM only.
*5	Polio:	The number of drops comprising the proper dose depends on the manufacturer's recommendations and will be given orally.
*6	Influenza:	Dosage may be varied with the recommendations and guidance of the manufacturer or medical authority. Worldwide geographic variations in seasonal influenza outbreaks increase potential morbidity rates in alert forces by flu. The requirement for mandatory vaccination of Army personnel will be further augmented by the mandatory requirement that all personnel in CMA/IMA will receive the flu vaccine regardless of program requirements in order that maximum protection may be afforded against influenza in the worldwide environment. Maximum effort will be given to immunize personnel during the October-November time period; however, the program will not be curtailed at the end of that period.

NOTE: Live viruses: There should be a 30-day separation period when giving more than one live virus for the best immunity reaction. If necessary, two live viruses may be given on the same day, but at different sites. Once a live virus has been administered, no other live virus will be administered until the 30-day separation period has elapsed. The receiving individual should be afebrile and in good health. He must not be receiving any of the following: steroids, alkylating drugs, anti-metabolites, immunosuppressive agents, or radiation therapy. Pregnant women will not receive any live viruses except polio.

20-12. TECHNIQUE OF SOAP MAKING.

a. Ingredients.

(1) Method one: Two #10 cans of animal fat, two #10 cans of water, and one #10 can of lye.

(2) Method two: Two #10 cans of animal fat and two #10 cans of water poured through ashes.

(3) Optional ingredients: One-half cup borax, one-half cup liquid washing ammonia, and two tablespoons of granulated sugar.

b. Technique.

(1) Cut the fat into small strips and place into a pot to melt - moderate heat.

(2) Slowly add the lye and water (or the water that has been poured through the ashes) to the melted fat and stir until the mixture is about the consistency of honey. The optional items may be added during this procedure.

(3) Pour the thickened mix into a container to cool. After standing a few hours, the soap may then be cut into the desired sizes.

(4) This type of soap is excellent for both laundry and hands.

CHAPTER 21

VETERINARY MEDICINE

21-1. FOOD PROCUREMENT, INSPECTION, AND PREPARATION.

a. Dangers from food sources.

(1) Physical - contamination of food by arthropods, metal fragments, glass, radioactive particles, etc.

(2) Chemical - contamination of food with chemical agents, industrial chemicals, and other adulterating chemicals (zinc, copper, cadmium, pesticides, etc.).

(3) Biological - contamination of food by pathogenic microorganisms (bacteria, fungi, virus) or unacceptable levels of spoilage microorganisms.

b. Semiperishable rations (canned and dried food products). Freezing and extreme heat can change semiperishables both chemically and physically; therefore, protect rations from environmental extremes. It is necessary to periodically monitor rations for condition of product and packaging as well as for arthropod infestations. Discard moldy grain products (ergotism). Cans with swelling and/or leaking cans should not be used. Rust on cans and dented cans can be used as long as product in can is unaffected.

c. Perishables.

(1) Fresh fruits and vegetables should be procured from an inspected source; however, cooking (to 116°F.), immersing in boiling water 30 min, or 100 ppm. chlorine disinfectant solution (1 1/2 oz. of 5% bleach in 5 gallon H_2O) will destroy <u>most</u> pathogenic organisms.

(a) If possible, avoid night soil grown vegetables. Always wash, peel, and disinfect (or cook) if in doubt.

(b) Acid foods should not be stored or served in galvanized containers (zinc toxicosis).

(c) Edibility and nutrition of unfamiliar plants are best determined by observing their use by the native people and animals (always cook).

(2) Eggs and dairy products.

(a) Eggs should always be cooked (salmonellosis). Blood and meat spots are acceptable in eggs (not rotten or cracked).

(b) Unpasteurized dairy products must be pasteurized or boiled for at least 15 seconds (TB, Q fever, brucellosis, and other).

(3) Shellfish and fish.

(a) <u>Cooking is essential for all</u> seafood (hepatitis,

bacteria), and freshwater fish (tapeworm, fluke, other).

(b) Some shellfish toxins (i.e., during red tides) are heat stable; therefore, it is best to avoid all shellfish.

(c) Some saltwater fish have heat stable toxins. Judge what is toxic by what the native population eats.

(d) Seafood spoils quickly; therefore, avoid if there are off-odors, sticky or pitting flesh, sunken eyes, or scales that come off easily. Remember, local ice can contaminate the product.

(4) Meat and meat products.

(a) If cooked well (to avoid trichinosis, tapeworms, other), fresh meat from healthy animals is safe to eat. Carcass meat offers less chance of potential contamination than visceral meat and therefore is preferred as a food source.

(b) Antemortem exam. Briefly follow outline as given under Animal Health section - animal exam in paragraph 21-3b. Be attentive especially to:

1. Posture and gait; reject deformed or "down" animals.

2. State of nutrition; reject if very poor (chronic disease).

3. Reaction to environment; reject if very lethargic (ill) or hyperexcitable (rabies, tetanus).

4. Appetite, rumination, feces; reject if disease is indicated.

5. Respiratory system; reject if breathing is labored or coughing is severe.

6. Vulva, mammary gland; reject if signs of infection are noted.

7. Hide, skin, hair; reject if there are diffuse lesions.

8. Temperature; reject if elevated (may recheck later).

NORMAL PHYSIOLOGIC VALUES

	Rectal T. (F.)	Heart rate	R. rate	Daily feces lbs	Daily urine ml./kg.	W.B.C. x103	HCT%
Horse	100.5	23-70	12	30-50	3-18	6-12	39-52
Cow	100.5	60-70	30	30-100	17-45	4-12	24-48
Sheep	103	60-120	19	2-6.5	10-14	4-12	24-50
Goat	104	70-135			10-14	6-16	24-48
Pig	102	58-86		1-6.5	5-30	11-22	32-50
Dog	101.5	100-130	22	0-1.5	20-100	6-18	37-55
Cat	101.5	110-140	26		10-20	8-25	24-45
Rabbit	102.5	123-304					

(c) Humane slaughter, field methods, and dressing.

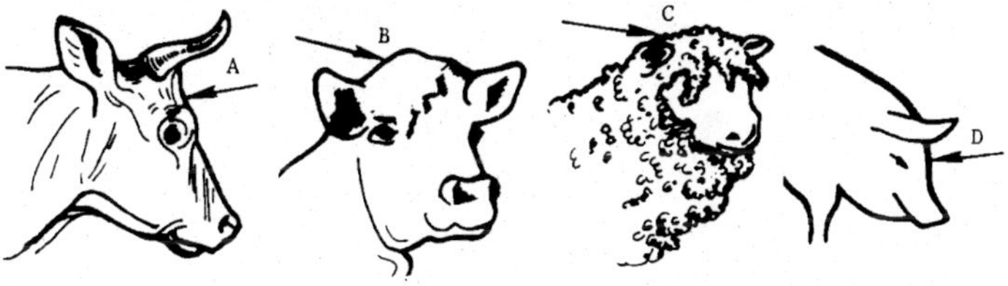

FIRING POSITION WITH HUMANE KILL.

A - Cattle B - Calves

C - Sheep D - Pigs

1. Bleed promptly; cut throat at point A. If head is to be mounted for trophy, insert knife at point B, cutting deeply until blood flows freely. In case of wound that bleeds freely or internally, bleeding may not be necessary. But it is far better to follow the sticking "ritual."

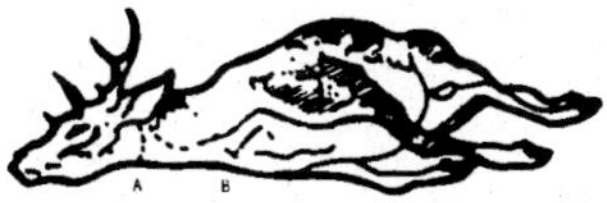

2. Remove genitals or udder. Prop carcass belly up; rocks or brush may be used for support. Cut circular area shown in illustration. Musk glands at points A and B may be removed to avoid tainting meat. Glands cease to function at time of death.

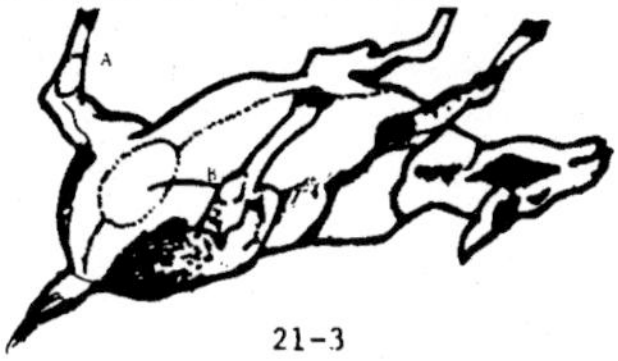

3. Split hide from tail to throat. Insert knife under skin, but do not cut into body cavity. Hide may be peeled back several inches on each side to keep hair out of meat. Cut through pelvic bone. Turning carcass downhill will cause viscera to sag into rib cavity. This will decrease chance of puncturing viscera while cutting through bone. Large intestine can then be cut free from pelvic cavity but not severed from viscera.

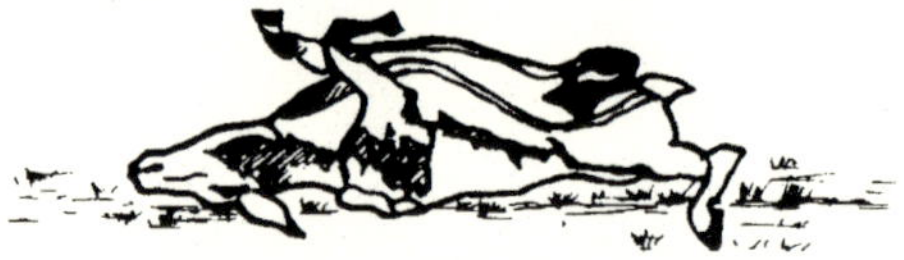

4. Open carcass by cutting through length of breastbone and neck into exposed windpipe. Turn carcass head uphill. Free gullet and pull viscera toward rear. An alternate method is to leave head downhill and strip viscera from rear out over the head.

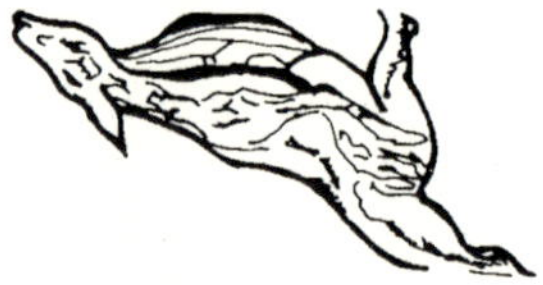

(c) Postmortem exam. Should be done immediately after slaughter. Be attentive for:

1. State of nutrition; reject emaciated animals.

2. Bruising; cut off bruised area if local.

3. Swelling in joints, muscle, bones; cut out if local, reject if found in more than one body area.

4. Edema; sign of disease, reject unless localized.

5. Inflammation, adhesion, or abcessed pleura, peritoneum, or viscera; sign of septicemia--reject carcass.

6. Cut through tongue, cheek, diaphram, lung, liver, and several lymph nodes (thoracic and mesenteric lymph nodes most important) to check for parasitism and/or signs of other infections.

Caseated areas (cheeselike hardened abcesses) call for rejection (possible TB).

(5) Poultry.

(a) Antemortem. Check as in red meat with emphasis on alertness of bird, signs of respiratory problems, and level of nutrition.

(b) Slaughter by ringing neck, dislocation of neck, or beheading.

(c) Postmortem. Check eyes, gonads, and visceral organs for tumors or skin lesions. Emaciated birds may indicate TB and therefore should be rejected. Generalized inflammation or abcesses (septicemia) also warrant rejection. Also reject jaundiced birds, birds with severe arthritis, ascites, or maggots (not lice).

(d) Poultry is a potential source of salmonellosis; therefore, use fresh, refrigerate, or freeze.

21-2. STORAGE AND PRESERVATION. Storage and preservation are best accomplished by cold. Other methods include smoking, curing, making jerky and pemmican, salting and pickling, canning and using sugar solutions, and antibiotic treatment.

a. Smoking. The process of smoking meat as a means of preservation and as a taste enhancer is extremely old. Although it has largely been replaced by more modern, faster methods of food preservation, it is still a viable procedure for the SF medic in a field environment during UW operations. There are several acceptable methods, and the one outlined below should not be considered as the only safe method. There are also variations in the step-by-step instructions, depending on the type of meat. Regardless of the type of meat, there are several basics for smoking meat that do not change.

(1) No matter what type of meat is smoked, a smokehouse will be needed. This can be any type of building that has a roof vent (or have one installed), that is otherwise fairly well sealed, and that has a floor that will take a firepit. The firepit (or box) should be centered in the floor and be about 2 feet deep and 2 feet wide, depending on the amount to be cured at one time and the size of the smokehouse.

(2) The wood used for the fire should be from deciduous trees (shed leaves in winter) and preferably green. Do not use conifers (needle leaf), such as pine, firs, spruces, cedars, as the smoke these woods produce gives the meat a disagreeable taste. Start the fire and let it burn down to coals only, and then stoke it with green wood. The fire should be a "cold smoke" fire (less than 85°F.) that has only coals, not flames, during the smoking process. The meat should then be placed in the smokehouse and hung from the rafters.

(3) The rafters should be wooden poles of green wood to prevent burning and should run the length of the smokehouse. Suspension line or string may be used to connect the meat to the rafters. When hung, the bottom of the meat should be at least 4 feet but no more than 5 feet from the top of the firepit. All meat should hang free (not touching any other meat or the walls of the smokehouse) so it will smoke evenly and prevent spoilage from contact. Usually meat is smoked a minimum of 4-5 days,

depending on the size of the smokehouse and the number and size of pieces of meat being smoked. After the meat is smoked, it should be stored in the smokehouse if feasible.

(4) Preparing meat for smoking varies with the type of meat.

(a) Beef.

1. Remove the large bones, especially the joints, to prevent souring during the smoking process.

2. Trim the fat from the outer surfaces of the meat. The fat should be kept for making pemmican and candles.

3. Section the meat into manageable pieces, always cutting across the grain, not with the grain. This makes for more tender meat and helps speed up the smoking process.

4. Cut a hole in the meat and string it with heavy twine, suspension line, etc. The hole should be placed so as to prevent the string ripping through the meat during the smoking process.

5. Hang the meat in the smokehouse and fill out a smoking record. The record will enable you to follow the same procedure the next time you smoke meat.

(b) Pork.

1. Pork smoking is much like the beef process. Hot water can be used to help remove the hair from the skin of the animal.

2. Do not remove the layered fat or the bones except ball and socket joint bones. Do not scrape off the rendered fat (fat oozing from the pork during smoking).

3. Follow steps 3, 4, and 5 above.

(c) Smoked meat will generally stay in good shape for up to 1 year, depending on how well the instructions are followed, the climate, insect and rodent control, the condition of the meat prior to smoking, and other factors. If the meat should appear sour around a bone area, section the meat to expose the sour area for 24 hours. If the sour appearance clears up, the meat is generally safe. If it does not clear up, dispose of the meat. If moisture patches or small holes appear on the surface of the meat, it is going sour. If the area can be cut out and the remainder appears to be good, it can be kept. If the holes or moisture is throughout, it is ruined and must be disposed of--if in doubt, throw it out.

b. Curing. One way to keep meat fresh in conjunction with smoking is by curing it. This process works well by itself, but is best used with smoking. Various spices, sugar, salt, and brines may be used, but the method described below is a dry salt (coarse, not table) treatment. Like smoking, curing is a simple process.

(1) A work/storage area protected from insects and rodents is important in this method. The initial step is the same as step 1 in the beef smoking process. After this step has been completed, rub salt into

the meat to prepare it for the salt box (a wooden container large enough to hold the sectioned salt-covered meat). Cover the bottom of the salt box with salt. Place the salted meat in the salt box. If more than one piece of meat is placed in the box, be sure that the pieces do not touch each other. Cover the meat with salt. This procedure should be repeated in 2 days and repeated again 2 days later. The salt should be changed for each repetition. On the sixth day, remove the meat from the salt box. Place a layer of green pine straw, hay, etc., on the ground or floor (again in an area protected from rodents and insects), cover the hay with salt, and place the meat on the layer of salt. Cover the meat with salt and place a layer of straw on the salt-covered meat.

(2) The meat may be left in this manner until used or up to 1 year, depending on the same factors as for smoked meat. It should be inspected regularly.

(3) It is generally recommended that the meat be smoked. If smoking and curing are to be done, curing should be done first.

(4) When the meat is to be used (if cured), it should be washed thoroughly and inspected. Again, if in doubt as to quality, throw it out. If the meat is still very salty, soak it in water for 2-3 hours, changing the water every 30 minutes.

(5) If possible, salt should be stored in a tightly sealed container. Do not reuse the salt. If sugar or other spices are to be used as well as salt, they should be added during the "rubbing" stage while curing. If a brine is to be used, it should not be used in a wooden or metal container. For adequate preservation, the brine should be a 10% salt solution (1 lb of salt to 9 pints of water) or stronger.

c. Meat preservation records. Records should contain the following information:

(1) Type of meat prepared.

(2) Source and date the meat was obtained.

(3) Weight and cut of meat.

(4) Time cured, time smoked, as applicable.

(5) Type and amount of wood used (for smoking).

(6) Approximate temperature of smoke.

(7) Type and amount of salt (for curing).

(8) Type and amount of seasoning, if any (for curing).

(9) Color and texture of meat when completed.

(10) Overall assessment.

d. Jerky. For field-prepared food that is light and nutritious, jerky fits the bill. Red meat (beef, venison, etc.) should be used.

(1) To prepare jerky--

(a) Trim the fat from the meat.

(b) Cut the meat with the grain of the muscle into 12-inch-long strips no more than 1 inch thick and 1/2 inch wide.

(c) Pack the meat in dry salt for 10-12 hours with each strip completely covered with salt and no contact between strips.

(d) Smoke the meat.

(2) The meat may also be sun dried (sprinkle liberally with pepper to cut down on insects and store above the insect line, 20 feet or higher) or dried over slow coals, as with smoking, also sprinkled liberally with pepper.

(3) If salt cured, wash thoroughly before eating.

e. Pemmican. Pemmican is also light and nutritious and can be made in the field. The two basic ingredients needed are lean meat--sun, wind, or smoke-dried (not salt-cured)--and rendered fat.

(1) Render fat by placing ground-up (preferred) or cut-up fat into a container. Boil the fat and pour off the tallow to use in pemmican. (Tallow can also be used to make candles.) The fat residue, called cracklings, can be eaten. One ounce of beef cracklings provides 207 calories; one ounce of pork cracklings, 219 calories.

(2) You need about 6 pounds of meat to make about 1 pound of pemmican.

(a) Dry, pound, and shred the meat.

(b) Prepare a casing, such as an intestine, by cleaning and tying one end.

(c) Lightly place (do not pack) the shredded meat in the casing.

(d) Pour hot tallow into the casing, heating the meat and filling the bag. The mixture in the casing should be about 60% fat (tallow) and 40% meat.

(e) Seal (sew or tie) the casing, then seal further by pouring tallow on the sealing.

(f) Allow the pemmican to harden.

(3) Pemmican will stay safe for consumption for approximately 5 years, depending on the type of tallow used.

f. Salting and pickling. Dry salt meat or immerse in a salt solution. Use 10:1 table salt and saltpeter (potassium nitrate) for both. With pickling, mix 50 pounds of salt and 5 pounds of saltpeter with 20 gallons of water.

g. Canning. Heat is used to destroy harmful microorganisms but this is not as good as above since thermophilic bacteria may remain stable. Canning is better with fresh fruit and vegetables.

h. Sugar solutions and antibiotic treatment of meat is suggested for preservation, but again this process is not as effective as those listed above.

21-3. ANIMAL HEALTH.

a. The association of men and animals may be viewed as threefold: Animals are often intimately associated with man's livelihood, such as work or food animals; they often have religious significance or are companions; and they have diseases that can be transmitted to man. With reference to animal health, consider the following:

(1) Animal care may reduce zoonotic reservoiring of human disease, increase food production capabilities, and in general increase the standard of living of the people concerned.

(2) Treating animals or advising on animal husbandry gains rapport and shows a caring attitude.

(3) Veterinary care with immediate observable results is best for short-term operations.

(4) Programs with distant goals must be approached with an appreciation for what is acceptable to the local population.

b. Animal examination: Approach the exam as you would with humans except use adequate caution and restraint.

(1) Allow owner and/or native population to handle and restrain the animal as much as possible. Restraint is probably the most difficult part of treating large animals. Following are a few simple methods of restraint that may be helpful. A rappelling rope may be used.

(a) Temporary rope halter (horse or cow). Fasten a rope loop around the animal's neck with a bowline knot. Pull a bight of the standing part of the rope through the loop from rear to front and place it over the animal's nose. Pull tight when in use.

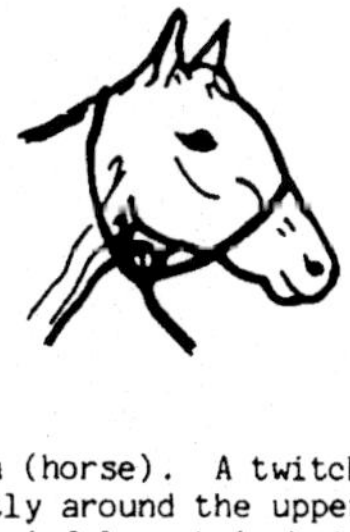

(b) Twitch (horse). A twitch is a small loop of rope or smooth chain twisted tightly around the upper lip of the horse to divert its attention while less painful work is being done on some other part of the body. A metal ring or rod or a stick may be used as a handle to wind-tighten the rope loop on the animal's nose.

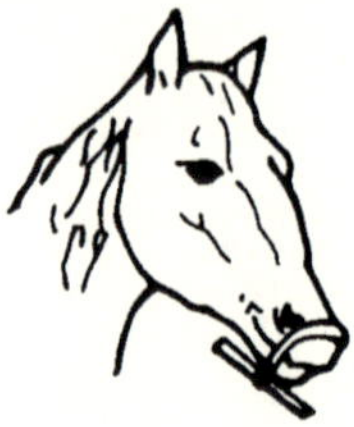

(c) Burley method of casting (cow). Use approx 40 ft

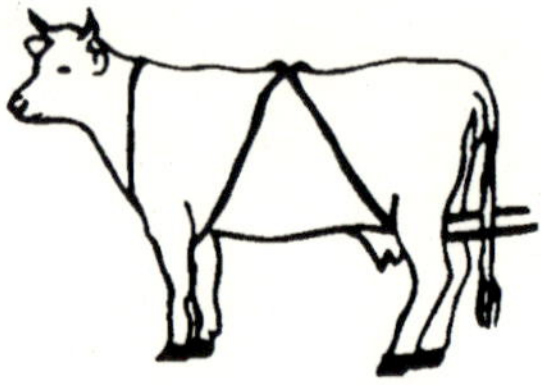

of rope with the center of the rope over withers. Place the rest of rope as pictured above. While the cow is being held by a strong halter at the head, pull the ends of the rope and the cow will fall. To tie the rear legs, keep both ropes taut and slide the uppermost one along the undersurface of the rear leg to the fetlock. Flex the leg and make a half hitch around the fetlock. Then carry end around the leg and above the hock, across the cannon bone and back around the fetlock. Tie the leg with several such figure "8s."

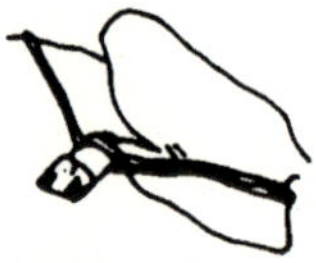

TYING THE COW AFTER CASTING.

Tying all four feet together is a good method of restraining after the animal has been cast. A rope is tied to one leg below the fetlock. The other legs are tied to this one alternately, first a front leg, then a rear one, etc.

(d) Strap hobble (horse). A strap with a "D" ring may be used to raise one foreleg. The leg is bent at the knee and the pastern is brought towards the upper arm. The strap is placed around the arm and pastern, and the end of the strap is brought through the "D" ring, pulled tight, and secured with a half hitch.

(e) Tail restraint (cow). The tail of a cow may be bent up sharply at the base, by an assistant, when it becomes necessary to distract its attention from another part of the body. Keep both hands at the base of the tail (grasping it like a baseball bat) to avoid breaking the tail. Stand to the side to avoid being kicked.

(2) SOAP approach to animal exam.

S. Subjective - use HAAA SEMAN LHL.

1. H - history - individual and herd.

2. AAA - activity, attitude, appetite.

3. S - skin - lesions, color, texture, state of hydration.

4. E - eye, ear, nose, and throat - look in the mouth if possible.

5. M - musculoskeletal system - palpate legs; watch the animal move.

6. A - abdomen - palpate, auscultate.

7. N - neurologic exam - coordination, cranial nerves, segmental reflexes.

8. L - lungs - auscultate, rate, dyspnea.

9. H - heart - auscultate, rate.

10. L - lymph nodes - palpate submandibular, cervical and prescapular, inguinal and popliteals.

O. Objective - use VUFL.

1. V - vital signs - see normal values (Antemortem Exam).

2. U - urinalysis - odor, color, pH, sp.gr., bacteria, etc.

3. F - fecal exam - blood, excessive mucous, diarrhea, parasites, etc.

4. L - other lab data - blood count, serology, etc.

A. Assessment - use DAMN - IT.

1. D - degenerative disease.

2. A - anomaly/allergic disorder.

3. M - metabolic disorder.

4. N - nutritional/neoplastic disorder.

5. I - infection/infestation.

6. T - traumatic/toxicosis.

P. Plan - use TAEP.

1. T - treat, if feasible (with allergies, malnutrition, infections, infestations, and trauma/toxins).

2. A - advise (nutrition, culling of carriers, animal husbandry practice).

3. E - education (on herd health, preventive medical actions that the owner or community can take themselves).

4. P - public health (zoonosis potential in animals, human nutrition from animal protein source).

c. Remember that the types of diseases of animals fit the same categories as those of humans; therefore, without detailed instruction in veterinary medicine, one can only make a diagnosis on his level of knowledge. Seek advice if needed and use the Merck Veterinary Manual if one is available on specific diseases.

CHAPTER 22

PRIMITIVE MEDICINE

22-1. GENERAL.

a. This chapter covers a number of primitive treatments using materials that are found worldwide. It does not cover herbal medicines because specific herbs (plants) are difficult to identify and some are found only in specific areas of the world. This does not mean, however, that they should not be used. To get information concerning types and uses of herbal medicines in a particular area, talk to the natives. But remember, it is preventive medicine (PM) that must be stressed. Proper hygiene, care in preparation of food and drink, waste disposal, insect and rodent control, and a good immunization program can greatly reduce the causes and number of diseases.

b. All of us--patients and doctors alike--depend upon wonder drugs, fine laboratories, and modern equipment. We have lost sight of the "country doctor" type of medicine--determination, common sense, and a few primitive treatments that can be lifesaving. Many areas of the world still depend on the practices of the local witch doctor or healer. And many herbs (plants) and treatments that they use are as effective as the most modern medications available. Herbal medicine has been practiced worldwide since before recorded history, and many modern medications come from refined herbs. For example, pectin can be obtained from the rinds (white stringy part) of citrus fruits and from apple pomace (the pulp left after the juice has been pressed out). If either is mixed with ground chalk, the result will be a primitive form of Kaopectate.

c. Although many herbal medicines and exotic treatments are effective, use them with extreme caution and only when faced with limited or nonexistent medical supplies. Some are dangerous and, instead of treating the disease or injury, may cause further damage or even death.

22-2. PRIMITIVE TREATMENTS.

a. Diarrhea is a common, debilitating ailment that can be caused by almost anything. Most cases can be avoided by following good PM practices. Treatment in many cases is fluids only for 24 hours. If that does not work and no antidiarrheal medication is available, grind chalk, charcoal, or dried bones into a powder. Mix one handful of powder with treated water and administer every 2 hours until diarrhea has slowed or stopped. Adding an equal portion of apple pomace or the rinds of citrus fruit to this mixture makes the mixture more effective. Tannic acid, which is found in tea, can also help control diarrhea. Prepare a strong solution of tea, if available, and administer 1 cup every 2 hours until diarrhea slows or stops. The inner bark of hardwood trees also contains tannic acid. Boil the inner bark for 2 hours or more to release the tannic acid. The resultant black brew has a vile taste and smell, but it will stop most cases of diarrhea.

b. Worms and intestinal parasites. Infestations can usually be avoided by maintaining strict preventive medicine measures. For example, never go barefooted. The following home remedies appear to work or at least control the degree of infestation, but they are not without danger. Most work on the principle of changing the environment of the gastrointestinal tract.

(1) Salt water. Four tablespoons of salt in 1 quart of water. This should be taken on a one time basis only.

(2) Tobacco. Eat 1 to 1 1/2 cigarettes. The nicotine in the cigarette kills or stuns the worms long enough for them to be passed. If the infestation is severe, the treatment can be repeated in 24 to 48 hours, but no sooner.

(3) Kerosene. Drink 2 tablespoons. Don't drink more. The treatment can be repeated in 24 to 48 hours, but no sooner.

(4) Hot peppers. Put peppers in soups, rice, meat dishes or eat them raw. This treatment is not effective unless peppers are made a steady part of the diet.

c. Sore throats are common and usually can be taken care of by gargling with warm salt water. If the tongue is coated, scrape it off with a tooth brush, a clean stick, or even a clean fingernail; then gargle with warm salt water.

d. Skin infections.

(1) Fungal infections. Keep the area clean and dry, and expose the area to sunlight as much as possible.

(2) Heat rash. Keep the area clean, dry, and cool. If powder is available, use it on affected area.

(3) The rule of thumb for all skin diseases is: "If it is wet, dry it, and if it is dry, wet it."

e. Burns. Soak dressings or clean rags that have been boiled for 10 minutes in tannic acid (tea or inner bark of hardwood trees), cool, and apply over the burns. This relieves the pain somewhat, seems to help speed healing, and offers some protection against infection.

f. Leaches and ticks. Apply a lit cigarette or a flaming match to the back of the leach or tick, and it will drop off. Covering it with moistened tobacco, grease, or oil will also make it drop off. Do not try to pull it off; part of the head may remain attached to the skin and cause an infection.

g. Bee, wasp, and hornet stings. Inspect the wound carefully and remove stinger if present. Apply baking soda, cold compress, mud, or coconut meat to the area. Spider, scorpion, and centipede bites can be treated the same way.

h. Chiggers. Nail polish applied over the red spots will cut off the chigger's air supply and kill it. Any variation of this, e.g., tree sap, will work.

22-3. MAGGOT THERAPY FOR WOUND DEBRIDEMENT.

a. Introducing maggots into a wound can be hazardous because the wound must be exposed to flies. Flies, because of their filthy habits, are likely to introduce bacteria into the wound, causing additional complications. Maggots will also invade live, healthy tissue when the dead tissue is gone or not readily available. Maggot invasion of healthy tissue causes extreme pain and hemorrhage, possibly severe enough to be fatal.

b. Despite the hazards involved, maggot therapy should be considered a viable alternative when, in the absence of antibiotics, a wound becomes severely infected, does not heal, and ordinary debridement is impossible.

(1) All bandages should be removed so that the wound is exposed to circulating flies. Flies are attracted to foul or fetid odors coming from the infected wound; they will not deposit eggs on fresh, clean wounds.

(2) In order to limit further contamination of the wound by disease organisms carried by the flies, those flies attracted to the wound should not be permitted to light directly on the wound surface. Instead, their activity should be restricted to the intact skin surface along the edge of the wound. Live maggots deposited here and/or maggots hatching from eggs deposited here will find their way into the wound with less additional contamination than if the flies were allowed free access to the wound.

(3) One exposure to the flies is usually all that is necessary to insure more than enough maggots for thorough debridement of a wound. Therefore, after the flies have deposited eggs, the wound should be covered with a bandage.

(4) The bandage should be removed daily to check for maggots. If no maggots are observed in the wound within 2 days after exposure to the flies, the bandage should be removed and the wound should be re-exposed. If the wound is found to be teeming with maggots when the bandage is removed, as many as possible should be removed using forceps or some other sterilized instrument or by flushing with sterile water. Only 50-100 maggots should be allowed to remain in the wound.

(5) Once the maggots have become established in the wound, it should be covered with a bandage again, but the maggot activity should be monitored closely each day. A frothy fluid produced by the maggots will make it difficult to see them. This fluid should be "sponged out" of the wound with an absorbent cloth so that all of the maggots in the wound can be seen. Care should be taken not to remove the maggots with the fluid.

(6) The period of time necessary for maggot debridement of a wound depends on a number of factors, including the depth and extent of the wound, the part of the body affected, the number of maggots present in the wound, and the fly species involved. In a survival situation, an individual will be able to control only one of these factors--the number, and sometimes not even that; therefore, the exact time to remove the maggots cannot be given in specific numbers of hours or days. However, it can be said with certainty that the maggots should be removed immediately once they have removed all the dead tissue and before they have become established in healthy tissue. When the maggots begin feeding on normal, healthy tissue, the individual will experience an increased level of pain at the site of the wound as the maggots come into contact with "live" nerves. Bright red blood in the wound also indicates that the maggots have reached healthy tissue.

(7) The maggots should be removed by flushing the wound repeatedly with sterile water. When all the maggots have been removed, the wound should be bandaged. To insure that the wound is free of maggots, check it every 4 hours or more often for several days. Any remaining

maggots should be removed with sterilized forceps or by flushing with sterile water.

(8) Once all of the maggots have been removed, bandage the wound and treat it as any other wound. It should heal normally provided there are no further complications.

22-4. SUMMARY. The treatments discussed in this chapter are by no means all of the primitive treatments or home remedies available for use. Most people have their own home remedy for various problems. Some work, some don't. The ones presented here have been used and do work, although some can be dangerous. The lack of modern medicine does not rule out medical treatment. Common sense, determination to succeed, and advice from the natives in the area on primitive treatments can provide the solution to a medical problem. Just keep one thing in mind: "First I shall do no harm."

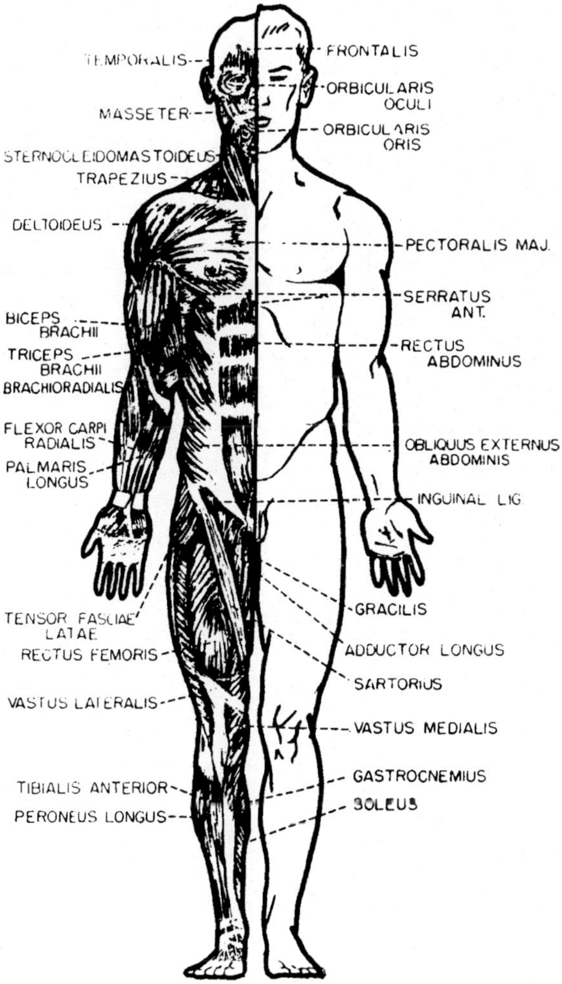

Figure 1. Important superficial muscles, anterior view.

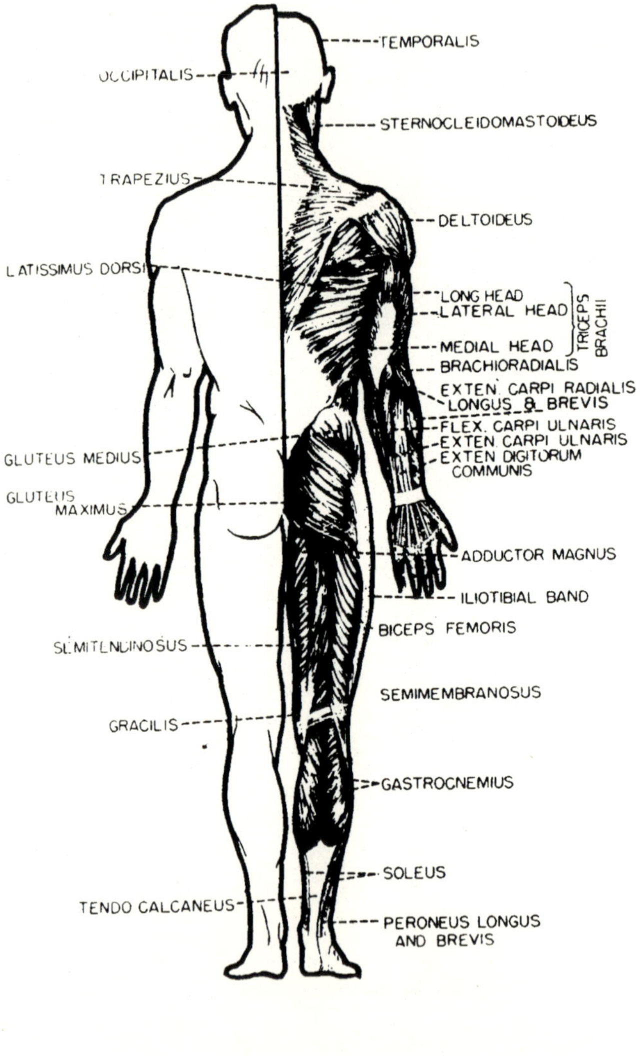

Figure 2. Important superficial muscles, posterior view.

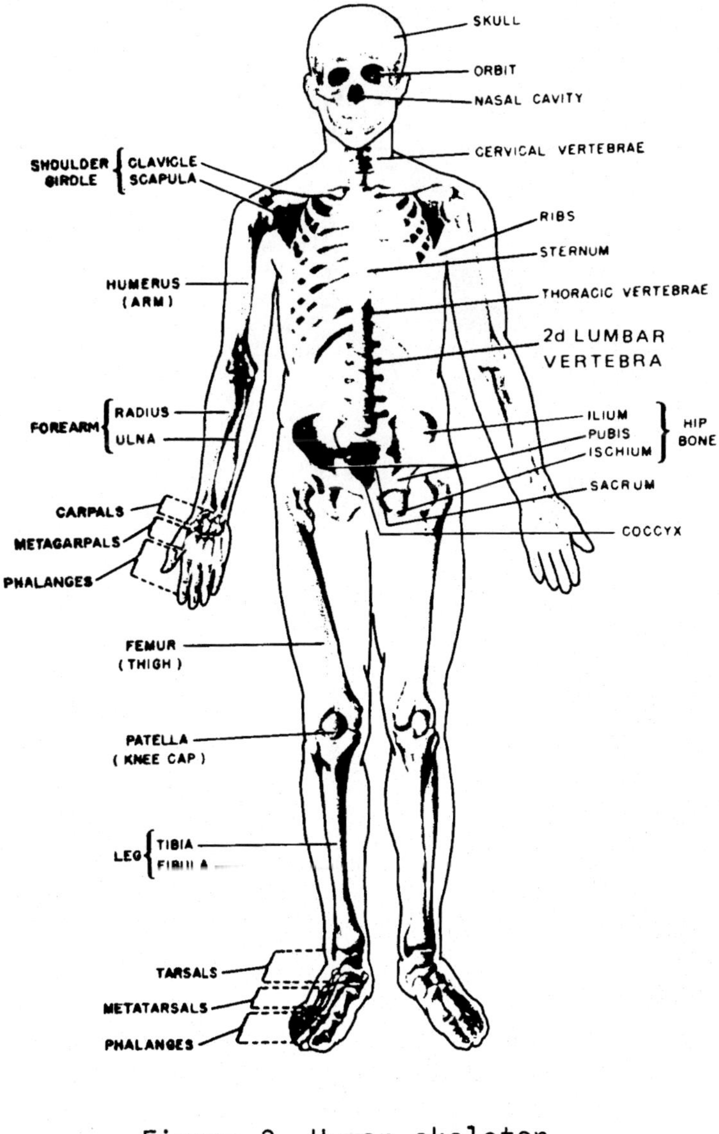

Figure 3. Human skeleton.

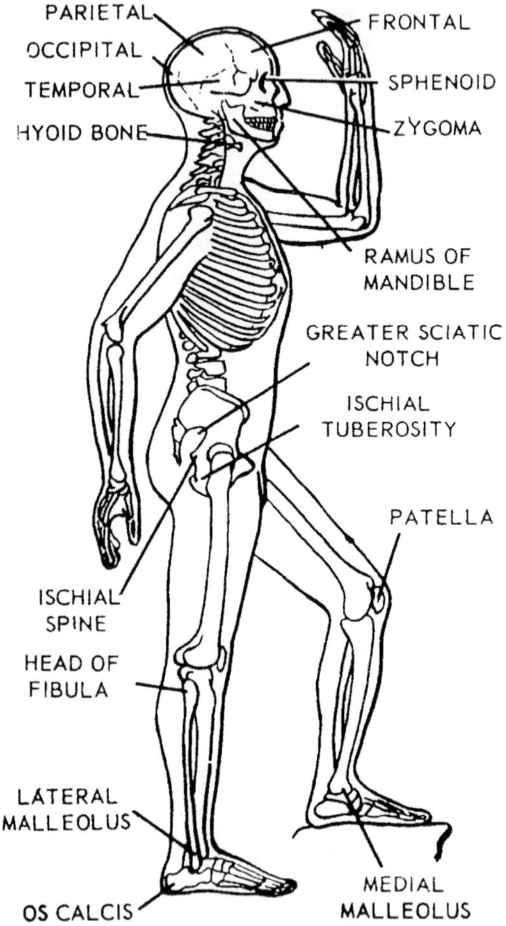

Figure 4. Lateral view.

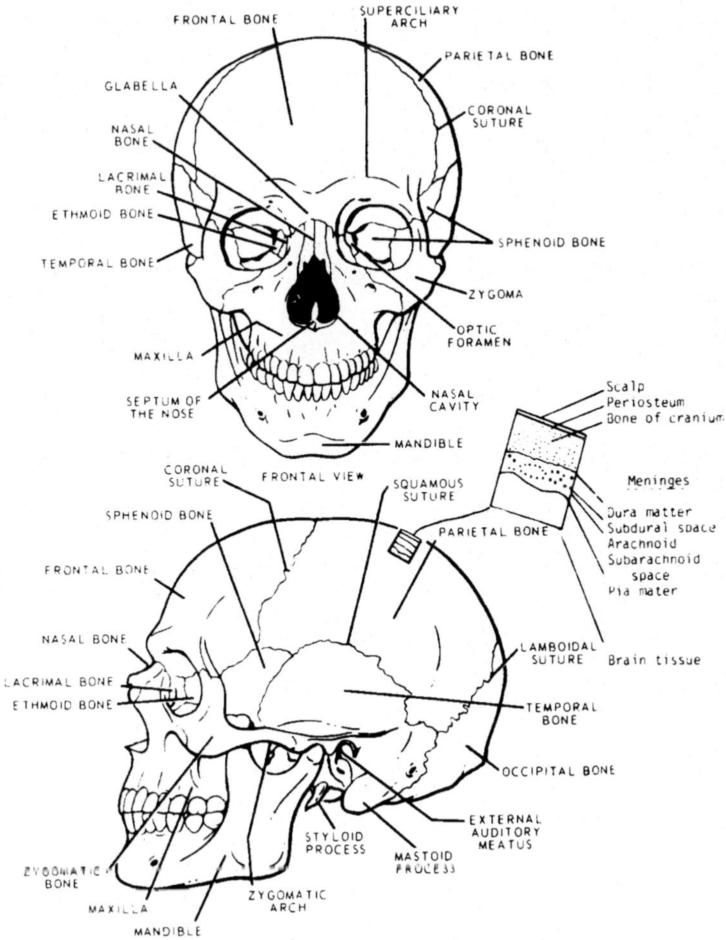

Figure 5. The skull.

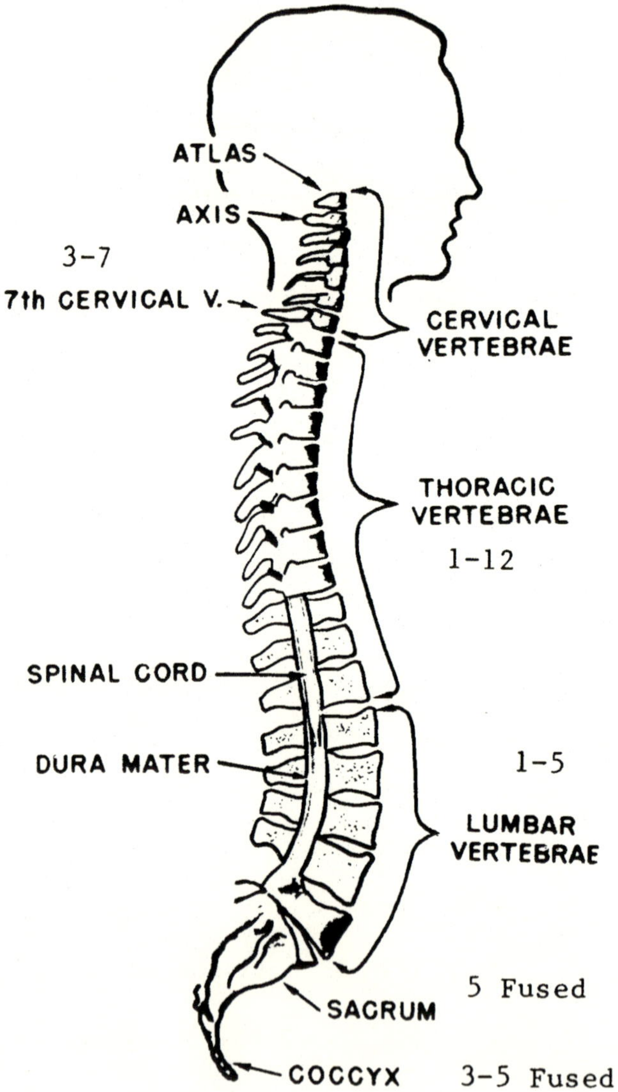

Figure 6. Vertebral column.

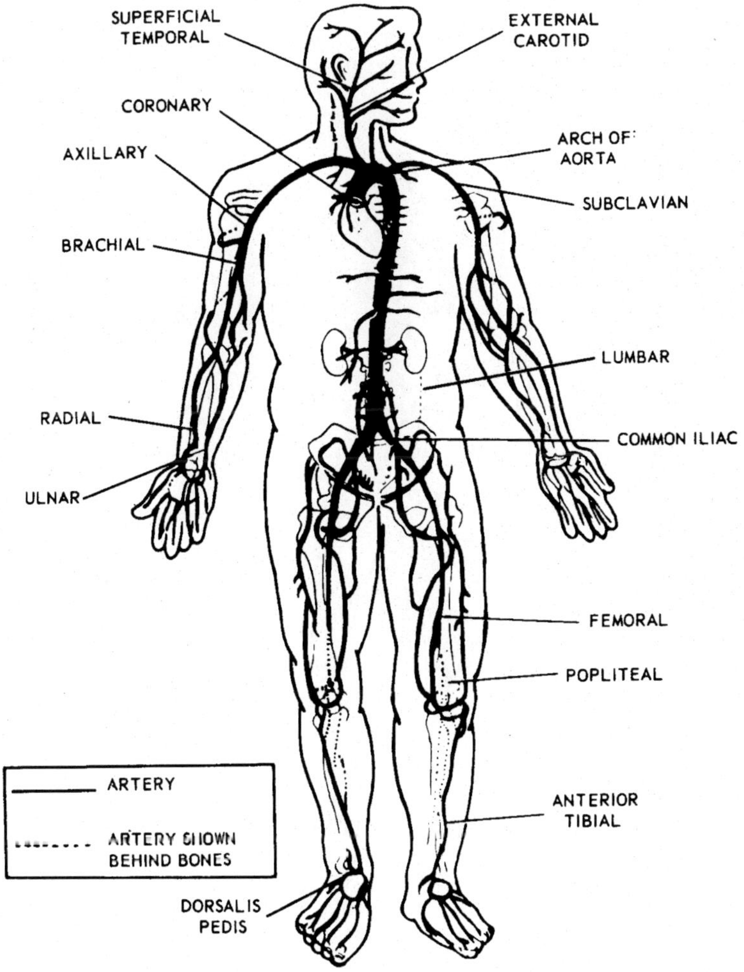

Figure 7. Large arteries of the systemic circulation.

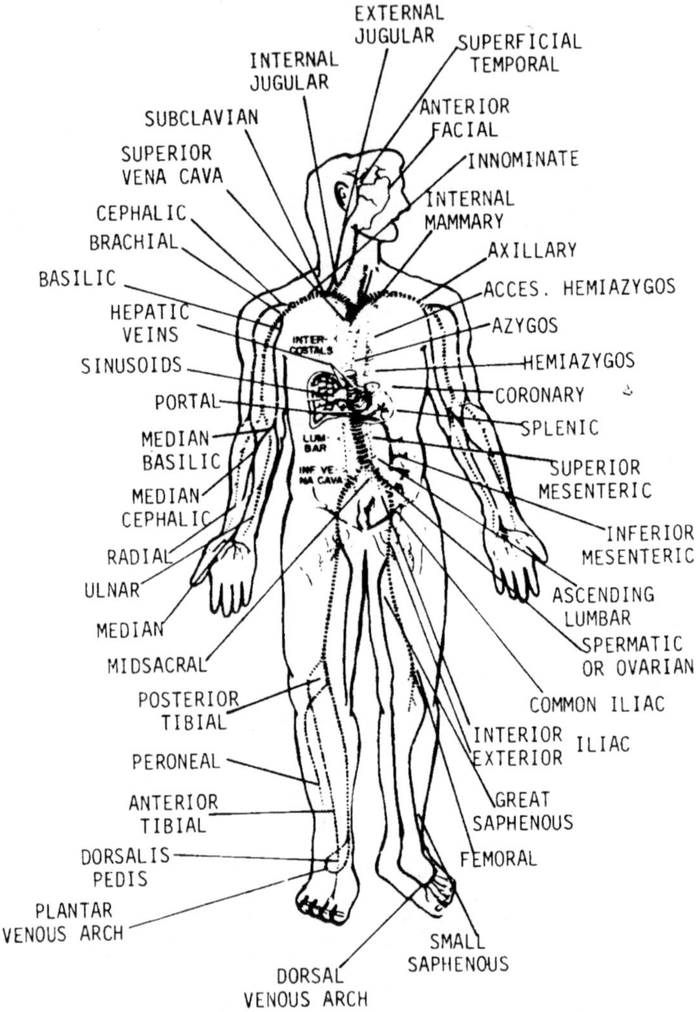

Figure 8. Large veins of the systemic circulation.

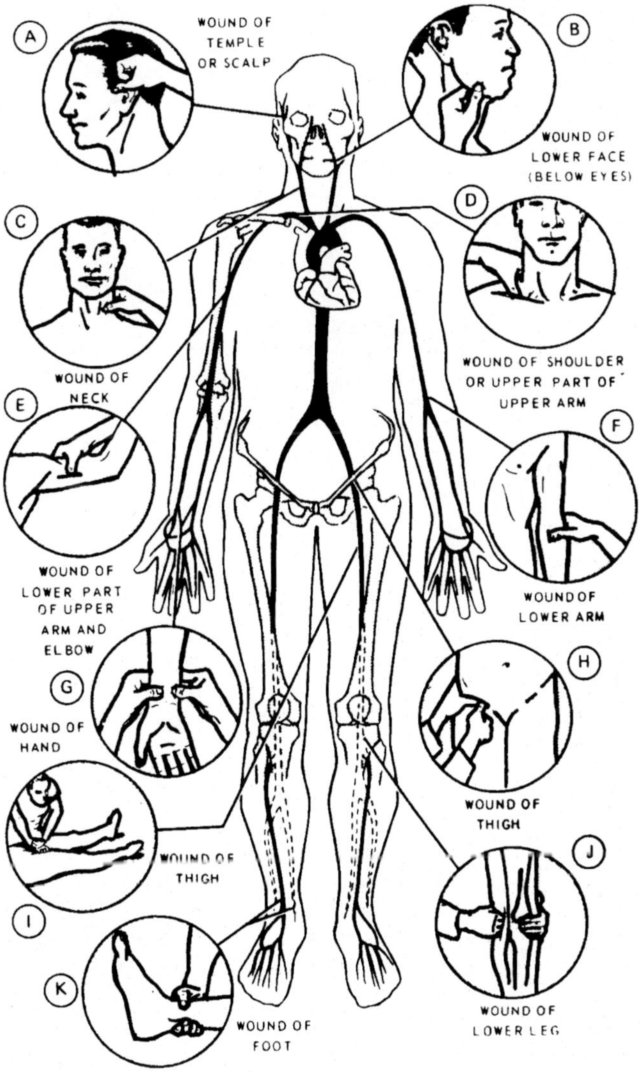

Figure 9. Pressure points for hemorrhage control.

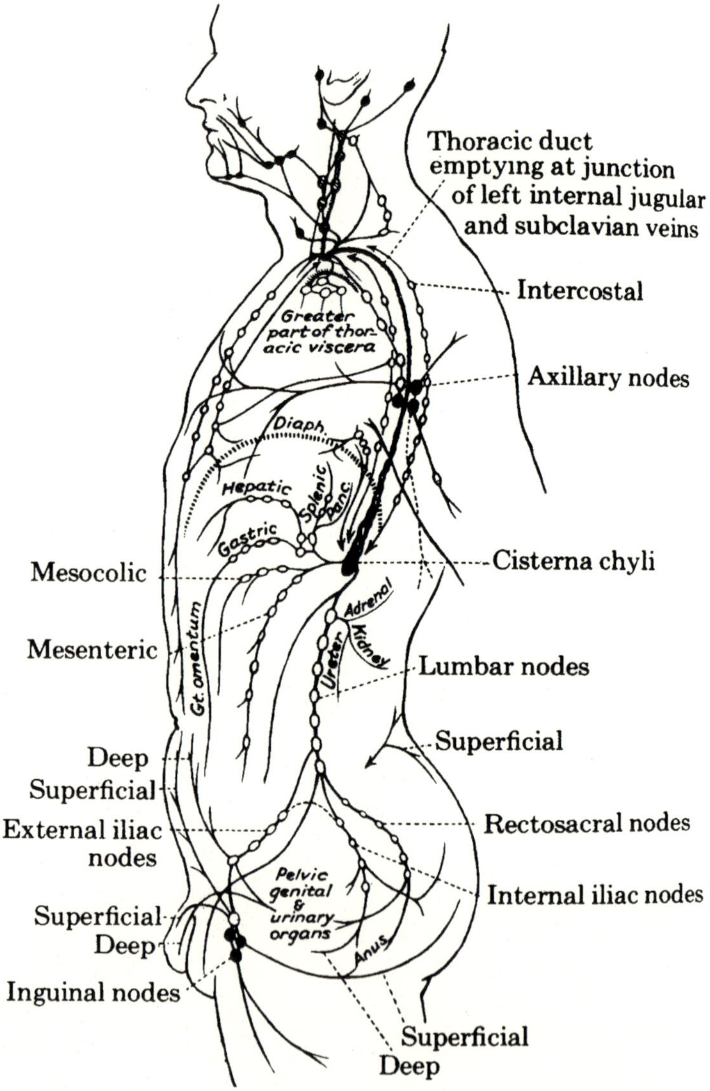

Figure 10. Lymphatic drainage of the body.

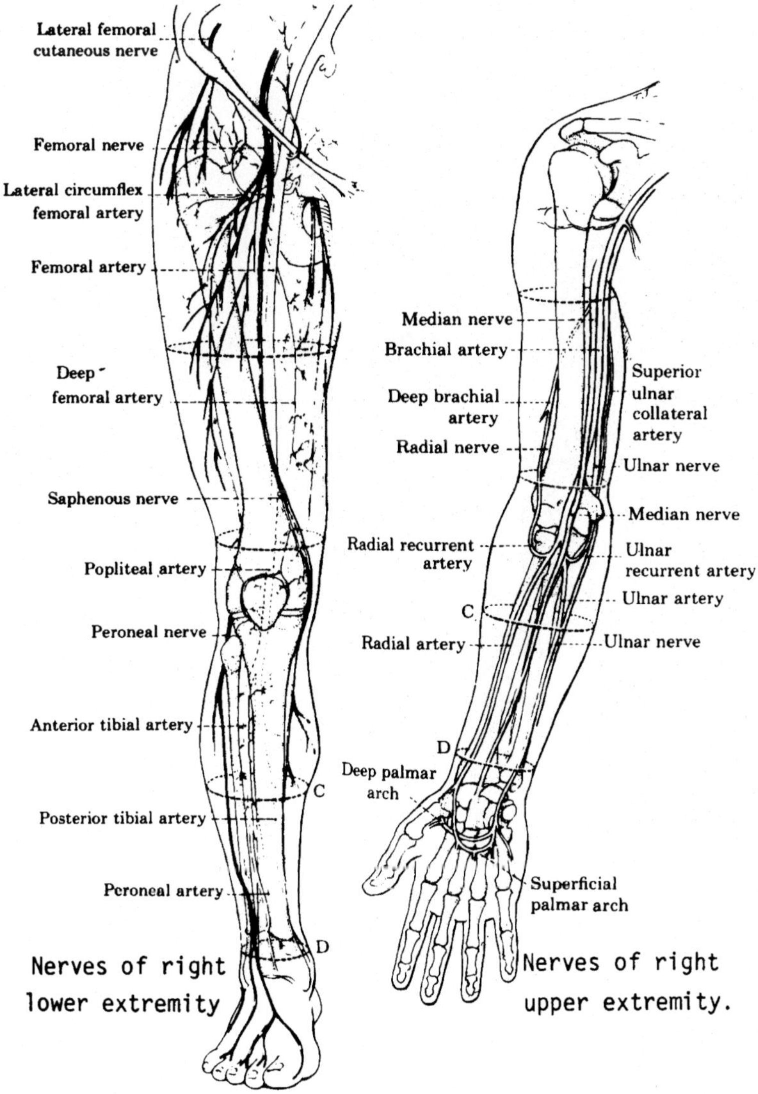

Figure 11. Nerves of the extremities.

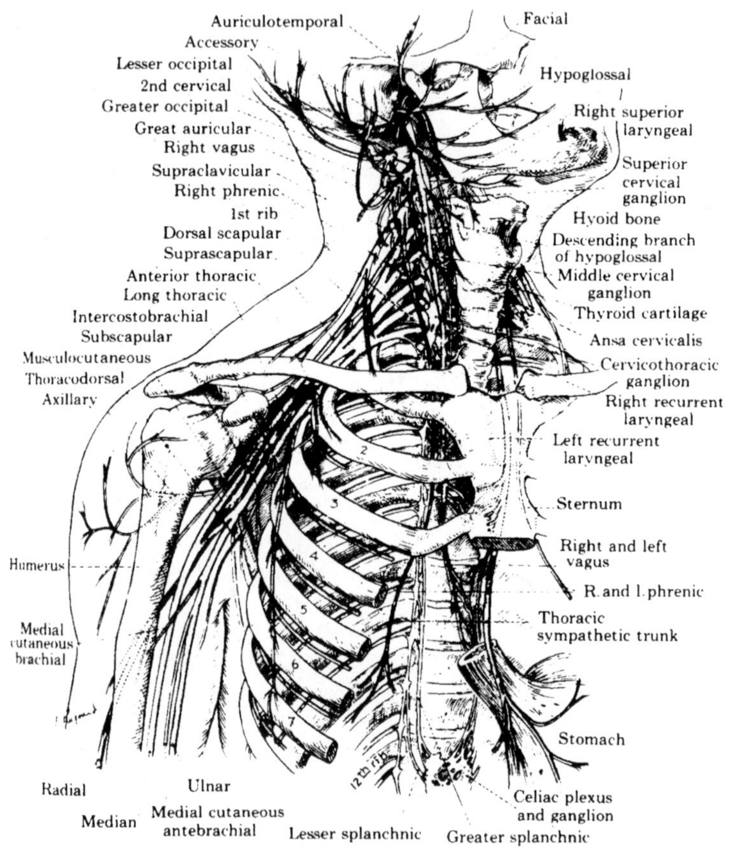

Figure 12. Deep nerves of neck, axilla, and upper thorax.

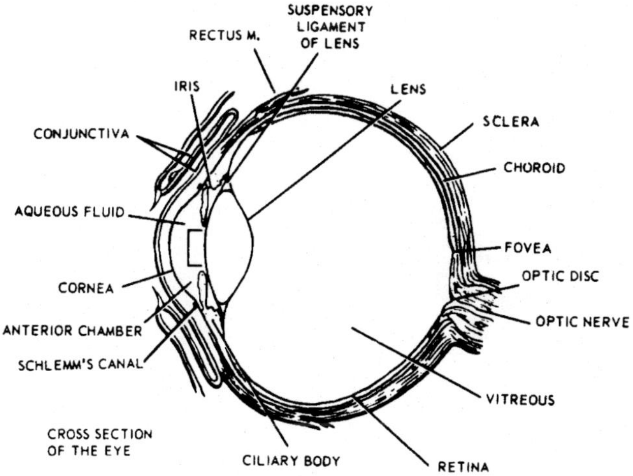

Figure 13. The eye.

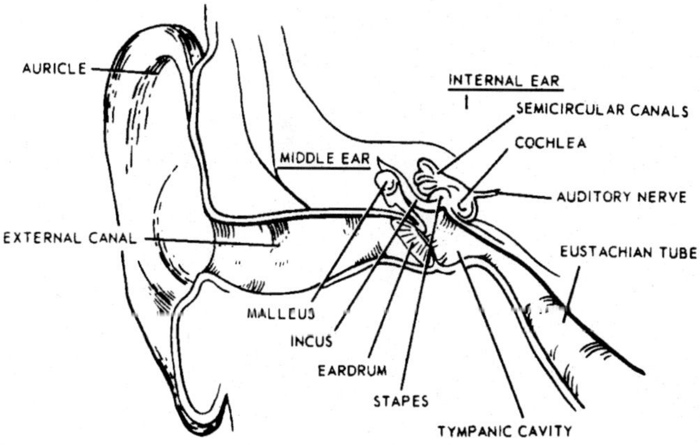

Figure 14. The ear.

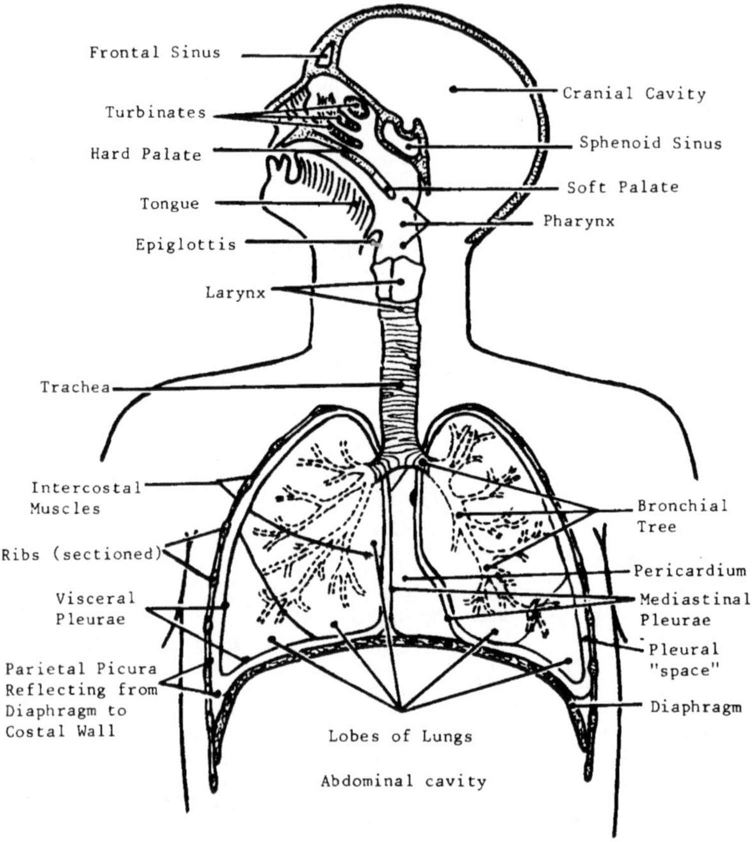

Figure 15. Schematic of the tract.

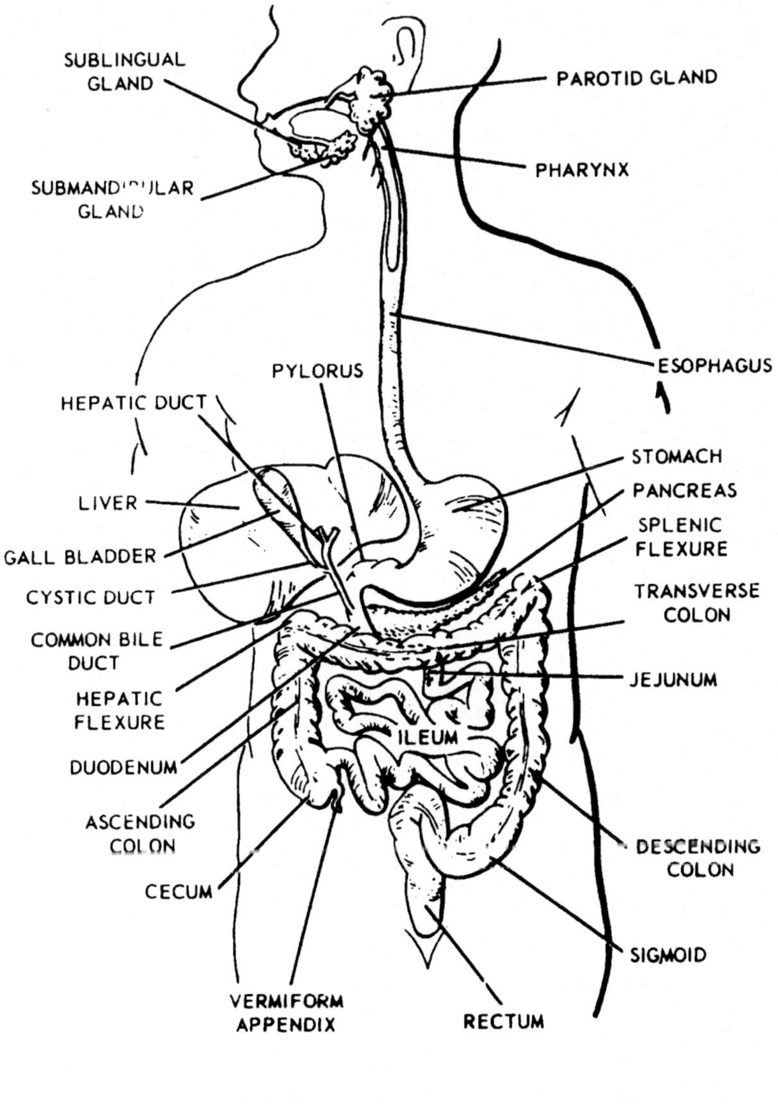

Figure 16. Digestive system.

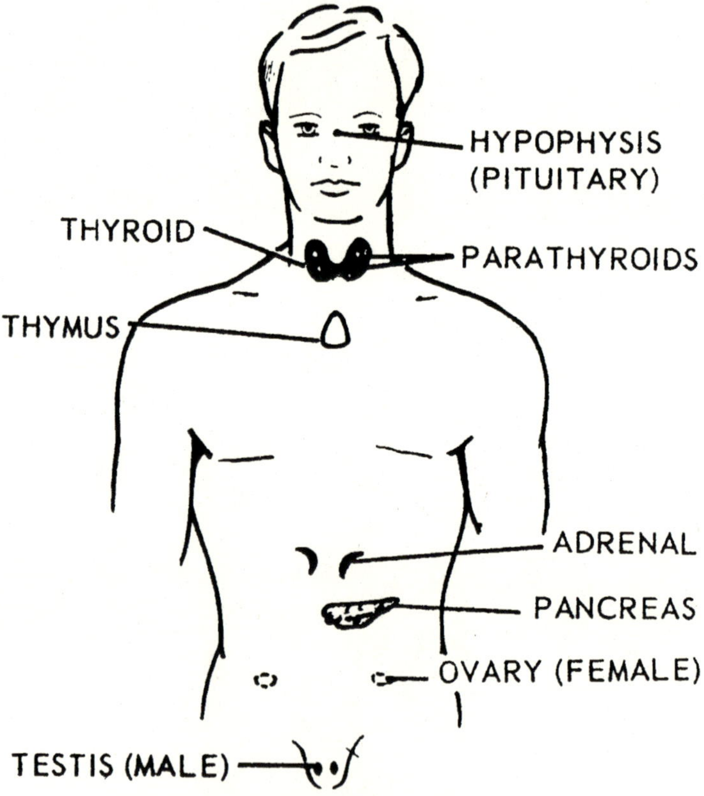

Figure 17. Endocrine system.

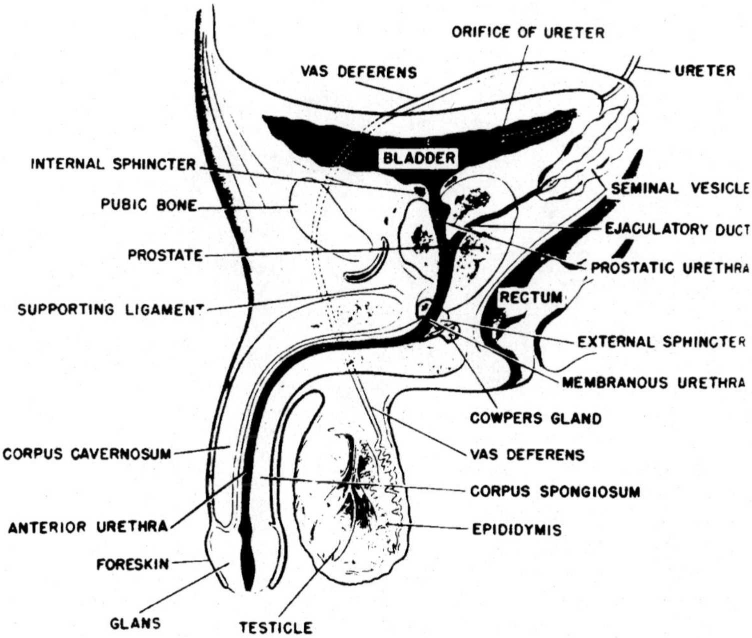

Figure 18. Male genital organs.

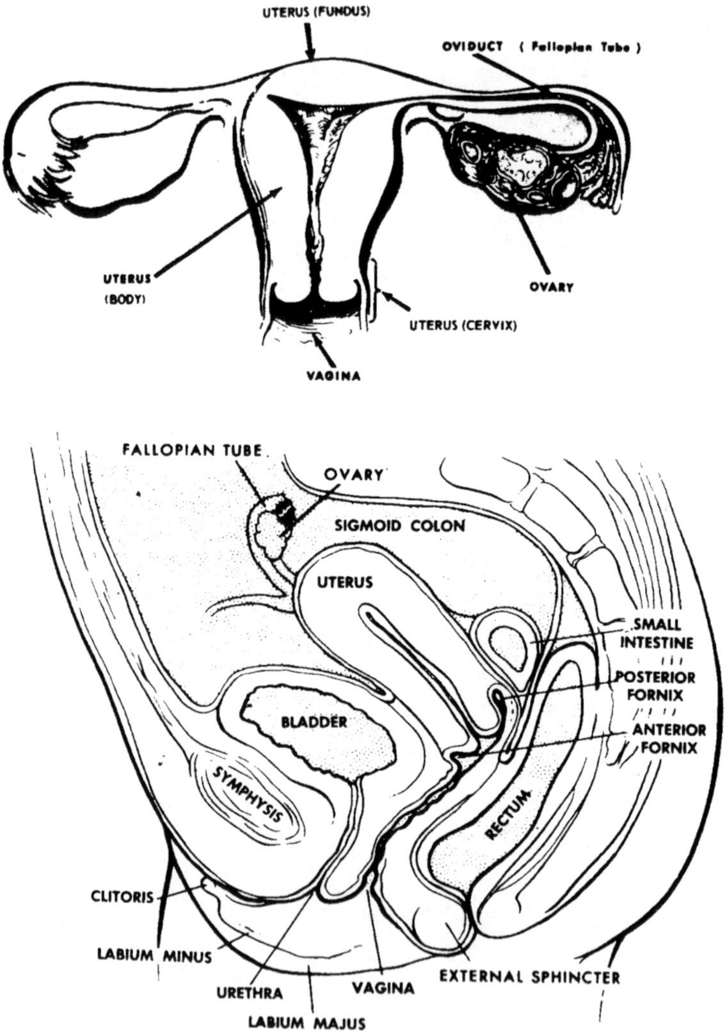

Figure 19. Female genital organs.

Appendix B

Bacteriological and Parasitic Plates

B-1 Bacteriological

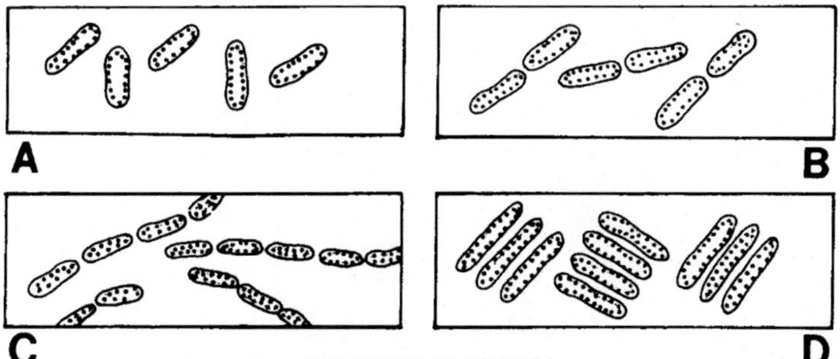

ARRANGEMENT OF BACILLI

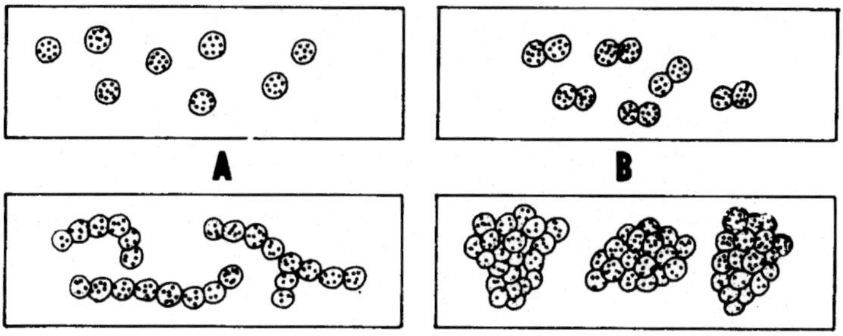

C

D

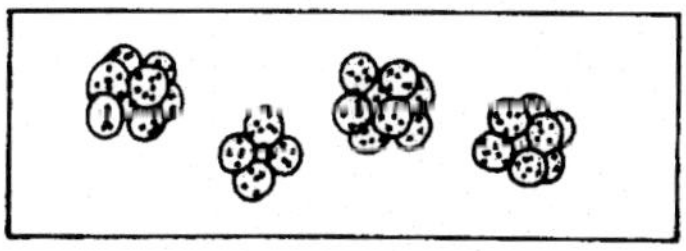

E

ARRANGEMENT OF COCCI

ARRANGEMENT OF BACTERIAL CELL

Arrangement	Terminology
COCCUS	
single	(A)......coccus
pair	(B)......diplococcus
chain	(C)......streptococcus
cluster	(D)......staphylococcus
four	(E)......tetrad (gaffkya)
eight	(E)......cube (sarcina)
BACILLUS	
single	(A)......bacillus
pair	(B)......diplobacillus
chain	(C)......streptobacillus
palisade	(D)......palisade

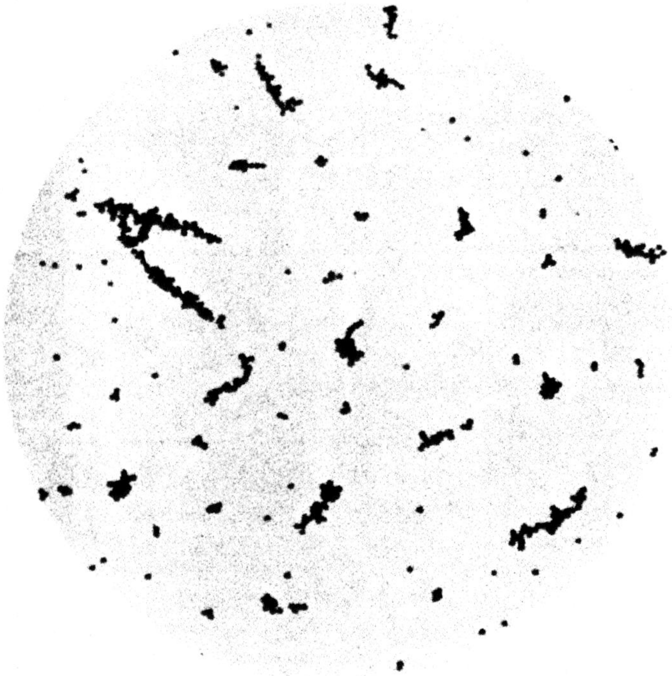

Figure 1. Gram-stained smear of Staphylococcus.

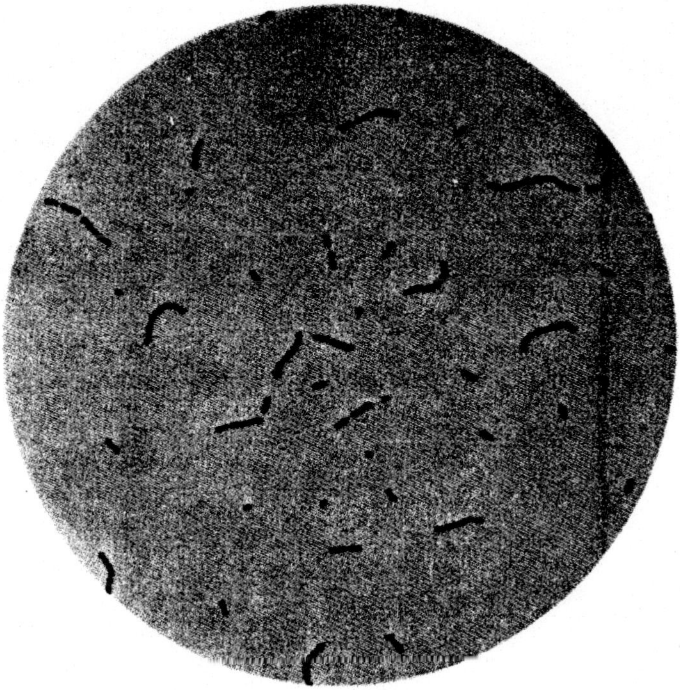

Figure 2. Gram-stained smear of Streptococcus.

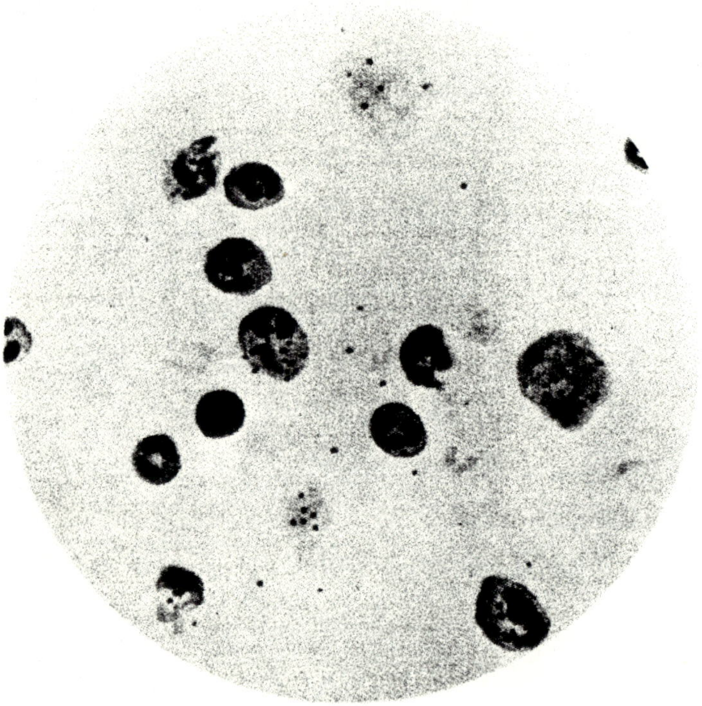

Figure 3. Gram-stained smear of Neisseria gonorrhea from urethral exudate.

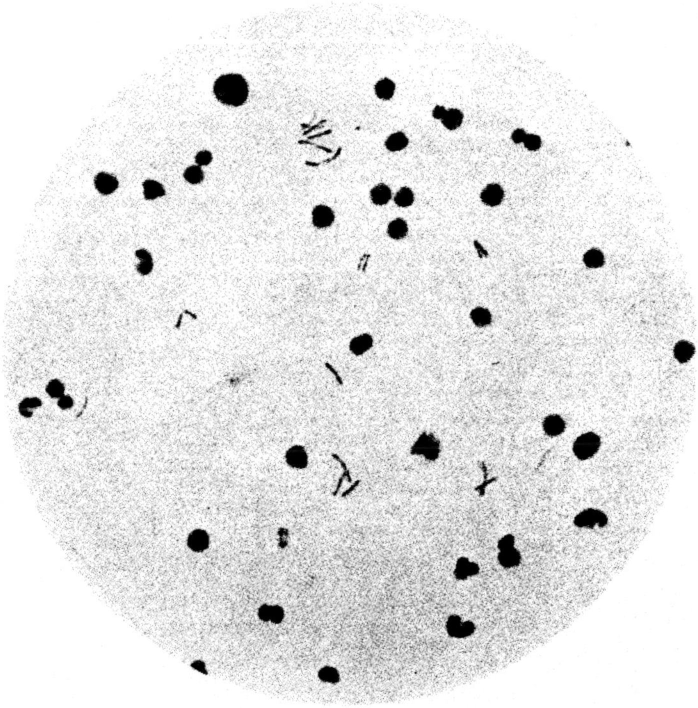

Figure 4. Acid-fast stained smear of Mycobacterium tuberculosis in sputum.

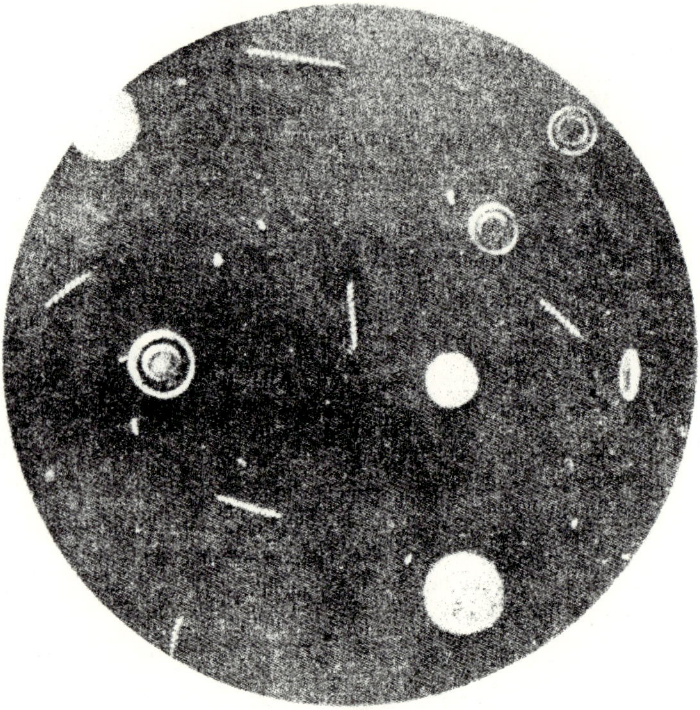

Figure 5. Dark-field mount of Treponema pallidum in exudate from penile lesion.

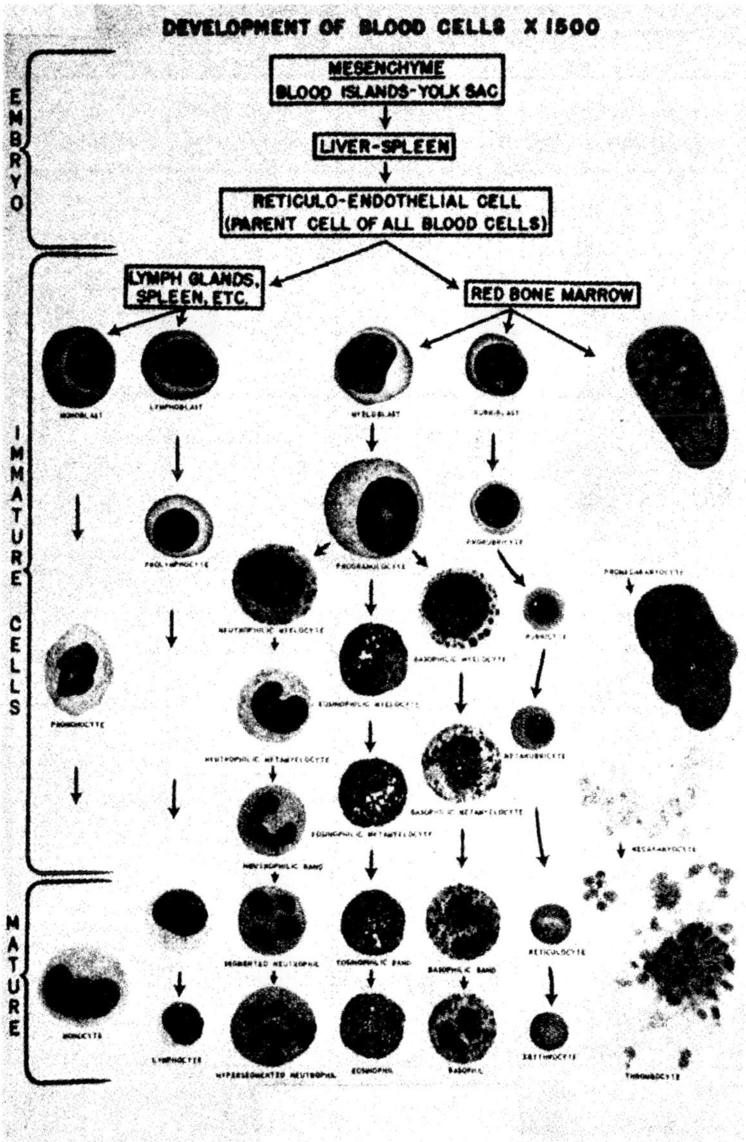
DEVELOPMENT OF BLOOD CELLS X 1500
EMBRYO
MESENCHYME
BLOOD ISLANDS-YOLK SAC
LIVER-SPLEEN
RETICULO-ENDOTHELIAL CELL
(PARENT CELL OF ALL BLOOD CELLS)
IMMATURE CELLS
LYMPH GLANDS, SPLEEN, ETC.
RED BONE MARROW
MATURE

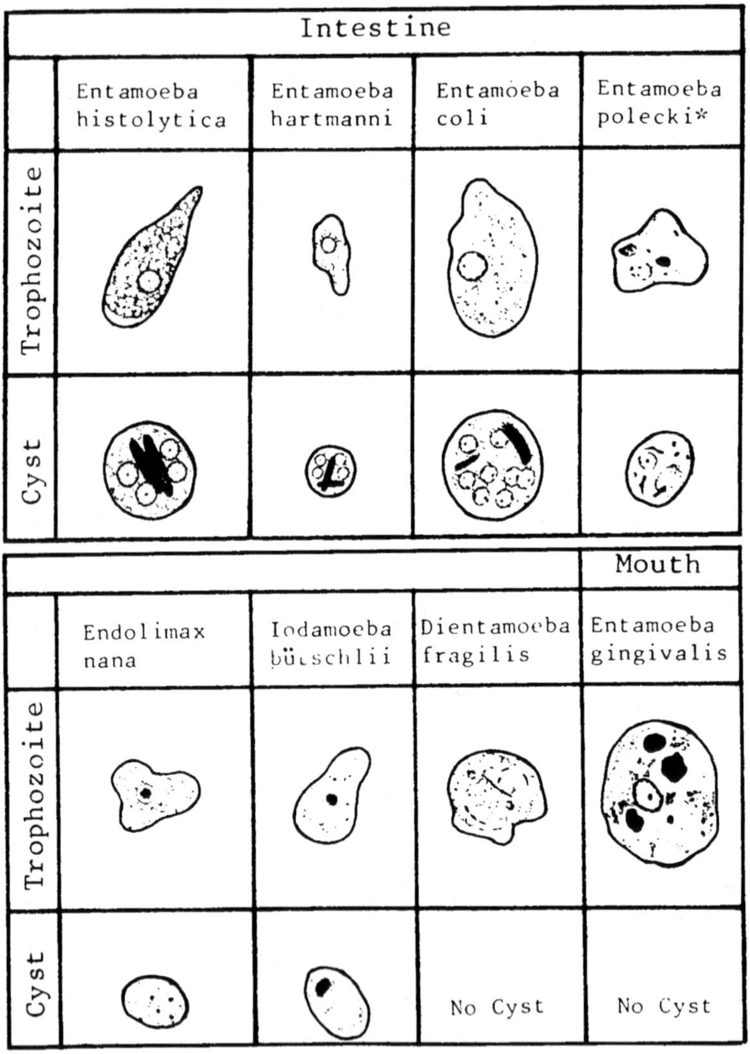

Figure 7. Intestinal protozoa and related species in man: Amebae.
Iron-hematoxylin stain.

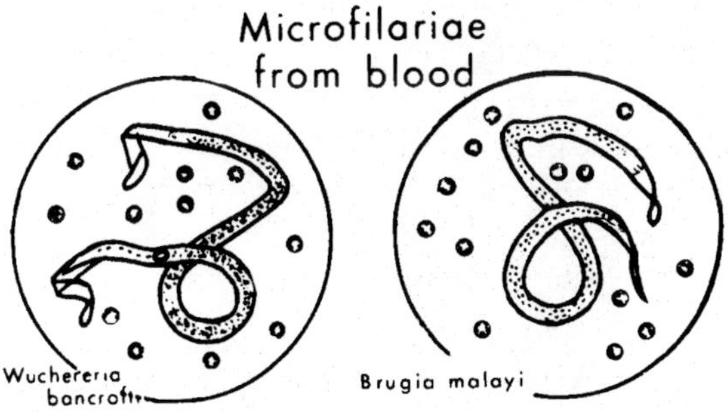

Filariasis

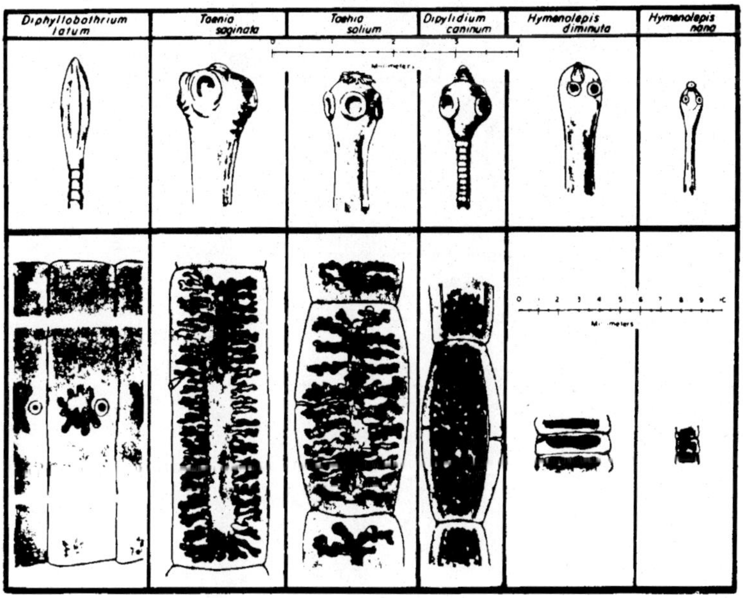

Figure 8. Scoleces and gravid proglottids of the cestode parasites commonly found in humans.

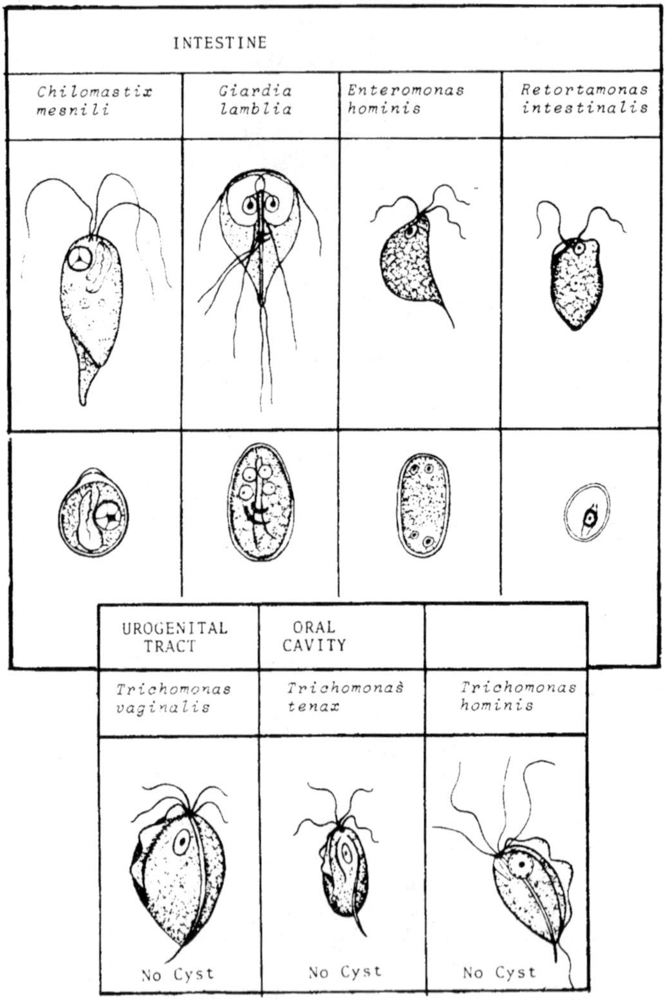

Figure 9. Intestinal protozoa and related species in man: Flagellates. Iron-hematoxylin stain.

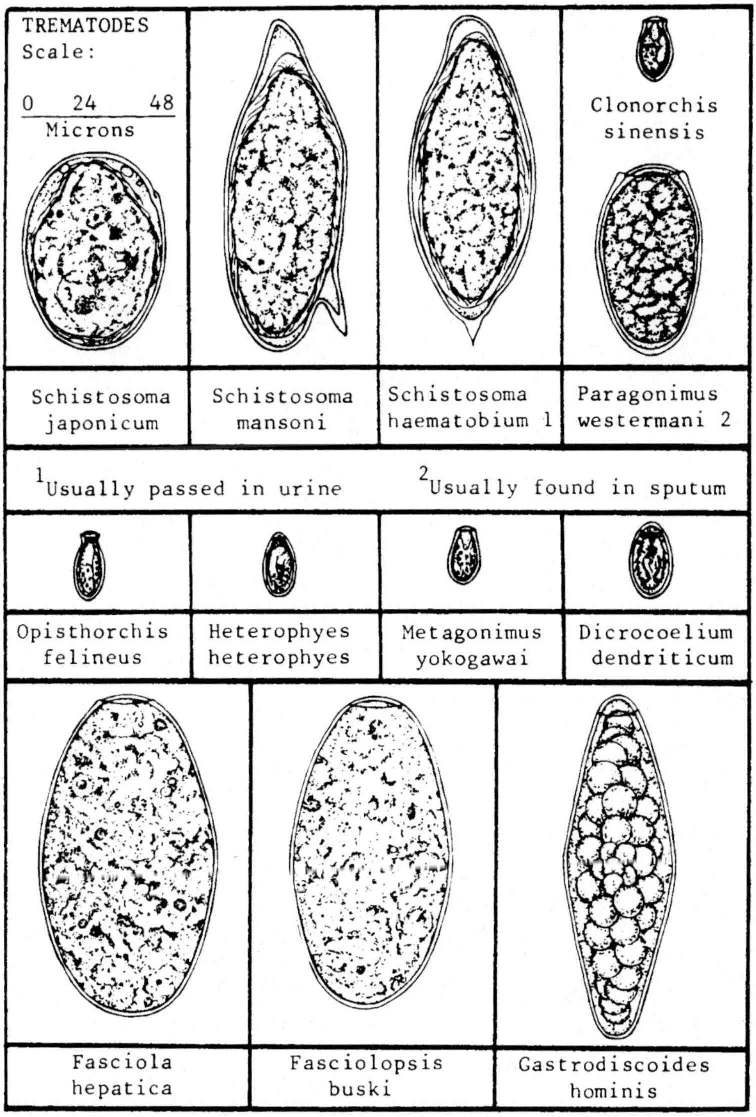

Figure 10. Trematode eggs found in humans.

(Adults)

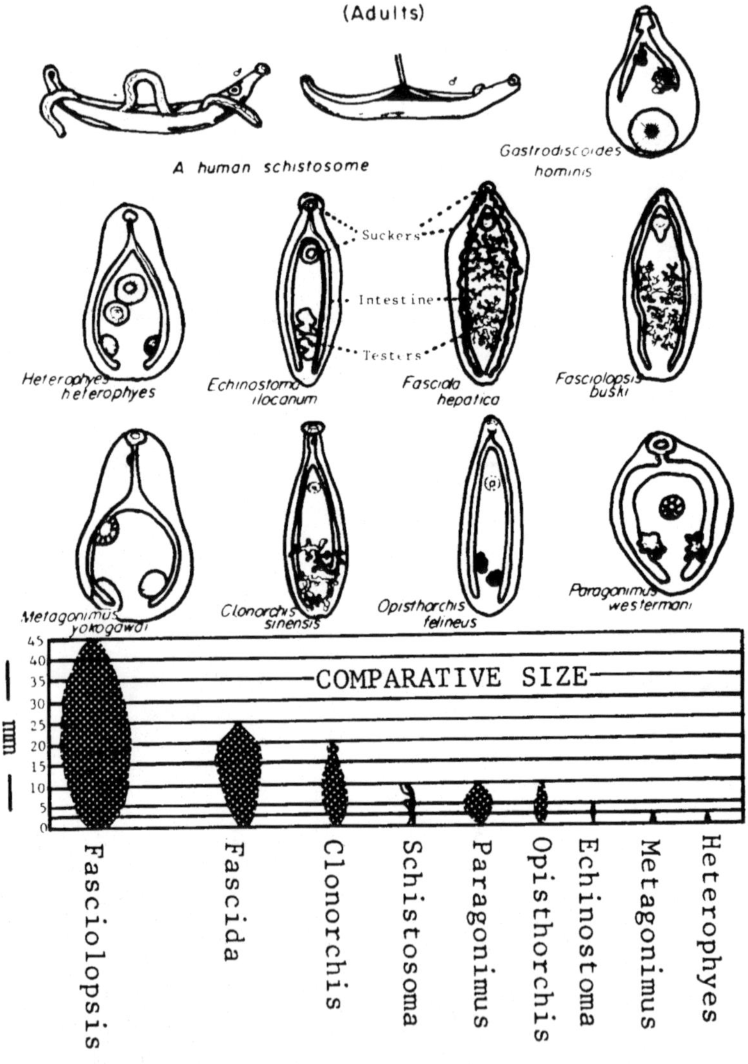

Figure 11. Different morphology of adult trematodes infecting humans.

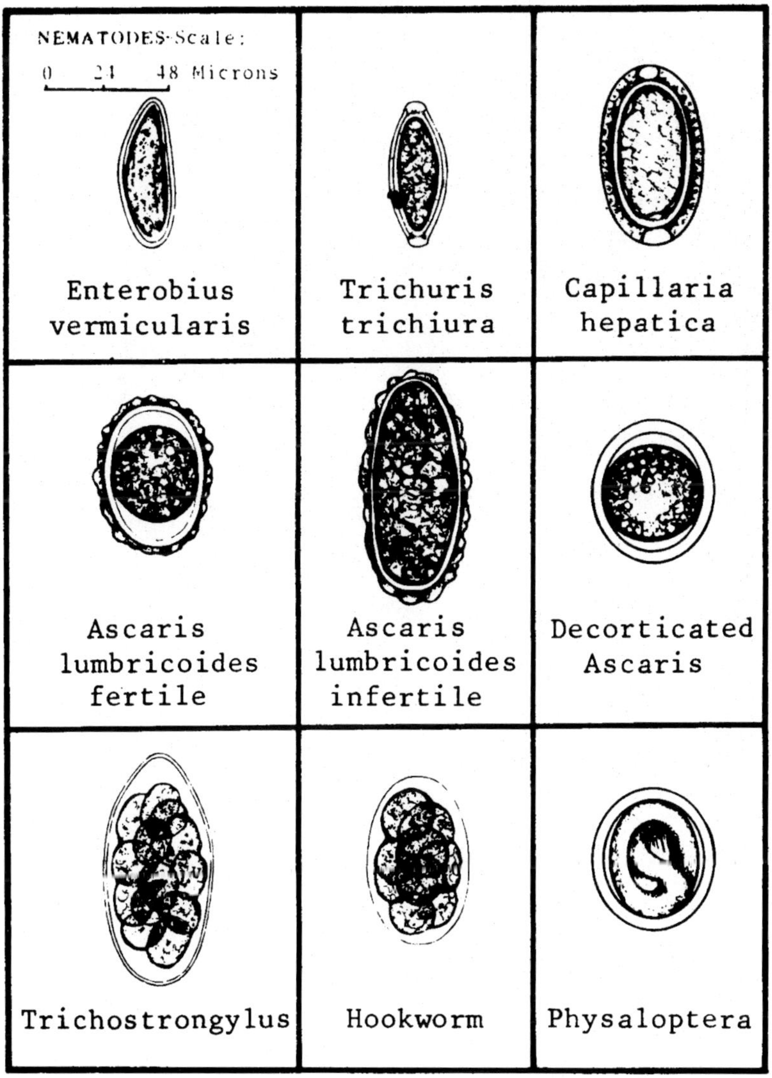

Figure 12. Nematode eggs found in humans.

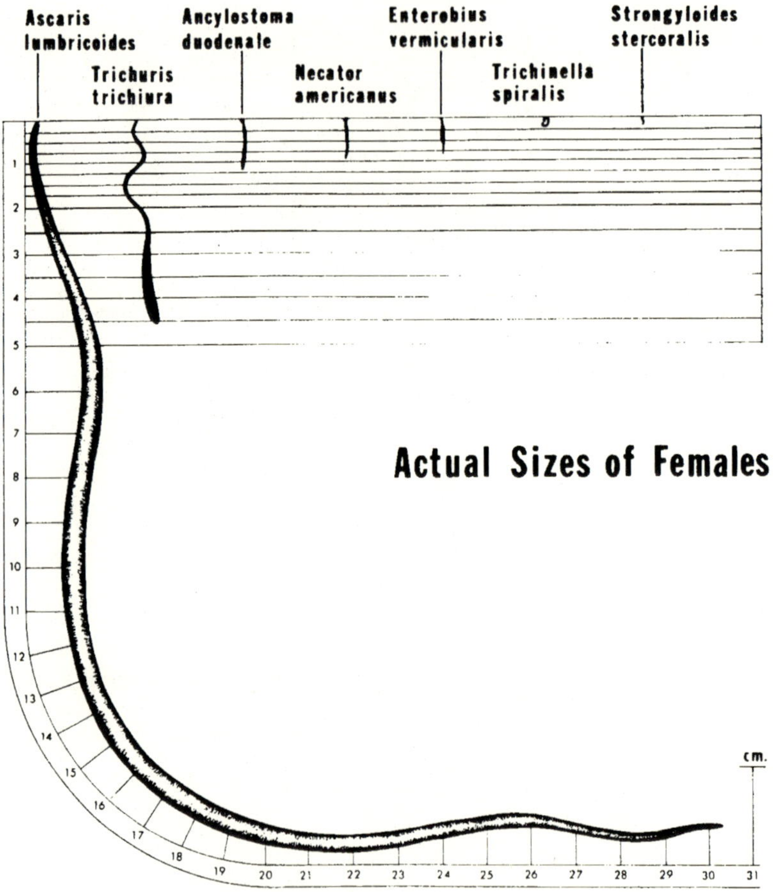

Figure 13. Relative sizes of intestinal roundworms.

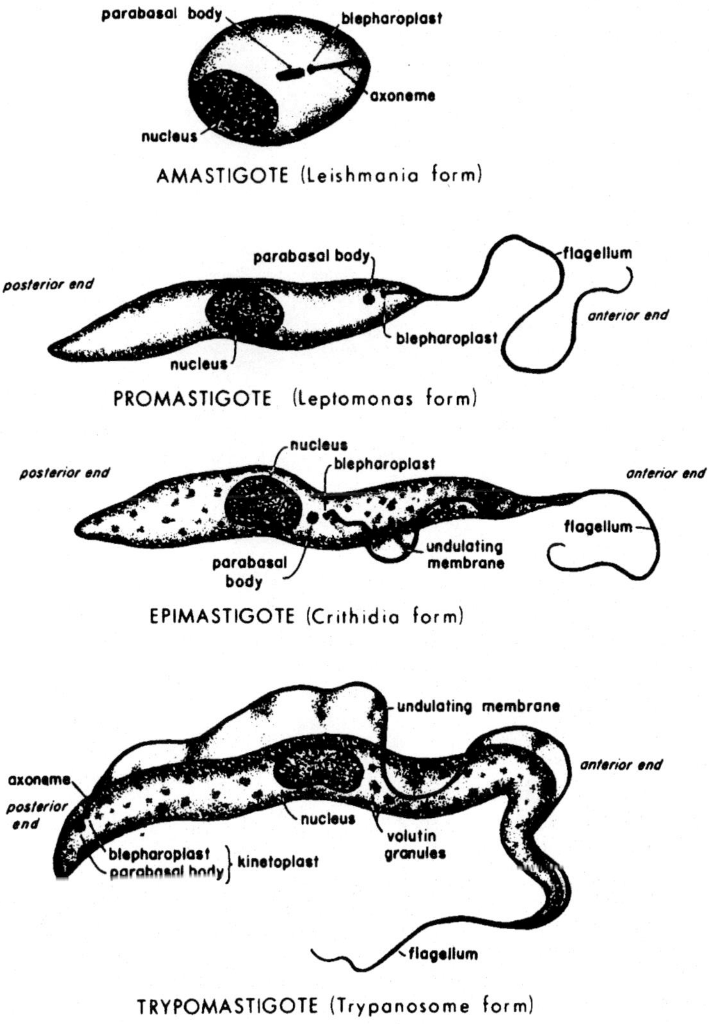

Figure 14. Morphological forms of hemoflagellates. Giemsa's stain. Greatly enlarged.

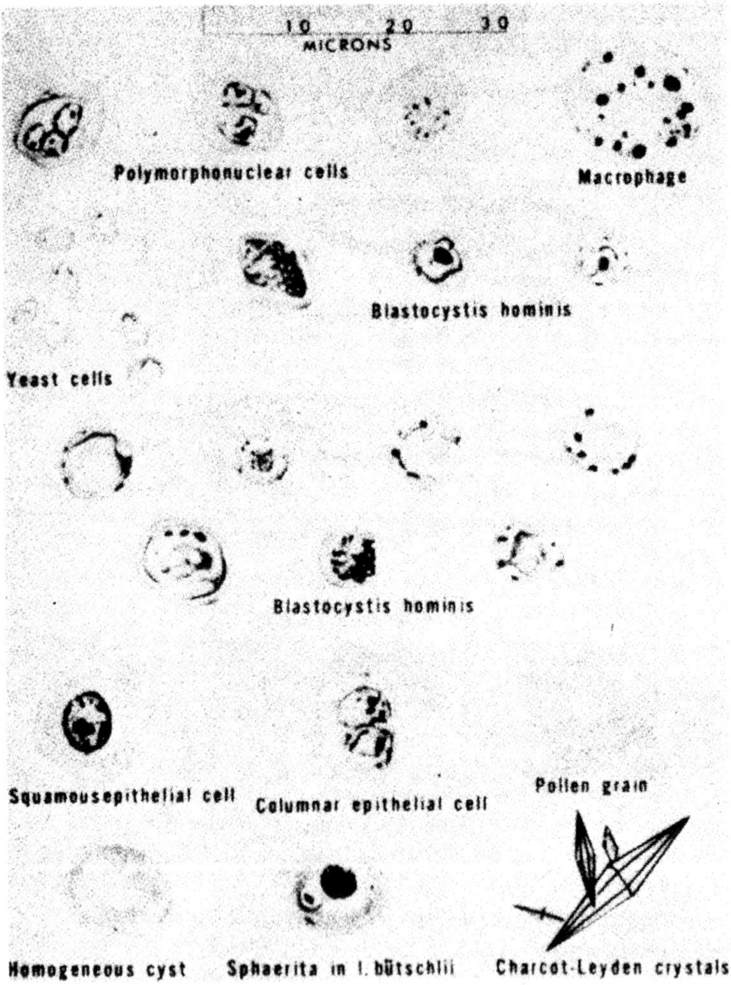

Figure 15. Objects in feces resembling protozoans.

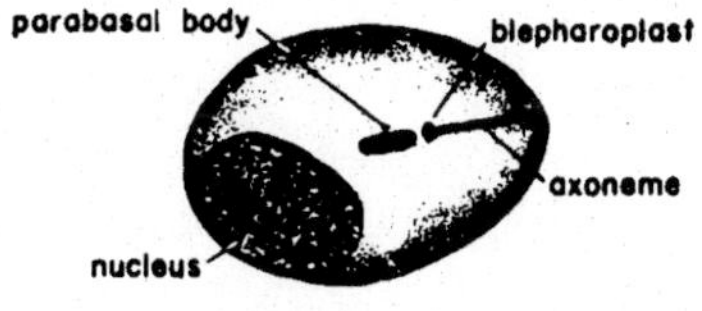

AMASTIGOTE (Leishmania form)

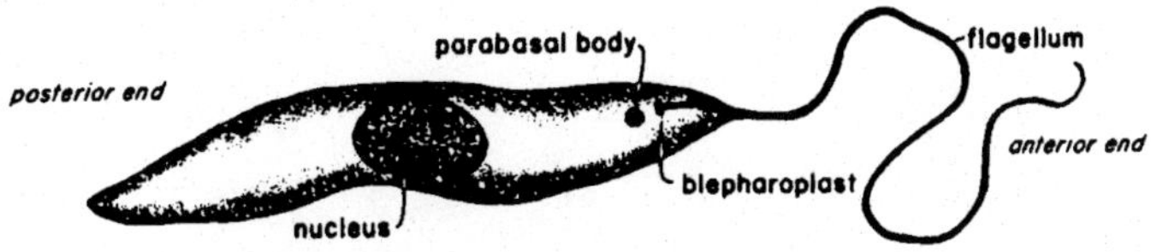

PROMASTIGOTE (Leptomonas form)

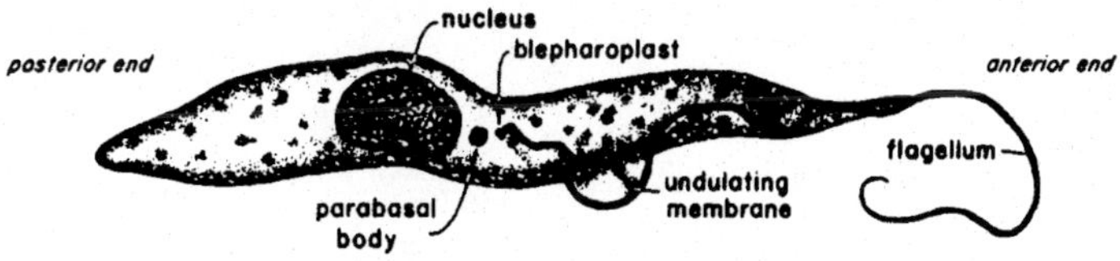

EPIMASTIGOTE (Crithidia form)

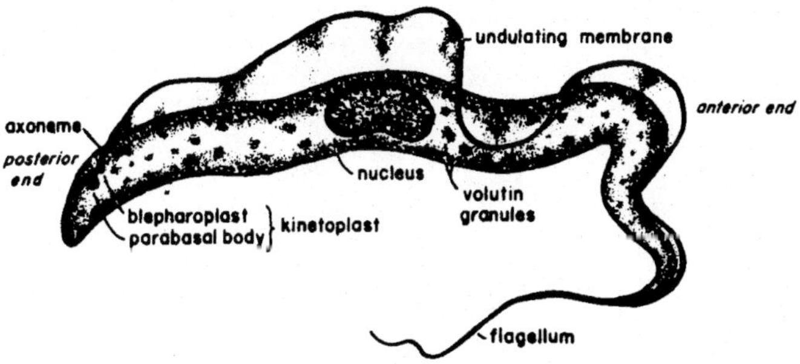

TRYPOMASTIGOTE (Trypanosome form)

Figure 14. Morphological forms of hemoflagellates. Giemsa's stain. Greatly enlarged.

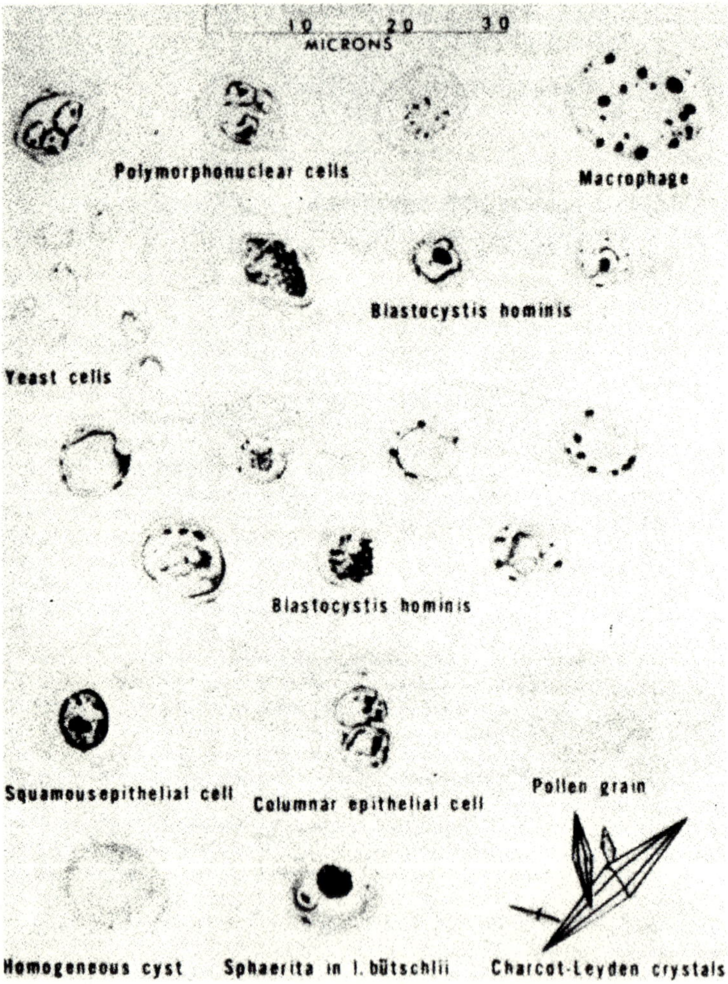

Figure 15. Objects in feces resembling protozoans.

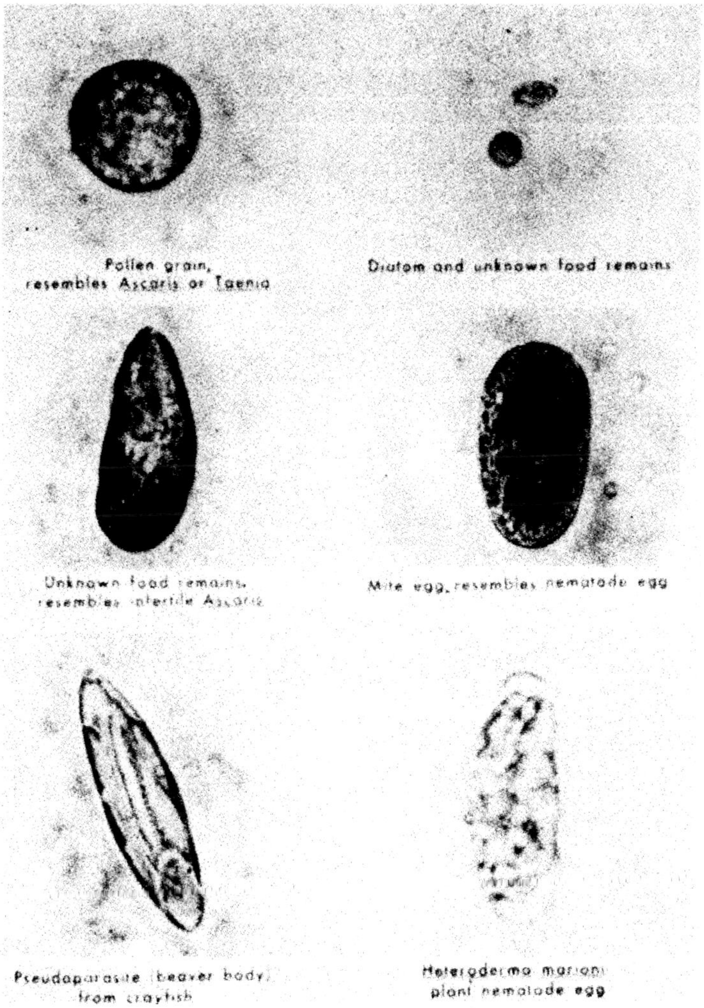

Figure 16. Objects in feces resembling the eggs of the helminths that parasitize humans.

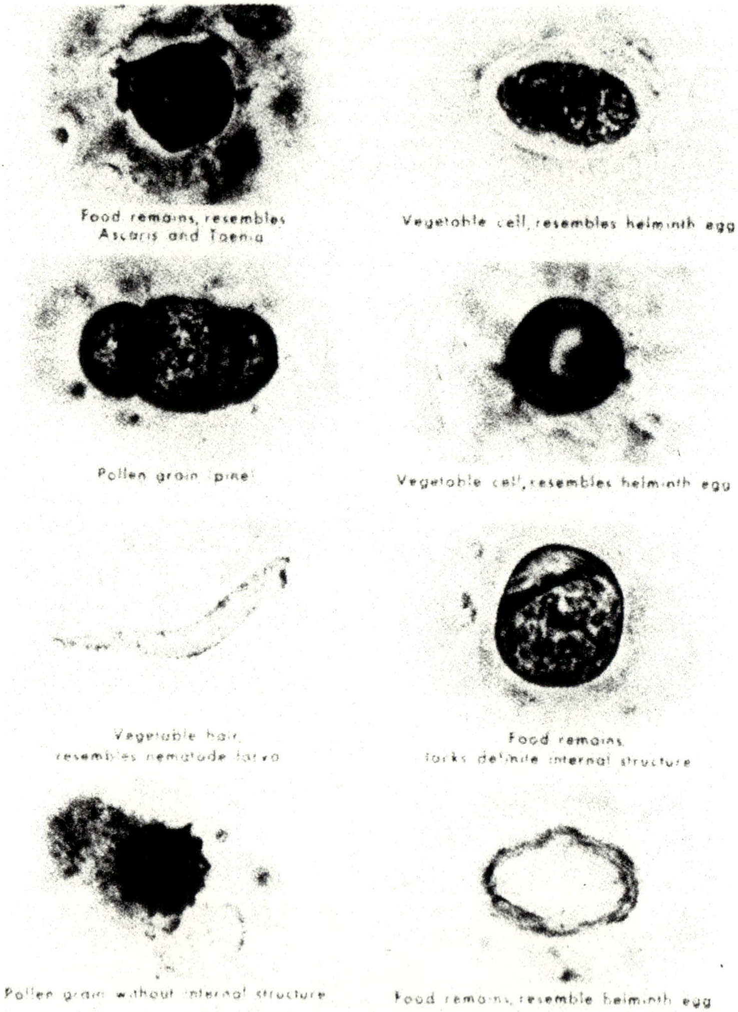

Figure 17. Objects in feces resembling the eggs of the helminths that parasitize humans.

F- Ring stage trophozoite.
G- Older ameboid trophozoite in process of development.
H- Mature trophzoite.
I- Mature trophzoite with chromatin in process of division.
J- Young schizont showing early division of chromatin.

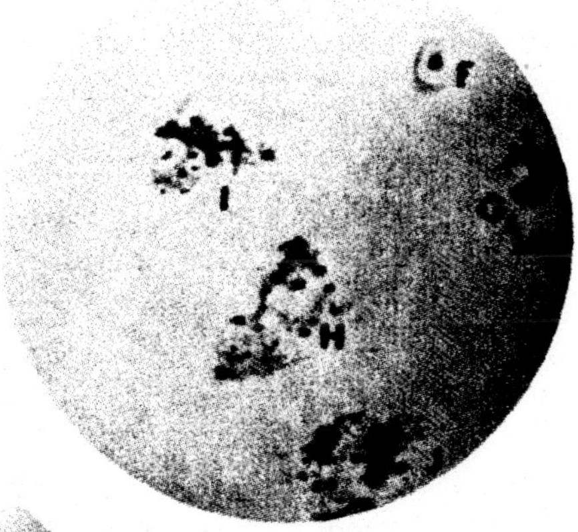

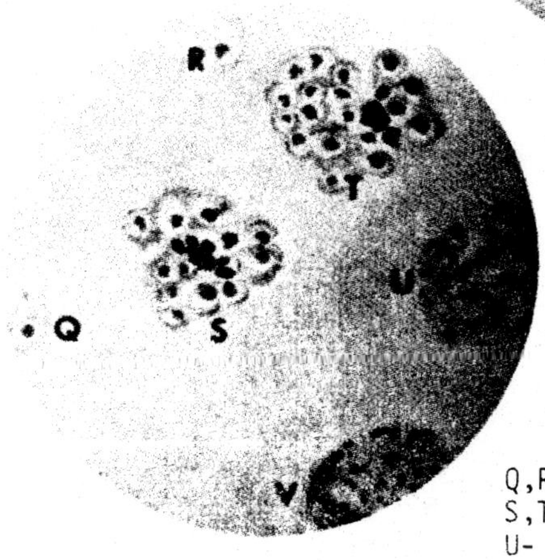

Q,R- Young rings.
S,T- Mature schizonts
U- Mature microgametocytes
V- Mature macrogametocytes

Figure 18. Plasmodium vivax. Giemsa's stain.

A,B,C, - Single nucleus ring forms
D,E - Double nucleus ring forms
F,G,H - Platelets
I- White blood cell

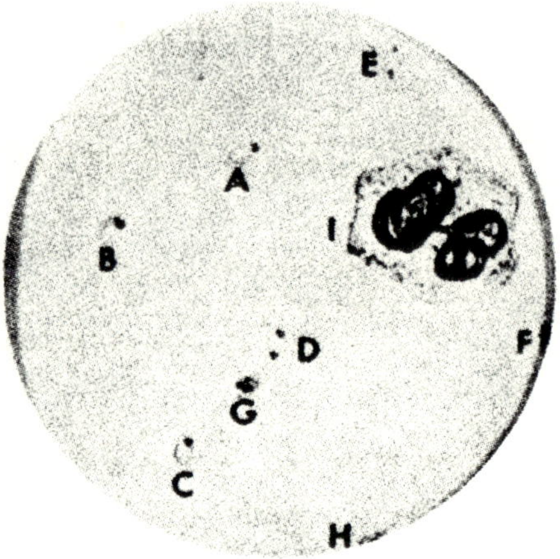

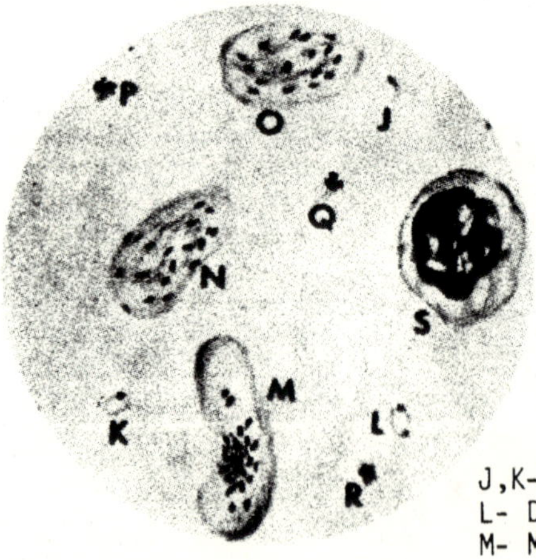

J,K- Single nucleus ring form
L- Double nucleus ring form
M- Mature macrogametocyte

Figure 19. Plasmodium falciparum. Giemsa's Stain.

A,B,C- Ring forms
D,E- Developing trophozoites
F- First stage schizont
G,H,I- Blood platelets
J- White blood cells
K,L,M,N- Ring forms

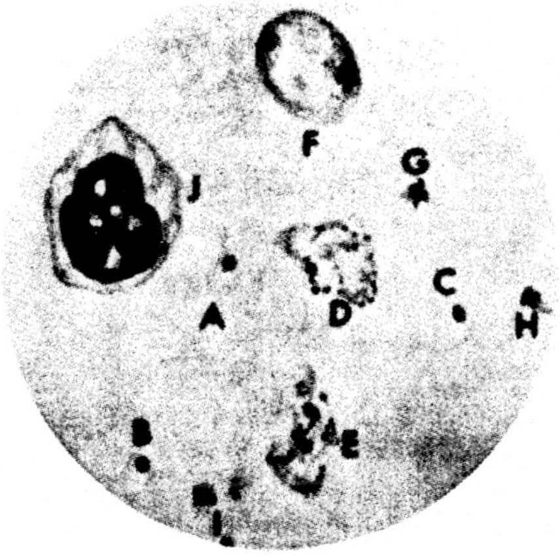

O,P,- Platelets
Q- Immature schizont
R- Mature schizont
S- Mature macrogametocyte
T- Mature microgametocyte

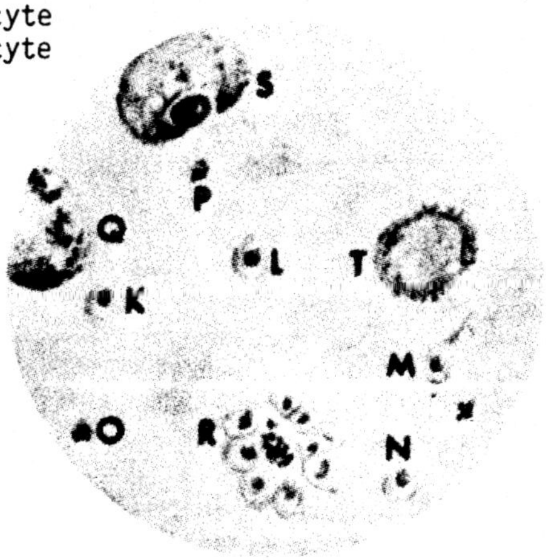

Figure 20. Plasmodium malariae. Giemsa's stain.

A- Young ring-shaped trophozoites
B,C,D- Older ring-shaped trophozoites

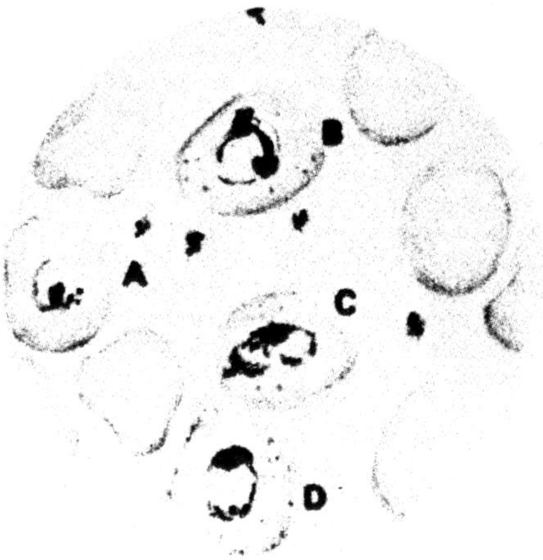

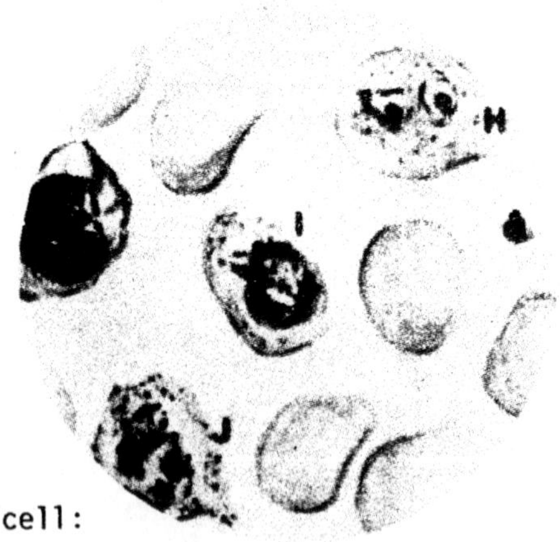

H- Doubly infected cell:
trophozoites
I- Developing schizont
J- First stage of the schizont

Figure 21. Plasmodium ovale. Giemsa's stain.

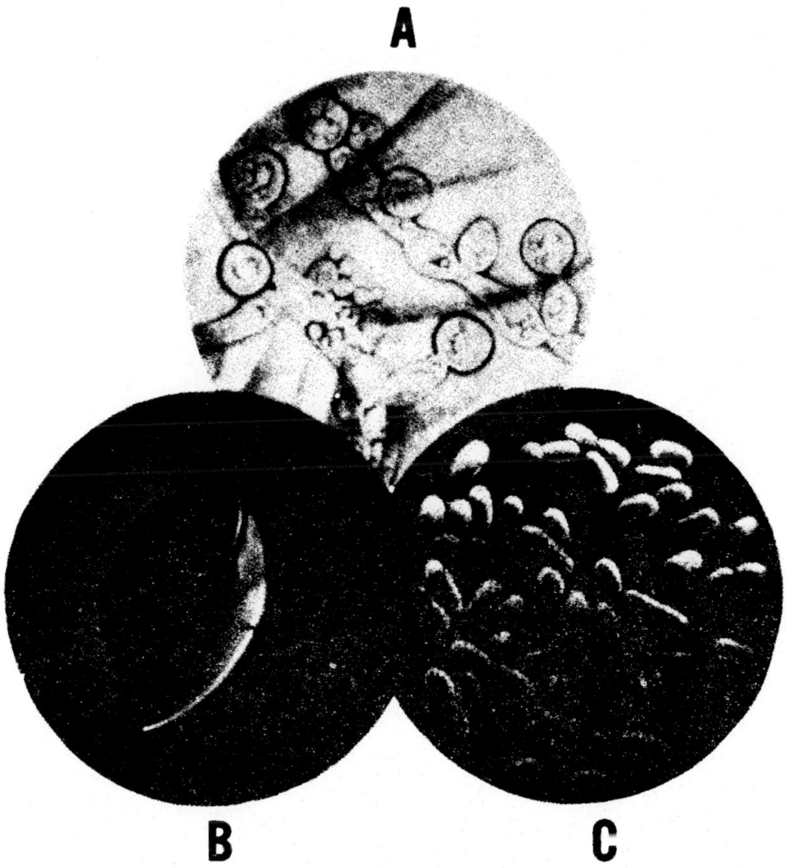

A-Candida albicans mycelia
B-Trichomonas vaginalis
C-Clue Cells,Hemophilus vaginalis

Figure 22. Causative agents of vaginitis.

APPENDIX C

LABORATORY PROCEDURES

C-1. NORMAL VALUES FOR URINE.

Color: Straw - yellow - amber.

Appearance: Clear - hazy - cloudy.

Reaction (pH): 4.6 - 8.

Specific gravity: 1.003-1.030 (for 24-hr specimen, specific gravity will range 1.015-1.025).

If there is a delay in analysis, add 4 drops of formalin to 100 cc. of urine to preserve specimen. Do not use if sugar concentration is to be determined. To obtain specific gravity when an insufficient amount of urine is present to float the weighted meter:

a. Dilute with distilled water and measure specific gravity of dilute mixture.

b. Multiply the numbers after decimal point by total volume of urine and water.

c. Divide by volume of urine diluted.

d. Add 1.

Example: 20 cc. of urine is diluted with 30 cc. of distilled water.

The specific gravity of this diluted mixture is 1.006; therefore, the undiluted urine is $\frac{.006 \times 50}{20} + 1 = 1.015$

C-2. STAINING TECHNIQUES.

a. Gram's stain.

(1) Dry thoroughly (air dry).

(2) Heat fix.

NOTE: Specimen is fixed to slide and may be stained at a later time without deterioration.

(3) Crystal violet (1 min).

(4) Wash with water.

(5) Gram's iodine (1 min).

(6) Wash with water.

(7) Spray with decolorizer (3-5 sec).

(8) Wash with water.

(9) Safranin (30 sec).

(10) Wash with water.

(11) Air dry.

b. Wright's stain.

(1) Air dry slide.

(2) Wright's stain (2 min).

(3) Add D/water (buffer) (4 min).

(4) Wash with water.

(5) Air dry.

NOTE: The times recommended for staining and buffering are approximate and should be adjusted with each fresh batch of stain.

C-3. DIRECT WET SMEAR. In the microscopic examination of fecal specimens for ova and parasites, the most simplified method is the direct wet smear method.

a. Materials needed:

(1) Medicine dropper.

(2) Physiological saline.

(3) Coverslips.

(4) Slides.

(5) Applicator sticks.

b. Technique:

(1) Place 1 drop of saline in center of slide.

(2) Select a small portion of feces and mix on slide with the 1 drop of saline that has been previously placed there.

(3) Add cover slip to the mixture and examine first using low power, then switch to high power for better observation of suspicious objects.

Adding a drop of Lugol's solution to a small portion of feces may be used as a rapid screening technique.

C-4. FORMALIN ETHER SEDIMENTATION METHOD. This method is excellent for recovery of cysts and helminth eggs.

a. Materials and equipment:

(1) Physiologic saline.
(2) Gauze.

(3) Formalin (10%).
(4) Ether.
(5) Applicator sticks.
(6) Slides.
(7) Beaker or specimen container.
(8) Funnel.
(9) Pointed centrifuge tubes.
(10) Stopper for centrifuge tubes.
(11) Coverslips.
(12) Iodine solution.

b. Technique:

(1) Take small portion of feces and mix in 10-12 cc. of saline in a beaker.

(2) Pass mixture through two layers of wet gauze, using funnel, into a pointed centrifuge tube.

(3) Centrifuge for 2 min at 1,500-2,000 rpm.

(4) Pour off supernate and resuspend sediment in fresh saline.

(5) Centrifuge again at 1,500-2,000 rpm for 2 min.

(6) Pour off supernate, resuspend sediment in fresh saline.

(7) Centrifuge again 1,500-2,000 rpm for 2 min.

(8) Pour off supernate.

(9) Repeat steps 6 and 7 until supernate is relatively clear.

(10) Add 10 cc. of 10% formalin to sediment.

(11) Mix thoroughly (1 min).

(12) Let stand for at least 10 min.

(13) Add 3 cc. of ether.

(14) Stopper the tube.

(15) Shake vigorously until thoroughly mixed (1 min).

(16) Centrifuge at <u>1,500 rpm</u> for 2 min.

(Four layers should result in tube: A small amount of sediment containing most of the protozoan cysts and ova, a layer of formalin, a plug of detritus just on top of the formalin, and a topmost layer of ether.)

(17) With applicator stick ream centrifuge tube to loosen fecal plug and pour off supernate.

(18) Quickly decant (pour off) the top three layers leaving the sediment undisturbed.

(19) Swab inside of centrifuge tube to clean all residue to

prevent contaminating sediment when pouring.

(20) Using applicator stick, mix remaining sediment in the tube with fluid that will drain back from the sides.

(21) Place drop on slide, add a drop of iodine, mix thoroughly, add coverslip, and examine using low power.

(22) Switch to high power to confirm findings.

All fecal specimens should be put in MIF solution prior to examinations. This will save space, cut down on stench, and preserve specimen (walnut size portion of specimen is all that is needed for lab findings).

Taking portions of specimen plus 3 times portion of MIF is the proper way to store or send specimen from field.

Formula for MIF: Lugol's solution - 10 parts, formaldehyde - 12.5 parts, tincture merthiolate - 77.5 parts.

Formula for Lugol's solution: Iodine (powdered crystals) 5 gm, potassium iodine (KI) 10 gm, distilled water 100 cc.; mix thoroughly and filter. This solution will remain satisfactory for months.

C-5. "DIXIE CUP" TECHNIQUE.

a. This technique is a variation of the formalin ether sedimentation method. It is faster, materials are a little cheaper, and it is thought to cause less damage to the ova, making them easier to recognize under the microscope. The technique is especially good for making a diagnosis in a low density infestation.

b. Technique:

(1) Add 50 ml. of MIF solution to about 25 ml. of feces.

(2) Stir and filter through two layers of gauze into a small paper cup (Dixie cup).

(3) Let it stand for 5 min and pour off the top layers of fluid, leaving about 10 ml. of material in the cup.

(4) Pour this 10 ml. of material into a test tube and add 3 to 5 ml. of ether.

(5) Centrifuge for 2 min at 1,500 rpm.

(6) Pour off the top layers of fluid (supernatant). Put a drop of the residue on a slide for microscopic examination.

C-6. TUBES ("VACUTAINERS"). Tubes to be used if sending specimens to hospital lab and if the following tubes are available:

a. Gray stopper tube.

(1) Sugar.

(2) Bun.

(3) NPN.

(4) Ammonia.

(5) Iron.

b. Purple stopper tube.

(1) Hematology (W.B.C., etc.).

(2) Alcohol.

(3) Carbon dioxide.

(4) Carbon monoxide.

(5) Oxygen.

c. Red stopper.

All procedures requiring clotted blood.

C-7. STOOL GUAIAC FOR OCCULT BLOOD.

a. Reagents:

(1) Hydrogen peroxide (3%).

(2) Glacial acetic acid.

(3) Saturated solution of gum guaiac in 95% ethyl alcohol.

b. Procedure:

(1) Smear small bit of feces on filter paper.

(2) Add:

(a) 1 drop guaiac solution .

(b) 1 drop glacial acetic acid.

(c) 1 drop hydrogen peroxide.

c. Interpretation of results:

(1) Positive reaction is when a blue or dark green color appears in 30 sec.

(2) Other colors or delayed reaction are regarded as negative.

APPENDIX D

CELLULAR COMPONENTS OF BLOOD, NORMAL VALUES,

AND SIGNIFICANCE OF BLOOD TEST

D-1. ERYTHROCYTES (RED BLOOD CELLS).

a. Erythrocytes comprise the majority of all blood cells; they are chiefly responsible for the color of blood. There are approximately 5 million erythrocytes in 1 cubic mm. of blood.

b. Normal red cell is a biconcave disk; red cell in normal blood has no nucleus.

c. Their principal function is to transport oxygen (accomplished by iron-containing hemoglobin). There are 15 grams of hemoglobin per 100 ml. of blood.

d. Red blood cells are produced in red bone marrow, which also provides most of the blood's leukocytes and all its platelets. Red cells of normal adults are found in short and flat bones--ribs, sternum, skull, vertebrae, bones of the hands and feet.

e. Bone marrow requires a number of nutrients, including iron, vitamin B_{12}, folic acid, and pyridoxine for normal erythropoiesis (formation of red cells).

g. Normal life expectancy of a red cell is between 115 and 130 days. It is then eliminated by phagocytosis in the reticuloendothelial system, predominately in the spleen and liver.

D-2. LEUKOCYTES (WHITE BLOOD CELLS).

a. Leukocytes normally are present in a concentration of between 5,000 and 10,000 cells in each cubic millimeter of blood (1 white cell for every 500-1,000 red cells).

b. Leukocytes have a nucleus and are capable of active movement.

c. Major categories of leukocytes include the granulocytic series, lymphocytes, monocytes, and plasma cells.

d. Leukocytosis--white cell count over 10,000.

e. Leukopenia--white cell count below 5,000.

f. Granulocytes--leukocytes produced in the marrow.

(1) Comprise 70% of all white cells.

(2) Called granulocytes because of the abundant granules contained in their cytoplasm, or polymorphonuclear leukocytes since their nuclei, when mature, are of a highly irregular, multilobed configuration.

g. Lymphocytes--a variety of leukocyte that arises in the thymus gland and lymph nodes; generally described as nongranular and including small and large varieties.

(1) Responsible for the immunologic competence of an individual.

(2) Comprise about 25 percent of the circulating white cells.

h. Monocytes--derived from components of the reticuloendothelial system (particularly spleen, liver, and lymph nodes).

(1) Constitute a ready source of mobile phagocytes, congregating and performing their scavenging function at sites of inflammation and tissue necrosis.

(2) Account for about 5 percent of the white cell count.

i. Plasmocytes--formed in the lymph nodes and bone marrow.

(1) Are the main and probably sole source of the circulating immune globulins.

(2) Represent approximately 1 percent of the blood leukocytes.

D-3. PLATELETS (THROMBOCYTES).

a. Platelets are the smallest and most fragile of the formed elements; they are small particles (devoid of nuclei) that arise as a result of a fragmentation from giant cells called megakaryocytes in the bone marrow.

b. There are approximately 250,000-500,000 platelets per cubic millimeter of blood.

c. Their prime function is to halt bleeding--accomplished by congregating and clumping at all sites of vascular injury and by plugging with their own substance the lumen of the blood vessels. As they disintegrate they release a constituent (platelet factor 3) that initiates clot formation in their immediate vicinity, thereby checking the flow of blood through the leakage of blood from the lacerated vessel.

d. They cause blood clots to shrink (retract), the effect of which is to draw together the margins of vascular defects, reduce their size, and further stem the leakage.

D-4. HEMATOLOGY NORMAL VALUES.

a. Hematocrit--Men: 39-54%; Women: 36-47%.

b. Hemoglobin--Children: 12-14 gm%; Newborn: 14.5-24.5 gm%.

c. If one counted 100 W.B.C. randomly on a blood smear, the white blood cells present in normal blood, the breakdown would be as follows: Total W.B.C. = 4,500-10,000.

(1) Segmented neutrophils	45-75%
(2) Immature band neutrophils	0- 7%
(3) Lymphocytes	15-35%
(4) Eosinophils	0- 7%
(5) Basophils	0- 1%

(6) Monocytes 0-12%

d. Normal platelet counts are usually in the range of 180,000-400,000. A "shift to the left" is a term for an increase over normal in the number of immature or "band" neutrophils. This is usually seen in the early part of an infection. A "shift to the right" refers to preponderance of mature (segmented) neutrophils as seen in the later stages of an infection.

D-5. CAUSES OF EOSINOPHILIA (7% or more).

a. Allergic states: Hay fever, asthma, exfoliative dermatitis, erythema multiforme, and drug reactions.

b. Parasitic diseases: Intestinal forms (hookworm, roundworm) and tissue forms (Toxocara, Trichina, Strongyloides, Echinococcus).

c. Skin disorders: Pemphigus and dermatitis herpetiformis.

d. Neoplasms: Myeloproliferative disorders, Hodgkin's disease, and metastatic carcinoma.

e. Other disorders: Scarlet fever, polyarteritis, eosinophilic granuloma, tropical eosinophilia, and pernicious anemia.

D-6. CAUSES OF NEUTROPHILIA (W.B.C. 10,000 or more).

a. Infection: Due to bacteria (especially pyogenic), mycobacteria, fungi, spirochetes, and parasites. May be localized or generalized.

b. Metabolic disorders: Due to diverse causes resulting in uremia, diabetes, acidosis, gout, and eclampsia.

c. Neoplasms: Usually widely disseminated myeloproliferative disorders, lymphoma, and metastatic carcinoma.

D-7. CAUSES OF NEUTROPENIA (W.B.C. 5,000 or below).

a. Infections: Acute viral (rubeola, hepatitis), rickettsial, bacterial (typhoid, brucella), or protozoan (malaria). All grave infections (bacteremia, miliary tuberculosis).

b. Marrow aplasia: Due to chemical or physical agents that regularly produce aplasia (e.g., benzol, radiation) and other rarer causes (drugs).

c. Nutritional deficits: Folic acid and vitamin B_{12}.

d. Splenomegaly: Due to diverse causes (e.g., congestive, infiltrative).

e. Other disorders: Systemic lupus erythematosus, anaphylaxis, antileukocyte antibodies, immunodeficiencies, pancreatic exocrine deficiency, and cyclic neutropenia (familial and sporadic).

D-8. CAUSES OF LYMPHOCYTOSIS (Lymphocyte count >35%).

a. Acute infection: Infectious mononucleosis, infectious

lymphocytosis, pertussis, mumps, rubella, infectious hepatitis, and the convalescent stage of many acute infections.

b. Chronic infections: Tuberculosis, syphilis, and brucellosis.

c. Metabolic disorders: Thyrotoxicosis and adrenal cortical insufficiency.

d. Neoplasms: Chronic lymphatic leukemia, lymphosarcoma.

D-9. CAUSES OF MONOCYTOSIS.

a. Bacterial infections: Brucellosis, tuberculosis, subacute bacterial endocarditis, and, rarely, typhoid fever.

b. Rickettsial infections: Rocky mountain spotted fever, typhus.

c. Protozoan infections: Malaria.

d. Neoplasms: Monocytic leukemia, Hodgkin's disease and other lymphomas, myeloproliferative disorders, multiple myeloma, and carcinomatosis.

e. Connective tissue disease: Rheumatoid arthritis and systemic lupus erythematosus.

f. Other disorders: Chronic ulcerative colitis, regional enteritis, sarcoidosis, lipid-storage diseases, hemolytic anemia, hypochromic anemia, and recovery from agranulocytosis.

D-10. CAUSES OF BONE MARROW PLASMACYTOSIS.

a. Acute infections: Rubella, rubeola, varicella, infectious hepatitis, infectious mononucleosis, and scarlet fever.

b. Chronic infections: Tuberculosis, syphilis, and fungus.

c. Allergic states: Serum sickness and drug reactions.

d. Collagen-vascular disorders: Acute rheumatic fever, rheumatoid arthritis, and systemic lupus erythematosus.

e. Neoplasms: Disseminated carcinoma, Hodgkin's disease, and multiple myeloma.

f. Other: Cirrhosis of the liver.

APPENDIX E

HISTORY AND PHYSICAL EXAMINATION GUIDE

E-1. OUTLINE OF MEDICAL HISTORY.

a. Identifying data: Name, rank, service number, unit, birthdate, sex, occupation, race, religion, marital status.

b. Chief complaint: Concise statement of primary reason the patient seeks help.

c. Present illness: State of health prior to onset of illness, nature and circumstances of onset, location and nature of pain or discomfort, progression, treatment received and its effect.

d. Past history:

(1) Childhood diseases.

(2) Previous illnesses and injuries.

(3) Previous hospitalization and surgery.

(4) Review of systems.

e. Family history: History of diabetes, hypertension, tuberculosis, etc.

f. Social history: Marital status, occupational data, and habits (tobacco, alcohol, drugs).

E-2. OUTLINE OF PHYSICAL EXAMINATION.

a. Vital signs: Height, weight, blood pressure, pulse, respirations, temperature.

b. General: Posture, emotional state, state of consciousness, acuteness or severity of illness.

c. Integument: Skin, hair, nails.

d. Eyes: Lids, sclera, cornea, conjunctiva, pupil, lens, fundus, ocular mobility, visual acuity.

e. Ears: External ear, canals, tympanic membranes, acuity.

f. Nose: External nose, septum, turbinates, patency.

g. Mouth: Lips, teeth, gingivae, tongue, tonsils, throat, palate, floor of mouth.

h. Neck: Trachea, thyroid, pulses, lymph nodes.

i. Lungs: Chest shape, symmetry, expansion, percussion and auscultation.

j. Heart: Pulse, B.P., color, peripheral perfusion, palpation, percussion and auscultation.

k. Breasts: Symmetry, masses, tenderness.

l. Abdomen: Inspection, palpation, percussion, auscultation for liver, spleen, kidneys, bladder, hernia, lymph nodes, masses, tenderness, muscle tone, bowel sounds.

m. Genitalia: Penis and testes.

n. Rectum and prostate.

o. Extremities: Strength, range of motion, pulses.

p. Back: Curvature, mobility.

q. Neurological: Cranial nerves, sensory system, motor system, reflexes, mental status, meningeal signs.

APPPENDIX F

FIELD STERILIZATION AND DISINFECTION

1. GENERAL.

a. An article is sterile or not sterile. There is <u>no</u> in-between. If any doubt exists, it is <u>not</u>.

b. All materials to be sterilized must be clean, free from oil, and in good working condition.

c. Wrappers for sterile goods must be double thickness and free from holes.

d. Label packs <u>when packed</u>.

e. Packs should be packaged loosely but securely.

f. Packs are dated when removed from sterilizer and are outdated in 4 weeks (2 weeks if humidity is high).

g. Articles being disinfected by boiling or with chemical solution must be covered by solution and the solution covered.

2. METHODS OF STERILIZATION AND DISINFECTION.

a. Steam under pressure (autoclave).

(1) Method of choice.

(2) Any commercial pressure cooker can be used if an autoclave is not available.

(3) Kills all organisms including spores.

(4) Must reach a <u>minimum</u> of <u>15 psi</u> and <u>250°</u>F. (121°C.) for <u>15 minutes</u> for sterilization. <u>NOTE:</u> If <u>using pressure</u> cooker, maintain approximately 17 psi on gage. This will assure 250°F. minimum temperature.

(5) Allow 30 minutes for instrument packs and linen + 15 minutes for drying, 15 minutes for rubber goods + 15 minutes for drying.

(6) Maximum size for all packs is 12 x 18 inches.

(7) Always use autoclave tape <u>and</u> Diack control if available.

b. Dry heat.

(1) Can be done in an oven.

(2) Used for ointments, oils, waxes and powders; may also be used for glassware, instruments, needles, and dry goods. It is destructive to fabrics.

(3) Time: For oils, ointments, waxes, and powders 120 minutes at 320°F.; for glassware, instruments, needles, and dry goods: 60 minutes at 320°F.

c. Flame (incineration).

(1) Used for materials that can be burned (food, paper, dressings, etc.).

(2) Time: Until completely destroyed.

d. Sunlight.

(1) Use for clothing, bedding, and mattresses.

(2) Time: 6 hours or more in direct sunlight on each side.

e. Chemicals.

(1) Zephiran chloride.

(a) Make 1:750 solution.

(b) Time: 18 hours minimum.

(c) Does not kill spores or tubercle bacilli.

(2) Alcohol.

(a) Make 70% solution.

(b) Time: 18 hours minimum.

(c) Does not kill spores.

(d) Will maintain sterility after sterilization by other methods.

(e) Add 0.5% sodium nitrite to prevent rust of instruments.

(3) Formaldehyde-alcohol solution.

(a) Most active germicidal agent available and will kill spores.

(b) RX.

Ethyl or isopropyl alcohol 99%	700 ml.
Formaldehyde solution U.S.P. 37%	25 ml.
Sodium nitrite	1.0 gm
Sodium bicarbonate	1.0 gm
Distilled water Q.S.ad	1,000 ml.

(c) Time: Metal instruments, 3 hours; catheters, 18-24 hours.

f. Boiling.

(1) Start timing after water comes to boil.

(2) Add 5 minutes time for each 1,000 ft elevation above sea level.

(3) Do not boil blades, scissors, etc., except in emergency (rusts edges).

(4) Addition of sodium carbonate to make a 2% solution will increase effectiveness.

(5) Boil for 30 minutes at sea level.

(6) Boiling does not kill spores.

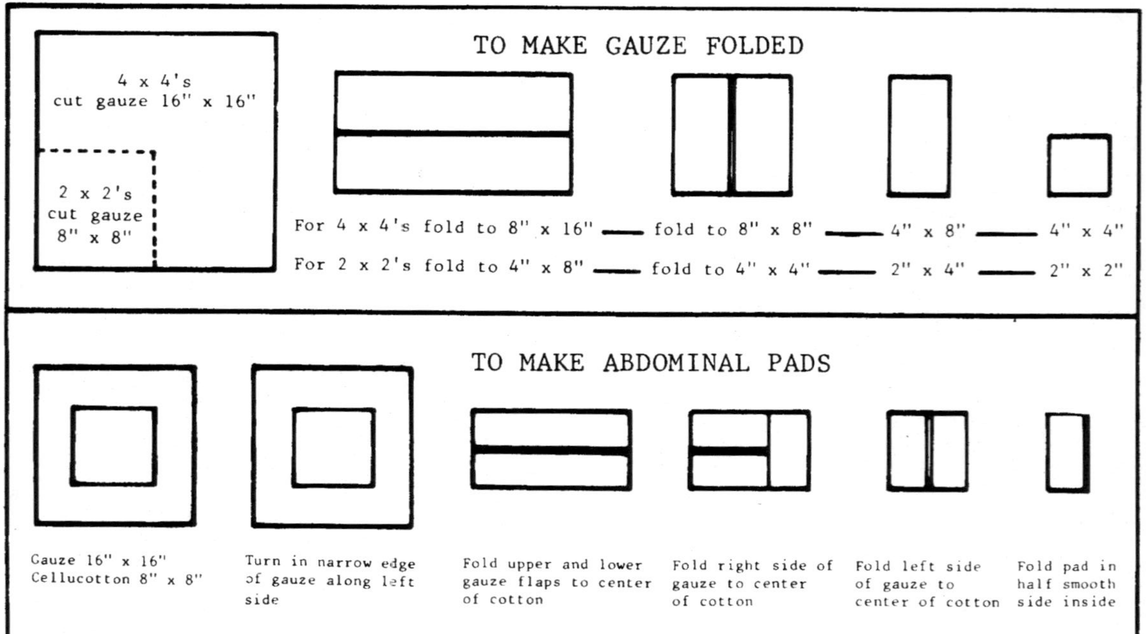

PREPARATION OF SURGICAL SUPPLIES

TO WRAP DRY GOODS

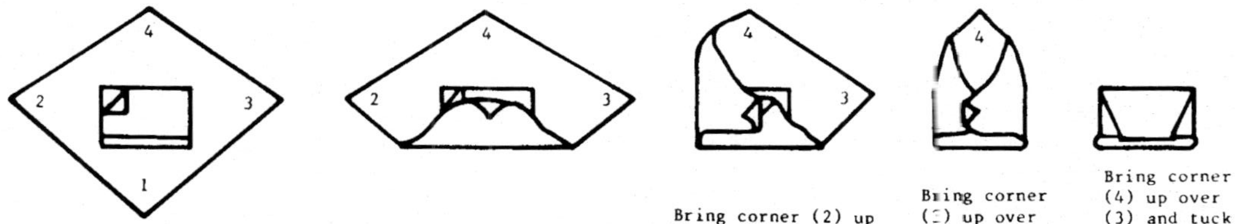

Place article to be wrapped on a double muslin or heavy paper

Bring corner (1) up over article; fold back flap

Bring corner (2) up over article; fold back flap

Bring corner (3) up over article; fold back flap

Bring corner (4) up over (3) and tuck under (2) and (3)

TO MAKE COTTON APPLICATORS

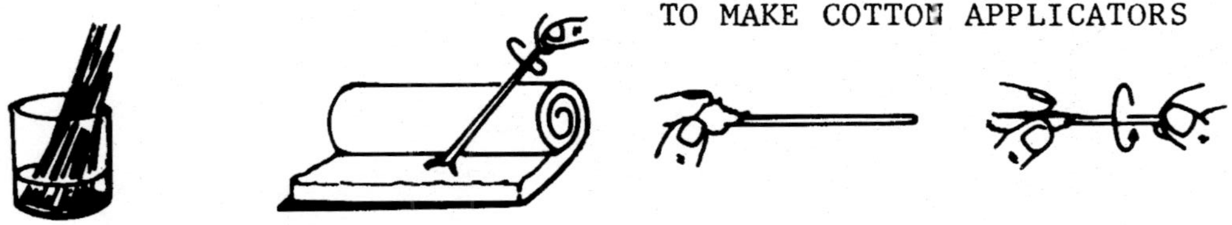

Place several applicator sticks in a small container of water.

Take applicator stick. Pick up small amount of cotton rotating stick.

Smooth cotton over end of stick; be sure tip is covered.

Wind cotton around stick.

PREPARATION OF SURGICAL SUPPLIES(CONT'D)

TO MAKE COTTON BALLS

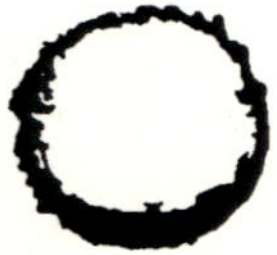

Take circular

piece of cotton

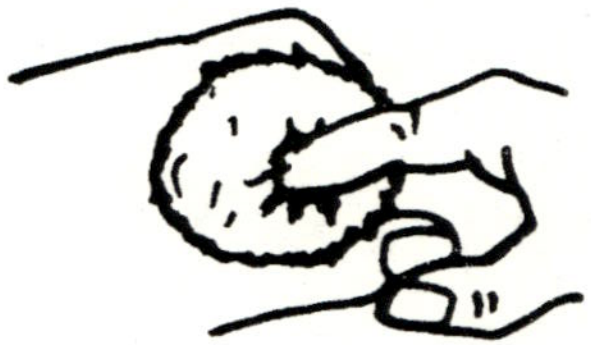

Place piece of cotton in circle formed by index finger and thumb; press in center of cotton.

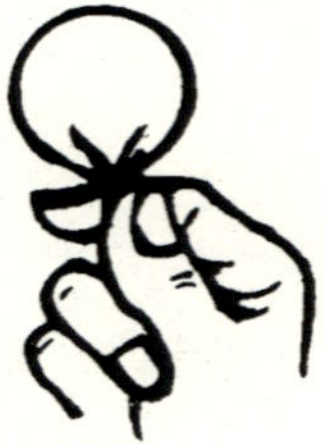

Moisten tips of index and middle finger, twist top of cotton together between fingers.

PREPARATION OF SURGICAL SUPPLIES(CONT'D)

APPENDIX G

DRUG OF CHOICE CHART

Infecting Organism	Drug of First Choice	Alternative Drugs
I. AEROBIC BACTERIA		
A. Gram-positive cocci		
1. Staphylococci		
a. Nonpenicillinase-producing	Penicillin	Cephalothin, vancomycin, erythromycin, lincomycin.
b. Penicillinase-producing	Penicillinase-resistant penicillin (e.g., methicillin, oxacillin)	Cephalothin, vancomycin, erythromycin, gentamicin, lincomycin.
2. Streptococci		
a. Pyogenic groups A, B, C	Penicillin	Erythromycin, cephalothin, ampicillin.
b. Viridans	Penicillin with or without streptomycin	Ampicillin, vancomycin with or without streptomycin, cephalothin, erythromycin.
c. Enterococci (group D)	Penicillin G with or without streptomycin	Ampicillin, chloramphenicol, tetracycline.
3. Pneumococcus (streptococcus pneumoniae)	Penicillin	Erythromycin, cephalothin.
B. Gram-negative cocci		
1. Neisseria catarrhalis	Penicillin	Tetracycline.
2. Neisseria gonorrhoeae	Penicillin	Tetracycline, ampicillin, spectinomycin.
C. Gram-negative bacilli		
1. Escherichia coli	Ampicillin, cephalothin	Kanamycin, tetracycline, gentamicin, chloramphenicol.
2. Aerobacter (Enterobacter) aerogenes	Kanamycin	Tetracycline with or without streptomycin, gentamicin.
3. Klebsiella species	Cephalothin	Kanamycin, polymyxin, chloramphenicol.
4. Pseudomonas aeruginosa	Gentamicin	Colistin, polymyxin, carbenicillin.
5. Proteus		
a. P. mirabilis	Ampicillin	Kanamycin, cephalothin, gentamicin.
b. Other Proteus	Kanamycin	Nalidixic acid, cephalothin, carbenicillin, gentamicin.

Infecting Organism	Drug of First Choice	Alternative Drugs
6. Serratia species	Gentamicin	Kanamycin, chloramphenicol.
7. Alcaligenes faecalis	Chloramphenicol or tetracycline	Penicillin G.
8. Salmonella typhi	Chloramphenicol	Ampicillin, cephalothin.
9. Hemophilus species		
a. H. influenzae	Ampicillin	Tetracycline, cephalothin.
b. H. ducreyi	Tetracycline	Sulfonamides, streptomycin.
10. Brucella species	Tetracycline	Chloramphenicol.
11. Pasteurella species		
a. P. tularensis	Streptomycin	Tetracycline.
b. P. pestis	Tetracycline	Streptomycin.
D. Gram-positive bacteria		
1. Bacillus anthracis	Penicillin	Erythromycin, tetracycline.
2. Corynebacterium species	Erythromycin	Penicillin.
3. Diphtheroid species	Penicillin	Ampicillin, erythromycin.
4. Mycobacterium tuberculosis	Isoniazid with or without streptomycin, with or without para-aminosalicylic acid or ethambutol.	Pyrazinamide, cycloserine, ethionamide, viomycin, kanamycin, capreomycin, erythromycin.
5. Listeria monocytogenes	Erythromycin	Penicillin.
II. MICROAEROPHILIC BACTERIA		
A. Gram-positive cocci		
1. Streptococci		
a. Hemolytic	Penicillin G	Ampicillin, tetracycline, chloramphenicol.
b. Nonhemolytic	Penicillin G	Ampicillin, tetracycline, chloramphenicol.
III. ANAEROBIC BACTERIA		
A. Gram-positive cocci		
1. Streptococcus species	Penicillin G	Ampicillin, tetracycline, chloramphenicol.
B. Gram-positive bacilli		
1. Clostridium species		
a. C. perfringens	Penicillin G and tetracycline	Cephalothin, erythromycin.
b. C. novyi	Penicillin G	Tetracycline, cephalothin.
c. C. histolyticum	Penicillin G	Tetracycline, cephalothin.
d. C. septicum	Penicillin G	Tetracycline, cephalothin.

Infecting Organism	Drug of First Choice	Alternative Drugs
e. C. sordellii	Penicillin G	Tetracycline, cephalothin.
f. C. sporogenes	Penicillin G	Cephalothin, tetracycline.
g. C. tetani	Penicillin G	Cephalothin, tetracycline.
C. Bacteroides species	Tetracycline with sulfadiazine	Chloramphenicol, Vibramycin.
IV. MISCELLANEOUS		
A. Actinomyces bovis	Penicillin G	Sulfadiazine.
B. Nocardia species	Sulfadiazine	Penicillin G.
C. Fusobacterium fusiforme	Penicillin	Tetracycline, erythromycin.
D. Calymmatobacterium granulomatis	Tetracycline	Streptomycin.
V. ACID FAST BACILLI		
A. Mycobacterium tuberculosis	Isoniazid with rifampin	Ethambutol; streptomycin; para-aminosalicylic acid (PAS); pyrazinamide; cycloserine; ethionamide; kanamycin; capreomycin.
B. Mycobacterium kansasii	Isoniazid with rifampin, with or without ethambutol	Streptomycin; an erythromycin; ethionamide; cycloserine; amikacin.
C. Mycobacterium aviumintracellulare complex	Isoniazid, rifampin, ethambutol, and streptomycin	Amikacin; ethionamide; cycloserine.
D. Mycobacterium fortuitum	Amikacin	Rifampin; doxycycline.
E. Mycobacterium marinum (balnei)	Minocycline	Rifampin.
F. Mycobacterium leprae (leprosy)	Dapsone with or without rifampin	Acedapsone; rifampin; clofazimine.
VI. ACTINOMYCETES		
A. Actinomyces israelii (actinomycosis)	Penicillin G	A tetracycline.
B. Nocardia	Trisulfapyrimidines	Trimethoprim-sulfamethoxazole; trisulfapyrimidines with minocycline or ampicillin or erythromycin; cycloserine.
VII. CHLAMYDIA		
A. Chlamydia psittaci (psittacosis; ornithosis)	A tetracycline	Chloramphenicol.

Infecting Organism	Drug of First Choice	Alternative Drugs
B. Chlamydia trachomatis		
1. (Trachoma)	A tetracycline (topical plus oral)	A sulfonamide (topical plus oral).
2. (Inclusion conjunctivitis)	An erythromycin	A tetracycline; a sulfonamide.
3. (Pneumonia)	An erythromycin	A sulfonamide.
4. (Urethritis)	A tetracycline	An erythromycin.
C. Lymphogranuloma venereum	A tetracycline	An erythromycin; a sulfonamide.
VIII. FUNGI		
A. Aspergillus	Amphotericin B	No dependable alternative.
B. Blastomyces dermatitidis	Amphotericin B	Hydroxystilbamidine.
C. Candida species	Amphotericin B with or without flucytosine	Nystatin (oral or topical); miconazole; clotrimazone (topical).
D. Chromomycosis	Flucytosine	No dependable alternative.
E. Coccidioides immitis	Amphotericin B	Miconazole.
F. Cryptococcus neoformans	Amphotericin B with or without flucytosine	No dependable alternative.
G. Dermatophytes (tinea)	Clotrimazole (topical) or miconazole (topical)	Tolnaftate (topical); haloprogin (topical) griseofulvin.
H. Histoplasma capsulatum	Amphotericin B	No dependable alternative.
I. Mucor	Amphotericin B	No dependable alternative.
J. Paracoccidioides brasiliensis	Amphotericin B	A sulfonamide; miconazole.
K. Sporothrix schenckii	An iodide	Amphotericin B.
IX. MYCOPLASMA Mycoplasma pneumoniae	An erythromycin or a tetracycline	
X. RICKETTSIA - Rocky Mountain spotted fever; endemic typhus (murine); tick bite fever; typhus, scrub typhus; Q fever	A tetracycline	Chloramphenicol.
XI. PNEUMOCYSTIS CARINII	Trimethoprim-sulfamethoxazole	Pentamidine.
XII. SPIROCHETES		
A. Borrelia recurrentis (relapsing fever)	A tetracycline	Penicillin G.
B. Leptospira	Penicillin G	A tetracycline.
C. Treponema pallidum (syphilis)	Penicillin G	A tetracycline; an erythromycin.
D. Treponema pertenue (yaws)	Penicillin G	A tetracycline.

Infecting Organism	Drug of First Choice	Alternative Drugs
XIII. VIRUSES		
A. Herpes simplex (keratitis)	Vidarabine (topical)	Idoxuridine (topical).
B. Herpes simplex (encephalitis)	Vidarabine	No alternative.
C. Influenza A	Amantadine	No alternative.
D. Vaccinia	Methisazone with or without vaccinia immune globulin	No alternative.

Made in United States
North Haven, CT
04 November 2026

21771713R00238